HOW NURSES' EMOTIONS AFFECT PATIENT CARE

Kathleen M. Gow, Ph.D. has expertise in the health care field that spans three disciplines: medical sociology, mental health (founding Director of the medical social work department at The Hospital for Sick Children, Toronto), and management studies. She has received seven awards for her contributions in these areas. Beyond this continent, Dr. Gow's research dates from 1957, when she was given a scholarship to undertake advanced work at the Tavistock Clinic, London, England and to conduct a 2-year study of health and social problems in Scandinavia, Central Europe, and the Middle East. Dr. Gow is internationally known as an author, educator, and consultant to government, educational institutions, and professional and hospital associations.

HOW NURSES' EMOTIONS AFFECT PATIENT CARE

Self-Studies by Nurses

KATHLEEN M. GOW, PH.D.

SPRINGER PUBLISHING COMPANY
New York

Copyright © 1982 by Springer Publishing Company, Inc.

Springer Publishing Company, Inc.
200 Park Avenue South
New York, New York 10003

83 84 85 86 / 10 9 8 7 6 5 4 3 2

Library of Congress Cataloging in Publication Data

Gow, Kathleen M.
  How nurses' emotions affect patient care.

  Bibliography: p.
    1. Nursing—Psychological aspects—Case studies.
  2. Nurse and patient—Case studies. I. Title.
  [DNLM: 1. Nursing care—Psychology. 2. Nurse-
  patient relations. WY 87 G722e]
  RT86.G68   610.73'01'9   81-9365
  ISBN 0-8261-3430-0   AACR2
  ISBN 0-8261-3431-9 (pbk.)

Printed in the United States of America

This project was supported (in part) by National Health Research and Development Project No. 6606-1350-42 of the Department of National Health and Welfare, Canada.

11-7-84

To Jill and Joe,
nurse and physician,
whose healing hands and hearts
are an inspiration
to all who are in their care

CONTENTS

III/CONCLUSIONS

FOREWORD

As professionals, nurses have accepted the importance of evaluating the emotional needs of their patients. Nurses understand that the physical condition of patients may be affected by emotions that are determined by the psychosocial, educational, and financial aspects of their lives—sometimes in a positive way, and sometimes in a negative way. Nurses, as well as other health care professionals, should consider these elements seriously while planning for their patients' present and future care.

The question arises whether or not nurses should become involved in the nonmedical areas of patients' lives. Nurses could insist that patients follow the suggested health care plans, regardless of any personal problems that may arise for them. Is it better for nurses to remain uninvolved and assume total control?

Nearly every nurse has been confronted by patients who refuse to accept nursing care. Some patients, even though desperately ill, may explode in anger at any attempts to provide that care. It is unlikely that nurses can remain uninvolved emotionally in such a situation, in spite of how hard they may try. The frustration and anger that can build up in a nurse, even though unexpressed, are certainly equal to those emotions that can build up in patients. Patients may complain that their needs are not always met, but neither are those of nurses. The patients have options that include accepting or rejecting the offer of care. What choices are available to the health care professionals?

Detachment is one option used by some health practitioners to protect themselves from sorrow, fear, anger, and guilt. This places an additional burden on the patient, who must find solace for himself. The message that a patient may get from the professional may be quite clear, though unspoken: "Keep your distance; do not distress or involve me in your problems. I am here, and you are there. Do not cross that line and enter my space!"

Nurses may try to find excuses to justify the distances they maintain between themselves and patients. True, often there are too few hours, too much work, and too much stress. Yet, none of these factors give legitimacy to nurses extinguishing empathic feelings.

The extent of involvement with a patient becomes a major factor in nursing care. If nurses are overwhelmed by *sympathy*, they tend to be immobilized and cannot be helpful to patients. If, however, they have *empathy* for patients, they can offer help in a therapeutic and professional way.

Nurses who follow the credo that it is unwise to show feelings to patients or families, shortchange themselves as well as those who rely on them for care. Recognizing the "self" in the practice situation enables nurses to respond more fully. It takes away the barrier between nurses and patients, allowing nurses to plan, implement, and evaluate care in a more meaningful way. What nurses bring of "self" to their situation makes the difference.

In *How Nurses' Emotions Affect Patient Care,* Dr. Kathleen Gow integrates research and clinical application in a way that is clear, thought-provoking, and useful to those who realize the importance of utilizing the "self" in nursing. Through meaningful comments and examples, she helps nurses explore emotions they have while providing care. She furnishes new insights into the ways in which nurses' feelings concerning their own inadequacies, fears, frustrations, anger, and even closeness can be acknowledged, and then used positively. She encourages nurses to be aware of their own responses, accept their own involvement of "self," and free themselves of their emotional discomfort in order to communicate their empathy in the very best spirit of nursing.

Gladys B. Lipkin, R.N.C., M.S., F.A.A.N.
Nurse Psychotherapist in Independent Practice
Bayside, New York

ACKNOWLEDGMENTS

I would like to extend my sincere appreciation to Anita W. O'Toole, R.N., Ph.D., Professor of Nursing, Kent State University for her thoughtful reading of the original manuscript. I would also like to formally acknowledge the work of the nurse data analysts whose commitment to scholarly research was outstanding. Further, this study is offered in deep appreciation of the nurses whose insightful self-accounts make this book a unique tool for their fellow travelers in the health professions, and for those who follow them. We owe them much.

HOW NURSES' EMOTIONS AFFECT PATIENT CARE

1
INTRODUCTION

Is there a nurse anywhere who has not asked herself, "How much do I care?" and "How much can I afford to care?"

This book is addressed to the realities of indifference and genuine concern in the professional practitioner-patient relationship. At the same time that practitioners in the so-called helping professions are required to be warm, open, sensitive, willing to share and risk themselves in meaningful relationships, they are reminded that one of the distinguishing characteristics of the mature, highly professionalized practitioner is emotional noninvolvement: affective neutrality. Is this conceptually valid? Is it humanly possible or realistic? Is it actually an option in the range of possible responses of a practitioner to her patient?

For their part, social scientists have tended to persevere in assuming that affective neutrality is a valid and indeed fundamental dimension of the practitioner-patient relationship. In fact, this theory is basic to a whole literature concerning the professions. Talcott Parsons (1951) in *The Social System* originally constructed the concept of affective neutrality and applied it to the doctor-patient relationship. Numerous others, including Eliot Friedson (1970) in *Profession of Medicine* and Bernard Blishen (1969) in *Doctors and Doctrines,* refer to this concept as a "given" in professional practice and proceed from that assumption. In empirical analyses of practitioner-patient interactions, the same untested concept is operative. Very often the implicit, if not explicit, assumption is that if the relationship was not helpful, it was because the professional became emotionally involved; if it was helpful, it was because he had not become emotionally involved. Yet, this assumption has received very little critical analysis or testing, particularly from the perspective of the practitioner. In fact, it may be argued with some validity that this concept has contributed—consciously or otherwise—to practitioners feeling them-

1

selves in a double-bind. Indeed, such tensions may be a major factor in the increasingly prevalent burn-out syndrome.

CRISIS IN IDENTITY

Nursing is a logical context in which to test these questions because the issue of emotional involvement (King, 1977) and related questions concerning sympathy, empathy, and rapport (Travelbee, 1971, pp. 119–155) are very much involved in nursing's intensive search to define its identity as a human service profession. Much of this concern is prompted by nursing's anxiety to establish itself as a colleague of the doctor, rather than a handmaiden: to establish nursing as a full-fledged profession among professions (Katz, 1969, pp. 54–81). The intensity of this anxiety and this search is vividly expressed in the following essay of a seasoned nurse who describes her view of the doctor-nurse game. (Through this text direct quotations are utilized from material written by graduate nurses, see p. 21 for detailed description of source. While the writers are not personally identified for reasons of confidentiality, their original papers are available on file.)

> Nurses are without open power. The nurse insinuates suggestions into a conversation with a doctor in such a way that the doctor thinks the ideas for better patient care originate with him, even though the nurses assess the patient 24 hours a day. Trying to get nurses to quit playing the game and assert themselves is one of the biggest problems I feel we must confront as women and professionals. When women are conditioned right from birth to be submissive and play the role of the manipulative subordinate [Bullough & Bullough, 1975], becoming actively engaged in the decision-making process is much easier said than done. . . . Nurses need to think and be educated as equals, rather than subservient to the doctor. We are immature as professionals because we have never had the chance to develop as autonomous human beings, free from the constraints put upon us by traditional female roles and the nursing profession to date. [Only as we free ourselves] will we attract [into nursing] creative, thinking people of both sexes.

Davis, Olesen, and Whittaker (1966) raise a related point:

> As college women prove more receptive to the possibility of combining a lifelong career with marriage and child-rearing, the very real danger is that other professions—medicine, law, engineering, architecture, social work, school counselling, college teaching, to mention a few—will suddenly appear more attractive to them than will nursing. To avoid this fate . . . nursing education must in the brief time

left it make of itself, of its relationship to the main body of nursing and of its role in the emerging pattern of health services, something much more vital, substantial and distinctive than it has up until now. (p. 175)

Solutions to this crisis in identity generally cluster around two distinct perceptions of the direction nursing should adopt. Some would argue that they are to some extent mutually exclusive: others would not (Churchill, 1977).

1. Increased professional identity lies in adopting the primary role of scientific colleague to the doctor: in developing a distinctive body of knowledge by doing research and/or developing advanced technical expertise in particular fields (Mulligan & Casse, 1965).

2. Increased professional identity lies in adopting the primary role of expressive specialist (in contrast to the doctor's primary role as instrumental specialist): developing specific knowledge of psychosocial dynamics and skill in therapeutic relationships—the "humanizer" of patient care (Johnson & Martin, 1966, pp. 206–211).

CONFLICTING RATIONALES

It is within the context of the latter role model that the issue of emotional involvement is most effectively tested. However, before proceeding to this focus, it may be useful to recognize some of the issues that are caught up in the adoption of this role model and the complexity of motivations involved in its consideration. (The rationales that are outlined subsequently are by no means exhaustive of those involved in adoption of this role model, nor are they mutually exclusive: this overview merely serves as background to the main study, not as a role study per se.) Characteristically, various and sometimes conflicting rationales are advanced in order to facilitate its adoption.

Most frequently advanced is what might be termed the *patient-oriented* rationale. It advocates an intensified focus upon the psychosocial needs of the patient *qua* patient. This is advocated not as a desirable extra in nursing care but even as the essence of it.

One of the events which we believe inspires faith and hope in a patient is the conviction that somebody cares about him. If this proves true, it implies that the quality of the nurse-patient relationship is a factor in the patient's recovery. Direct contact with a patient somehow increases his sense of being a worthwhile individual person, and this experience inspirits him—it does something to the body which helps it throw off illness. (Jourard, 1971, p. 206)

To be more specific, Jourard (1971) continues:

Man's phenomenal field [his perceptions, beliefs, ideals, imaginings, memories] in-cluding his self-structure, is a variable related both to behavior and to physiology. The content of a man's phenomenal field is a sensitive indicator of his total organ-ismic state—either well or ill—just as is the pulse, skin temperature, or blood chem-istry. . . . When the phenomenal field is not "checked" routinely in nursing . . . a crime of omission is committed, the gravity of which is no less serious than failure to make routine physiological checks. (p. 126)

A second theme, less publicized and perhaps even less consciously ad-mitted, is what might be termed an *organizational orientation*. Here the interpersonal orientation to patients appears to be at least primarily adopted as a means of ensuring maintenance of the hospital system *qua* system.

Most professions have emphasized the importance of "good interpersonal relation-ships" but careful study shows that what so-called interpersonal experts among nurses actually do is institute clever manipulations which make the patient do what he is supposed to do. In short, much of contemporary interpersonal competence seems to entail suaveness in getting patients to conform to the roles they are sup-posed to play in the social system of the hospital so the system will work smoothly, work will get done faster and the patients will be less of a bother to care for. It would seem that there has been a movement afoot in the nursing professions to train prac-titioners to teach patients how to become good "organization men"—whose be-havior will be good for the organization of a ward. (Jourard, 1964, p. 149)

A third rationale for advocating an interpersonal relations role model is *(nurse) status-oriented*. With expertise, nurses seek to buy their ticket to independence: to trade the deferrent, subservient role for one of author-ity—even superiority—over their medical colleagues in matters that per-tain to the patients' psychosocial field (see Shockley, 1975).

Finally, though by no means exhaustively, yet another note sounding in this interpersonal theme is the *public image-orientation*. Numbers of books, newspaper articles, and researched reports document the public's extreme dissatisfaction with the quality of the practitioner-patient rela-tionship (Pickering, 1973), and often point specifically to the dehumanizing aspects of nursing care (de Hartog, 1964; Lovegrove, 1979). Conscious of the waning image of the nurse as patient-oriented, and mindful of the power of the public to jeopardize efforts toward professionalization, the argument runs that personal rather than impersonal treatment will strike positively at one source of the latent hostility that the lay public holds for nursing.

Yet for all these arguments and more, within the context of the nurse-patient-hospital-community system, there is still considerable resistance to adopting the expressive specialist orientation as the primary function of nursing care (Friedson, 1970, pp. 63–66; La Sor & Elliott, 1977). Not only is the conflict generational, with older generations tending to adhere to older viewpoints, while more recently educated (or reeducated) nurses tend to put their faith in newer approaches (Strauss, 1966, pp. 60–108; Kramer, 1974, p. 234), but the conflict is often interdepartmental as well. Medical-surgical nursing is accused of lagging behind other specialties (such as pediatrics and psychiatry) in accepting the interpersonal approach as a keystone function.

Several decades ago, this was not a contentious issue. Nurses were not expected to enter the patient's world (Goffman, 1957). More specifically, they were instructed not to enter. Ironically, this also served to isolate and insulate the nurse from herself. She could don her uniform and "practice" nursing. So convinced was she that to become involved with patients' feelings and anxieties would not only intrude on the patient's privacy but also be a breach of professional etiquette, that she was able to rationalize her separateness as thoroughly professional.

This is not to imply, as some current literature might appear to do, that in the past nurses did not care about their patients as anything more than disease entities. Indeed, the image of the nurse as ministering angel (Jones and Jones, 1975, p. 156) came out of those days and is often sentimentalized by physicians (Deutscher, 1955) as the golden age when nurses really did care. However, there is a marked difference between the qualities of caring that were cited in the early days of nursing and those now cited as obligatory and characteristic of the therapeutic role. In earlier days, "the occupation crystallized around certain virtuous feminine themes: responsibility, motherliness, femininity, purity, service and efficient housekeeping. . . . 'Responsibility' meant orderliness, cleanliness, prudence, industriousness, self-discipline and sensibility" (Strauss, 1966, pp. 87–88). Now the therapeutic role demands "empathic understanding; unqualified giving, [that the practitioner be able] to sense or infer the conscious feelings and meanings underlying the other's outward communication. In a certain real sense, the other person's experience becomes alive in him also" (Barrett-Lennard, 1965).

Whether nurses in the past were more service-oriented than now is hardly the point. What is significant (at least in the model under discussion) is that the concept of service has changed. In general, what was once regarded as a rather simple intuitive matter is now perceived as deserving careful and conscious scrutiny. Where strong moral character and common sense once served, these are no longer considered to be sufficient. "Once the professions began to scrutinize the moral and psychological dimensions of nursing—began to convert the ethical feminine qualities into informed procedures—something of the ambiguity attending those psychological dimensions began to appear. Thoughtful nurses have wrestled ever since with pinning down those elusive dimensions" (Strauss, 1966, p. 93).

CONFLICTING RESPONSES

Indeed, the new concept of service has brought with it a host of self-incriminating questions. That the same nurse, in one situation, can be so open and sensitive to the feelings of her patient—and herself—that she carefully weighs the use of each word for its therapeutic value, and yet, in the next situation can be so closed and insensitive to her patient's feelings and the emptiness of her own words is surely the reason that self-awareness in the nurse-patient relationship has come to be recognized as such a problematic dynamic. Here a nurse of more than 10 years experience describes and very thoughtfully attempts to subjectively analyze the reasons for her very different use of self in two situations.

My patient was Mr. M, age 60, diagnosed as having terminal stages of carcinoma of the prostate. His wife and immediate family—a son, a daughter, and their respective mates—were fully aware of his critical condition and had seemingly accepted his inevitable death.

At the time the following interview took place Mr. M had slipped into unconsciousness. All formal treatment had been stopped and nursing care was directed toward the comfort and protection of his rights as a human being in his last hours. By 10:00 P.M. the family was alternating between pacing the corridors and clustering around his bedside, tormented by waiting, not knowing if they should leave or stay for the moment of death.

Relative: Do you think Father will last through the night, nurse? His condition hasn't changed. We've been here all day. I just don't know what to do.

I took this to be a direct request for help. I realized this must be one of the hardest times for relatives to cope with—too late for words, too early for separation, they probably wished they could take off or just get it over with; at the same time they were desperately clinging to something they were in the process of losing forever. They needed support in making a difficult decision. Having developed a close working relationship with the family in the past few weeks, and more importantly, having resolved my own feelings surrounding the eventual death of Mr. M, also partly through maturity gained from recent past experience, I felt comfortable and fairly competent in offering my assistance.

My Response: It's very difficult to say. He could leave us at any moment, but on the other hand he may still be with us tomorrow. He is resting comfortably. You've had a very long day. Perhaps it would be best if you all got some rest. Your father's in good hands and you've done all you can at the moment.

Realizing that relatives usually have a great many guilt feelings to deal with at this time, I tried to provide universal reassurance (''with us,'' ''resting comfortably,'' ''father,'' ''good hands''), taking some of the responsibility on myself by sharing their situation and yet still presenting a realistic picture (''could leave . . . but . . . still be''). There was really nothing more they could do for Mr. M now that he was unconscious and not likely to regain consciousness, but at the same time it was important for them to feel useful. Therefore I commented that they had done all that they could and then gently suggested an alternative.

Relative: Yes, we are tired but I hate to leave Father alone. If he should die . . .

They were still going through the agonies and guilt feelings of deciding whether to leave (''are tired but . . . ''). The sentence left hanging asked for immediate response.

My Response: I understand how you must feel. I'm sure if it were my father I'd feel the same way. Perhaps one of you could stay.

I felt I should acknowledge my acceptance of their feelings, again trying to create an atmosphere of ''oneness,'' all sharing the same crisis (''my father,'' ''feel the same''). But rather than throwing the problem back to them I should offer an alternative, introduced and softened with the indefinite ''perhaps.''

Relative: I'd like to stay. I'm not tired. I'm used to these hours and I'd certainly feel better staying.

She was a nurse and I knew she would probably feel the most comfortable in
the present situation.

Evaluation

I was satisfied with the outcome of the interview. A solution had been reached
that met everyone's needs. Those who felt too uncomfortable staying were assisted by alleviation of their guilt and by reassurance that someone would stay. They
could return home knowing their father didn't die alone yet not feeling ashamed
or guilty for having avoided a moment many people find difficult to face.

Mrs. G, a 47-year-old widow, had had extensive abdominal surgery. Complications of surgery, causing her to be bed-ridden for some time, had led to the development of a large vaginal fistula and several abdominal orifices, all of which
drained foul-smelling matter.

On trying to ambulate Mrs. G, the nursing staff found her to be extremely uncooperative and as days passed, conflict increased until she was labelled by all as a
difficult and hard-to-manage patient. Nursing staff began to isolate themselves
from her, fewer visits were made to her room, and from day to day she was passed
from nursing assignment to nursing assignment. Eventually it was decided that
Mrs. G warranted a team conference and the drawing up of a nursing care plan to
handle her nursing care problems. Armed with this I presented myself to give her
her morning care.

Nurse: G-o-o-d morning, Mrs. G, isn't it a lovely day! Let's just whip
through your bath and get you on those feet of yours—you must be tired of
staying in bed.
Mrs. G: I'm not getting out of bed today, so you needn't sound so cheerful.
I'll get up when I'm ready to.

I was a little taken aback—but only momentarily. I had studied the nursing
care plan—obviously this patient was just difficult and demanding. She had probably been used to getting her own way all her life—and she was one of those
private-patient, single-room women! Hadn't I tried to sound cheerful and optimistic? I thought, She must be just trying me out—I'll try again—after all, it's
for her own good.

My Response: Well, Mrs. G, you know you won't get better lying in bed.
Why don't we just take a little walk and see the lovely view from the window?
Mrs. G: I don't want to look out the window. I'm quite happy where I am,
thank you.

I was becoming frustrated and just a little angry. This interview wasn't going quite as I had planned. I thought, What's wrong with this woman anyway—surely she must realize it doesn't matter to me whether she gets up. And why doesn't she listen to me? After all, I'm her nurse—I know what's best for her.

My Response: Mrs. G, I haven't got all day—there are other patients a lot sicker than you who want to get better. If you don't help yourself, how can we be expected to help you?

Mrs. G: I don't care if I die—what have I got to live for anyway? I haven't even got a family—and I know you nurses can't stand the smell in here. Well, neither can I!

At this point it didn't matter what Mrs. G said, because I was no longer listening. I had closed her out. I responded in a self-righteous, defensive manner.

My Response: All right, Mrs. G, I've tried—no one can make you. I've got other patients to see. I'll come back and see you later.

Analysis and Evaluation

Obviously I had failed to meet or even recognize Mrs. G's needs. I had become involved in drawing up a nursing care plan so much so as to the exclusion of giving the nursing care. As a professional planner I was remote from Mrs. G's problem, guessing at her needs, oblivious to the fact that needs can be determined by asking the patient about them.

Perhaps this was partly due to my own vigorous training and indoctrination concerning what is good for the patient, but more likely it was due to my lack of self-awareness. I was unsure of myself and therefore when my authority was challenged I responded with anxiety, quickly converting it to indignant anger.

Mrs. G would remain a problem patient until I became secure enough to recognize my anxiety and carry out ways of responding that would promote reduction and redirection of it.

ANGER AND ANXIETY

In this connection—prompted by Becker's work on the dance band musician (1966, pp. 212–216)—an interesting question is raised by Vollmer and Mills (1966). Does it apply to the helping professions? "In occupations requiring much creativity, ought we to expect frequent hostility when the practitioner comes into close contact with consumers of his services?" (p. 225). At first reading, this would seem to be at best an academic point: at worst a travesty of the ethics of the professional relationship.

However, as one considers it in the light of specific documentation, it is not far from reality (Gow, 1967). But surely the key lies in the meaning of "expect." There is little argument that we should not expect, in the sense of condone, frequent outbursts of hostility—nurse to patient. But there is every indication that we should expect, in the sense of anticipate, hostility. This is one of the chief reasons that students in psychiatry, clinical psychology, and social work are required to devote a major proportion of their class and field study to the practice of self-awareness. That these practitioners without exception will harbor feelings of disgust, anger, or resentment toward some of their clients some of the time is accepted by their educators and colleagues in the field as axiomatic. That it will require considerable time and consolidated effort to learn how to understand and cope with their feelings in a professional manner is one reason that training in these fields usually requires an undergraduate degree prior to admittance to the professional school. Even then, trainees in these fields are introduced to face-to-face contact with their clients in highly sheltered contexts where they are responsible for a few carefully chosen clients/patients and are given intense supervision.

Furthermore, of all the helping professionals, the nurse is the one who, at least theoretically, is assigned to "live" with her patient for a full 8-hour tour of duty. It can be argued with validity that this places far more strain on her capabilities in interpersonal relationships than any other profession. Physicians, psychiatrists, social workers, lawyers, and clergy all relate to their patients by appointment—often singly, and if in groups, groups that have a more singular focus rather than a diffuse (physical-social-emotional-spiritual) treatment base.

> Total patient care prevokes emotions of such strength that psychological defenses are set up which greatly reduce the nurse's ability to engage in significant relationships with patients. . . . For the very reason that nurses receive so little help in *confronting* anxiety provoking experiences they do not develop the needed capacity to tolerate and deal more effectively with anxiety. As a consequence, they continue to suffer from a higher level of anxiety than is justified by the objective situation alone, while nursing care remains broken into small segments and entire areas of care go uncultivated. (Brown, 1966, pp. 196–197)

For the very reason that the nurse's fear, guilt, and hostility are neither accepted nor acceptable, Jourard (1971, pp. 179–188) explains, she may become ashamed and afraid of her real self. Consequently, she suppresses and represses her honest reactions and replaces them insofar as she is able with what she believes she "should" feel. In time, following the role models available to her, she becomes a nurse with a squelched real self and a contrived bedside manner. . . . I [have] noted that the "bedside manner" with its false jollity, or assumed omniscience, omnipotence and imperturbability, are special cases of "character armor" . . . donned by nurses and physicians to squelch their own feelings and to squelch self-disclosure in patients. (pp. 185, 197)

That nurses develop this character armor is clearly understandable (Reich, 1948). Some studies place major blame on the stripping technique (Dickinson-Taylor, 1960), which shears nurses of their identities and makes them over in terms of their function. "Patient care and patient cure must suffer in direct proportion to the effectiveness with which training and administrative procedures have stripped people, changing them from human persons into nurses" (Jourard, 1964, p. 150).

However, almost regardless of the causal framework, unless nursing realistically confronts its propensity for "armored" practitioners (Jourard, 1971, p. 184) very little progress can be made toward genuine consideration of the expressive role model. In fact Jourard goes further to propose that "a latent function of the bedside manner is to foster increasing self-alienation in nurses, thus jeopardizing their own health and well-being" (p. 184).

WHAT IS A PROFESSIONAL RELATIONSHIP?

In fact, upon close scrutiny, the nature of the professional relationship vis-à-vis the expressive role is not altogether clear. Indeed, the qualities of the ideal-type expressive practitioner tend to imply a certain inconsistency. In its concern to allow and encourage the nurse to be herself with patients, certain of the literature tends to simply leave the nurse there (Saupe, 1974). This "being oneself" approach is largely unconscious and varies with the personality, and, to carry it to its ultimate conclusion, with the particular mood of the nurse on any particular day. Yet other literature and professional codes of ethics directly imply that the nurse contracts to put the needs of the patient before her own. Put another way, especially where the psychosocial needs of the patient are emotionally demanding or threatening to the nurse, the nurse proposes in fact to be better than her natural self: that is, the professional role requires her in certain situations to be *more* than just herself. The professional use of self must be conscious, and while the mode of expression will vary with the individual, the commitment to make the relationship therapeutic for the patient should not. At the same time, detachment and nonemotional involvement are often cited as characteristic of the most highly professional.

The following account by a graduate nurse vividly illustrates the confusing messages regarding professionalism that exist in the literature and with which health professionals constantly struggle in their practices.

E. M. Jones [1962] tells us that when she was a student there seemed to be a motto, Don't Become Involved with Your Patients. She felt that this was a protective device to spare the nurse from emotional breakdown as a result of "painful, disturbing, and depressing problems of their patients." I agree that this attitude was supposed to protect the nurses, but it seems to me that as a result, both the nurse and the patient ended up suffering. A nurse who felt distressed over a patient's predicament would use defense mechanisms (such as avoidance of the patient) to keep herself from getting emotionally involved. However, by the mere fact that she was having these feelings she was already emotionally involved. Instead of admitting this, a process of denial went on, and the nurse never came to grips with her emotions; the patient suffered from loneliness and the feeling that the nurse was uncaring and coldhearted. The nurse was also useless in providing supportive care, since she required support herself, which she never received. Most of the articles that I read deal with the destructive effects of negative emotions. One article that was written by a doctor argued that, since nurses have to be clear-headed all the time, to deal with the unexpected, they should not have their judgment clouded by sympathy and pity. He maintained that callousness is part of the job and that bursting into tears and crying doesn't help the patient. He tried to back this up with the fact that doctors don't look after their own families, since they get emotionally involved and therefore cannot trust their judgment. [Edwards, 1957]

It is common knowledge that extreme emotions can cloud judgment. A high level of anxiety or stress will alter anyone's normal behavior if it is not controlled. However, if a nurse was ready to admit to these emotions and understand why she was feeling the way she did, her anxiety level would not reach this stage of clouded judgment, or if it did, she would admit this and deal with it or refer the patient to another nurse.

I find myself disagreeing quite vehemently with the remark that callousness is part of the job. How can a nurse possibly help the patient when the patient sees her as cold and heartless? This attitude destroys any attempt to create a therapeutic environment.

Since the patients are the reason for being, so to speak, let us look at what the patients say about nurses who emulate the doctor's stereotype. S. J. Bruce presents a very good study on what mothers want and need from nurses and how nurses respond to mothers in the highly emotional state of affairs connected to stillbirths. It seems that the mothers are supported best by nurses who care and show it by their actions, such as taking the time to sit and listen without rationalizing about what had happened or denying the feelings of the mother. Many of the nurses do not let the mothers cry because they can not handle emotion themselves. If the nurse accepts this emotional release as important to the recovery of the mother, she can encourage her to cry or even cry along if that is how she feels. The major area of care for such a mother is involved with the emotional adjustment to the loss of her child. But, a nurse can not help if she doesn't understand her own emotions. Some of the things the mothers in Bruce's [1962] study say are: "I was so lonely, I wanted to talk to anyone about anything"; "I wanted so much for them to say they cared"; "I wanted to be alone but not forgotten"; "One nurse let me cry and I bawled buckets. I felt much better doing this, and I was glad she stayed with me"; "Graduates must be trained not to show feelings. I liked the students best"; "I just wanted someone who looked like they cared. All they had to say was they understood and were sorry. I was so lonely."

The major problem here is that the nurses also grieve the mother's loss, but attempt to deny their feelings and respond by acting stiff and uncaring. The patients seem to need someone who will care. Caring involves emotion and it has to be sincere. People, and especially children, are able to tell if someone really cares or is just acting.

The issue of emotional involvement with patients boils down to the fact that nurses must come to terms with their own emotional needs before they can meet the needs of others.

As evident in this account, health professionals are increasingly concerned with identifying the dimensions of the practitioner-patient relationship and with furthering their skills in this direction. Recent emphasis on meeting the needs of the dying patient has focused this concern and deepened it (Gramzow, 1976). Practitioners who have operated under the assumption that emotional noninvolvement is an ideal and feasible mind-set as well as a viable activity are beginning to question themselves. They are asking whether, in fact, this concept has simply provided a model for legitimizing what is essentially a dehumanizing approach to patient care for both patient and nurse. It is true that there is a running commentary, if not controversy, in the literature concerning the concepts of sympathy and empathy, the components of each, and their appropriateness to rapport in the nursing role (Travelbee, 1971, chap. 10; Kalisch, 1973; Peplau, 1969). Leaders in the field point to recent articles by nurses such as "We used paperwork to hide from our patients" (Jones, 1978), "Speak out: Can I love them all?" (King, 1978), "Nurse, could you care more?'' (Lovegrove, 1979), and "Do I still care?'' (Sklar-Mathie, 1978) as evidence that these questions are of central significance to the practice of nursing. They point to studies that indicate that "given all the time in the world" to spend talking with patients without fear of neglecting other duties, nurses chose not to involve themselves in this activity (Davis, 1966, p. 191).

CURRENT RESEARCH

Whether one chooses to interpret the issue as one of conceptual confusion or even as a question of semantic distinctions, there is total agreement that the lack of research in this entire area of emotional involvement with patients is serious. For example, Kramer and Schmalenberg (1978b) offer this observation:

> Although empathic responses are basic to all communicative processes and are an essential element of the interpersonal process, little or no research has been done which examines the genesis of empathy in people. Sullivan, for example, fails to make explicit the problems posed by the empathic response, while Mead, who has provided the most complete and explicit theory of the social self, of social interaction and communication, of the nature of social integration, appears to have accepted empathic reactions as given (Cottrell & Dymond, 1949). (p. 75)

Yet the research in this area, however scanty, indicates that empathic reactions can in no way be considered a "given." In "Therapeutic Effectiveness of Counselling by Nursing Personnel: Review of the Literature," Peitchinis (1972) finds the evidence overwhelming that registered nurses are, by and large, low in those qualities associated with effective listening to patients' concerns and helpful facilitating responses. Building on the work of Matthews (1962), who defined a patient-centered response as one that "encourages the patient to disclose how he sees his world, what he is experiencing, and the meanings these experiences have for him" (pp. 154–162), Wallston, Cohen, Wallston, Smith and De Vellis (1978) rated the responses of working, professional nurses to simulated patients' statements. Utilizing the Person-Centeredness Coding Schema developed by Matthews, among other findings Wallston et al. conclude:

> Data . . . indicate[d] that, on the average, nurses were judged to be performing somewhere between a level "0" ("Does not elicit information but gives information") and level " + 1" ("Elicits information but limits patient response"). Few re-

sponses were judged to be actually counter therapeutic; but, at the same time, there was much room for improvement. (p. 158)

Another study of registered nurses conducted by LaMonica, Carew, Winder, Haase, and Blanchard (1976), which utilized the Index of Communication developed by Carkhuff (1969), found that "the subjects' scores lay almost at the mid-point between hurting another person and only partially responding to superficially expressed feelings" (LaMonica et al., 1976, p. 450).

This response behavior is not unique to nursing. Christine Maslach (1976), who studied physicians, poverty lawyers, social welfare workers, prison personnel, child care workers, psychiatric nurses, and others, asks this critical question:

> Hour after hour, day after day, health and social service professionals are intimately involved with troubled human beings. What happens to people who work intensely with others, learning about their psychological, social or physical problems? . . . our research indicates, they are often unable to cope with this continual emotional stress and burn-out occurs. They lose all concern, all emotional feeling, for the persons they work with and come to treat them in detached or even dehumanized ways . . . they tend to cope with stress by a form of distancing that not only hurts themselves but is damaging to all of us as their human clients. . . . like a wire that has too much electricity flowing through it, the worker just burns out and emotionally disconnects. (pp. 16, 19)

In referring to Mehrabian and Epstein's study (1972), which found that a distinct relationship exists between helping behavior and empathy, Kramer and Schmalenberg (1978b) focus on nursing:

> A study of the therapeutic relationships of various professionals indicates that a sample of 112 registered nurses scored lower on a measure of accurate empathy than ten other occupational groups with whom they were compared. (Truax, Altmann and Millis Jr., 1974). The only group who was less empathic than nurses were manufacturing plant supervisors. This same lack of empathy in nurses was also pointed out by Duff and Hollingshead [1968, pp. 225–240] who reported that 71 percent of nurses showed no evidence of empathy. (p. 76)

For my own part, I do not find these facts surprising. Nor do I believe that nursing should feel discouraged by them. Challenged, yes—but not inferior or guilt-ridden to the point of feeling impotent and immobile. After all no other profession requires of its practitioners—particularly those in the hospital ward situation—to physically care for, intellectually comprehend, and emotionally cope with such a variety, complexity, and unrelenting succession of all forms of human suffering as does nursing. Consider whether there is any other professional who is continuously on call to cope with such a wide range and simultaneous intensity of physical, social, emotional, and spiritual problems. While the nurse's function is not to be the superspecialist in each or all of these areas, it is her responsibility to be the generic specialist through whom absolutely critical data in all of these aspects is assessed and communicated. At times, this is a responsibility of almost superhuman proportions.

A NEW RESEARCH FOCUS

To date much of the literature on the nurse-patient relationship seeks to increase understanding of relationship skills through descriptive or conceptual approaches (Lewis, 1973; Aiken & Aiken, 1973), which may incorporate a workbook format to aid readers in application of these approaches (Merser & O'Connor, 1974) or samples of specific nursing care plans (Lambert & Lambert, 1979). Research studies are conducted in laboratory settings or in some cases are constructed so as to observe the nurse in interaction with patients. If and when actual nurse-patient dialogue is incorporated into the material the meaning of the dialogue is often analyzed and interpreted by a third, objective party. Such an analysis may provide valuable insights into where the nurse missed the cue and where she responded in less than a therapeutic manner (Lewis, 1973). However, a consistent limitation through these methods is that while the researcher can describe the practitioner's behavior, he/she can only infer what its meaning may be to that practitioner. How the nurse feels in a situation may be quite different—at times even opposed—to how she acts (Goffman, 1971). Moreover, one seldom feels one way. In fact, very often the salient response factors are of a conflicting nature. Depending upon which response factor(s) is/are given priority (which in turn is a psychological-sociological-situational decision-making process)—the external response (i.e., the conduct) is constructed—consciously or unconsciously. Rarely are we admitted into the practitioner's subjective view of the situation or the dialogue that passed between herself and the patient. And if we are, almost never does this view proceed beyond description of the interaction to include the subjectively understood reasons for the particular use that the practitioner made of her self at that particular moment. (For further discussion of these points, see chapter 16, Epilogue to the Researcher, pp. 305–313.)

In addition to various articles, notable exceptions to this are two books that incorporate first-person descriptions of the specific problems that nursing students face as they are socialized into the profession: *Becoming a Nurse* (Ross, 1961) and *The Silent Dialogue* (Olesen & Whittaker, 1968). A third, *Reality Shock: Why Nurses Leave Nursing* (Kramer, 1974) deals with the plight of the new nurse graduates and their shocklike reactions to the real work setting. These books and the subjective data they present are extremely instructive and, in terms of chronological development alone, document highly supportive background data to the present study. *Emotional Involvement in Nursing* does not deal with the undergraduate student or the new graduate nurse—but rather with the seasoned graduate nurse who documents not only her view of her conduct in the nurse-patient relationship, but also her accompanying thoughts and feelings. In terms of Kramer's typology of phases, the nurses in this study are in the conflict resolution phase and represent the various types of positive and negative conflict resolution Kramer (1974, pp. 159–166) describes.

While this empirical study involves graduate nurses, the basic research question is equally relevant and applicable to all health professionals who consider the practitioner-patient relationship to be a central focus in their practice. An in-depth analysis of actual practitioner response patterns as perceived by the practitioner is virtually nonexistent in current research. Yet practitioner definition of the situation is absolutely crucial to the quality of the practitioner-patient relationship. Many authors advocate that fundamental and lasting progress will only be accomplished if total patient care is approached from the subjective view of the nurse: that it is only as the nurse is encouraged to know herself that she can begin to know her patient (Jourard, 1964, p. 140). I believe that there are educational and administrative changes that must parallel increased practitioner skill in relationships in order for the latter to be allowed to be realistically operative. At the same time, it will be as more recognition is given to the perceived perspective and needs of the nurse, the way in which she internally constructs reality, and as more research and analysis are brought to bear on how she defines the situation that she will be freed to honestly confront the multidimensions of the expressive role in nursing. Only as these perspectives are incorporated can we begin to be a little more confident in specifying the nature of conflict and the meaning of conduct in relation to subjective meaning states. In essence, this is the dimension that must be examined if the concept of emotional involvement in the practitioner-patient relationship is to be empirically tested, at least from the view of the practitioner.

IN THE STUDY

2
THE STUDY

This book is a documentary given by 275 graduate nurses. They recount their own thought and feeling processes prior to and simultaneous with their outward actions in the nurse-patient encounter. These were seasoned graduate nurses who were enrolled in a public health certificate course in nursing at one of the larger North American universities. In order to qualify for admittance to this course (which was initially a full-time 9-month course and was subsequently divided into two full-time sessions of 4 months each, 1 year apart) the candidate was required to be a graduate of a diploma school of nursing who was a Registered Nurse or was eligible for registration. Completion of this course qualified the nurse for practice as a public health nurse. These practitioners ranged in age from 22 to 55 years old, the average age being 35–40. They varied in ethnic and religious background, length and nature of professional work experience. Most often prior work experience involved hospital employment in capacities such as ward nurse, assistant or head nurse or unit supervisor, in addition to a few who had already been practicing in the capacity of a public health nurse. Having a background both as a mental health specialist and as a medical sociologist, I was involved in teaching a unit on the meaning of illness.

Either directly or indirectly, the problem that these nurses most often raised was their concern that they had entered nursing because they had liked people and wanted to help them. Now they were questioning their skills in this area and their actual motives. In order to address these very real and human issues, I gave the following assignment:

Discuss two situations in which you were involved as a nurse (in any setting): (1) where you feel you were helpful in the situation; (2) where you feel you were not helpful in the situation.

*In your professional practice you draw upon knowledge, skills, attitudes, experi-
ence, community resources, etc. Central to these is the self factor. This assignment is given to help you assess this factor. Evaluation of your paper, therefore,
will not be based on your success or failure in the situations presented but upon
your ability to examine your use of self in each of them.*

Each year, class members expressed the view that this had been a difficult assignment, but the most revealing analysis in this area that they had
ever undertaken. "If only we had required to do this in our initial
training . . . "; "If only someone had shared nurses' self-accounts with
us such as the ones we've written . . ."

In the beginning I found it difficult to examine myself in preparing this essay. I
think this fact is significant in itself. It illustrates that I have not functioned to my
fullest capacity as a professional person. As a staff nurse, working on a medical or
surgical unit, I see now that I was really only concerned about completing medical treatments and assigned tasks—not in dealing with the emotional needs of
patients. One reason for this is the shortage of nurses and the heavy work load.
Another reason is the inadequacy one feels at times in trying to help people solve
problems. So one quietly "forgets" these problems. . . .

In writing this assignment, I have faced a reality that I have been denying. By
failing to evaluate my own use of self, how easily I have deceived myself into
believing that I'm OK and that it's the other person who's at fault. . . .

Along the road, there will be many backward steps because experience is our
primary teacher. It is hoped that with continual examination of past situations,
our relationships with people will progress toward being more helpful than unhelpful. I wish that I had started this process at the beginning of my career. . . .

DATA COLLECTION

It was really the nurses themselves who urged me to reproduce these accounts in casebook form. Meanwhile, it became apparent to me that in
addition to the educative value of the material, trends and apparent correlations were emerging that might have considerable potential within the
research frame. As a result of these two factors, and based on the rationale
outlined above, the present study evolved. Over the next 5-year period,
the data were collected. As usual, the nurses' accounts—which included
comments from me in my capacity as educator—were returned to each
member of the class. Then I asked that all information that could

possibly identify the nurse, patient, family, or institution be deleted from the case studies. These were returned to me with permission from the nurses to use all or any part of their (now anonymous) papers in possible subsequent published form. This was perceived as a potential contribution to professional literature and is congruent with the academic context in which we were situated.

Leading researchers rightly caution the social researcher to cultivate a reflective consciousness concerning the effect of one's role and status—even biographical characteristics—upon one's theoretical orientations, the respondents' material, and in turn upon the study's findings. For example, Solley and Murphy (1960) make a distinction between nonreflective and reflective consciousness. "Man is conscious of being conscious . . . it is at this level that the scientist operates; he is not merely nonreflectively conscious of a dial, he is reflectively conscious of his immediate consciousness in that he 'reads' the dial and it is his reflective-consciousness that he records, not 'immediate experience' " (p. 294). Accordingly, the sections in chapter 16 entitled "Relationship to the Study Group" and "Limitations of the Data" incorporate this perspective in considerable detail. This has been provided in order that the reader may be able to place and evaluate the study's findings relative to the precise environment—both cognitive and affective—in which the data were collected.

HYPOTHESES

1. There are distinct Helpful and Unhelpful factors that nurses themselves identify as regularized responses when they are in interaction with patients and colleagues.

2. There are distinct Situation factors that nurses themselves identify as regularized settings for their responses.

3. When the Situation factors cited by nurses are cross-tabulated with the Helpful and Unhelpful Response factors cited by nurses, regularized Situation-Response patterns may be identified.

4. The subjectively described thought and feeling processes of nurses prior to and simultaneous with their actions in the nurse-patient relationship will not include the Response factor of affective neutrality.

5. The preceding hypothesis will apply equally whether the nurse is describing a Situation in which she perceives herself as being Helpful or one in which she perceives herself as being Unhelpful.

PILOT STUDY

A pilot study involving 50 of the 550 cases was undertaken in order to determine the feasibility of a larger study. It was readily apparent that the material afforded two major forms of data.

1. Data concerning the Situations that the nurse cites as settings for her Helpful/Unhelpful Responses, e.g., death, birth of child, convalescence, etc.
2. Data concerning the factors that the nurse cites as contributing to her Helpful/Unhelpful Responses, e.g., "didn't want to understand," "afraid of breaking down and crying in front of patient," etc.

TREATMENT OF THE DATA

As discussed in the Epilogue to the Researcher, the basic theoretical framework of the study is symbolic interactionism. The approach to the data was not unlike the perspective discussed in Becker, Geir, Hughes and Strauss's *Boys in White* (1961), where the authors' major focus was on the concerns that their subjects brought forward, the matters that worried them the most, and those occasions of tension or conflict for them. Typical concerns of the nurses in this study are represented in the following:

"Be" rather than "seem." Who am I really, the person the world sees or the person my inner self knows? Until I can resolve this conflict, self-understanding is impossible and how can I understand another if I do not understand myself?

Sometimes I'd love to leave my self on the doorstep on my way to work, put on a mask, have a noninvolved day and pick self up again after 8 hours. But it doesn't work. To relate and be helpful we need to involve ourselves.

Consistent with the unique subjective nature of the material in this study, in the recording of the data a concerted effort was made to interpret or translate the nurses' statements as little as possible. Wherever feasible within the limitations that are necessarily involved in any classification scheme—however crude—the nurses' own words were used. (Having stated this, one is, at the same time, acutely aware that virtually all analysis is in fact secondary analysis and that in the coding of this data it is impossible to avoid interpreting and translating the material to some extent.) In most cases, the nurse's perception of the problem was clearly stated. For example, even though an adolescent patient was also convalescing, it was clear whether the nurse saw the problem as centered in adolescence or in convalescence. This is not to imply that the nurse's perception of the situation necessarily reflected all the dimensions of the actual situation. However, it is her definition of the problem situation that is of most salience to this study. With this as the definitive criterion, a content analysis was conducted on each of the 550 cases by a panel of three judges (myself and two data analysts). The two data analysts were eminently qualified to conduct the content analysis. (Both are Registered Nurses of 10–20 years experience including direct bedside care, teaching, and administration. One is currently director of nursing in a general hospital.)

To begin with, the three judges independently read and coded the same 50 cases (not those used in the pilot study). Both Situation and Response factors that had emerged in the pilot study were used as a starting point for categories; after reassessment, they were more clearly defined among the three judges, and finer distinctions made. For example, a difference was delineated between the nurse describing herself as "felt guilty, but could not communicate" (i.e., didn't know how to) and "felt guilty but would not communicate" (i.e., due to anger, hostility).

The percentage of coding agreement among the three judges—who read and coded the cases independently—had been set at 70%. Accordingly, the process of clarification in coding continued until this level of agreement had been reached and maintained on over 200 cases.

Following this process, all 550 cases were then coded as to:

1. Situation cited by the nurse
2. Case described as helpful or unhelpful by the nurse
3. Response factors cited by the nurse in each case

The material collected over the 5-year data collection period indicates no perceptible variation, that is, the data shows no evidence of being related to any particular features of individual classes from year to year. It is also significant in terms of reliability that, in each of these areas, the final categories confirmed those of the pilot study, incorporating only minimal additions (see appendix 1).

Problem Situations

1. Pregnancy/Birth
2. Adolescence
3. Interpretation of Condition
4. Professional/Personal Relationship
5. Psychiatric
6. Unmarried Mothers
7. Convalescence
8. Alcoholism
9. Elderly
10. Colleague Relationship
11. Cultural Adaptation
12. Death/Dying

Several categories require explication: Interpretation of Condition refers to situations where the nurse described the problem as her involvement in having to interpret a particular condition (e.g., a handicap, an operation). By contrast, Convalescence refers to the state of the patient as being the problem situation. Cultural Adaptation refers to situations where language, racial, or ethnic differences were cited by nurses as the principal barrier. Colleague Relationship refers to interactions that involved nursing personnel or other allied professional and paraprofessional colleagues. Professional/Personal Relationship refers to those situations where the nurse attempted to professionally treat a personal friend.

Table 2.1 illustrates the distribution of problem Situations and their percentages in relation to the total number of cases in the study. Table 2.2 illustrates the distribution of Helpful to Unhelpful cases in each problem Situation.

Helpful Response Factors

1. Took time to explain.
2. Was a sounding board.
3. Gave moral support.

TABLE 2.1
Distribution of Situations

	Number	Percentage
Pregnancy/birth	51	9
Adolescence	18	3
Interpretation of condition	112	20
Professional/personal relationship	22	4
Psychiatric	46	8
Unmarried mothers	10	2
Convalescence	116	21
Alcoholism	9	2
Elderly	31	6
Colleague relationship	43	8
Cultural adaptation	14	3
Death/dying	78	14
Total	550	100

TABLE 2.2
Percentages of Helpful and Unhelpful Cases in Each Situation

	Helpful Cases (%)	Unhelpful Cases (%)
Pregnancy/birth	59	41
Adolescence	32	68
Interpretation of condition	45	55
Professional/personal relationship	68	32
Psychiatric	59	41
Unmarried mothers	40	60
Convalescence	54	46
Alcoholism	44	56
Elderly	52	48
Colleague relationship	40	60
Cultural adaptation	29	71
Death/dying	49	51

4. Came to terms with own feelings; was able to enter into patient's problem (i.e., was difficult for nurse).
5. Initiated referral to another profession/resource.
6. Helped patient express feelings.
7. Liked the patient.
8. Not unduly influenced by negative opinions of other staff regarding the patient's personality.
9. Nonjudgmental.
10. Helped family members deal with the situation.
11. Wanted to understand how patient felt.
12. Looked beyond patient's outward response/behavior to underlying causes.
13. Made this case the basis for overall policy change/improvement.
14. Was trying to prove self to senior staff members.
15. Discussed religion with patient.
16. Used innovative rehabilitative procedure (i.e., departed from usual, normal).
17. Used physical closeness (e.g., held patient's hand).
18. Positively identified with patient due to similar life/professional experience.
19. Had received training in recognizing social-emotional needs of patients.
20. Was honest with patient/relatives.

Several categories require delineation.

Took time to explain refers to the response of explaining procedures that are being carried out in the course of the patient's care. This is in contrast to the problem Situation of Interpretation of Condition, where the nurse cites the basic problem as being her responsibility to interpret a particular condition. While both *was a sounding board* and *helped patient express feelings* involved the nurse in listening, the former was perceived by the nurses to be primarily initiated by the patient, whereas the latter was actively initiated by the nurse. *Gave moral support,* on the other hand, was characterized as more verbal on the part of the nurse, as she actively offered reassurance. *Came to terms with own feelings; was able to enter into patient's problem* was described in terms of the issue having been difficult for the nurse to resolve, one with which she had to consciously struggle.

Unhelpful Response Factors

1. Felt inadequate to enter into patient's problem because had not personally resolved the issue (i.e., tension in nurse's mind).
2. Felt guilty but could not communicate (i.e., wanted to but didn't know how).
3. Treated the condition, overlooking the patient.
4. Breakdown of interprofessional communication/cooperation.
5. Short staffed; too little time to devote to the patient.
6. Purposely disregarded significant cues in patient's statements/behavior.
7. Felt pressured (within self) into doing things rather than coping with feeling elements (tension present).
8. Negatively influenced by opinions of other staff members regarding personality of the patient.
9. Lacked training in recognizing social-emotional needs of patients.
10. Did not want to understand.
11. Afraid would break down and cry in front of patient.
12. Was disapproving, judgmental.
13. Failed to look beyond initial negative impression of patient's personality.
14. Avoided needs of family members.
15. Prejudiced toward group of which patient was a member.
16. Overidentified due to being similar age to patient.
17. Incapacitated by own fear of death.
18. Failed to seek authoritative advice regarding innovation.
19. Disregarded own judgment because wanted approval of senior staff members.
20. Rationalized actions and thoughts (e.g., "not my problem").
21. Self-image was threatened.
22. Disliked patient.
23. Lost professional role: patient became friend.
24. Felt guilty but still would not communicate (i.e., more hostile feeling than number 2).

Several categories require delineation. *Felt inadequate to enter into patient's problem because had not personally resolved the issue* is the corol-

lary to number 4 in the Helpful factors. *Felt guilty but could not communicate* is distinguished by participants from *felt guilty but still would not
communicate*. The reason behind the former is not knowing what to say;
the reason behind the latter is that hostility or anger is causing noncom-
munication.

The actual frequency of Helpful Response factors and Unhelpful Response factors to each problem Situation are tabled in appendix 2 (tables
A and B respectively). In Tables 2.3 and 2.4 these frequencies are translated in the form of percentages. (A particular Response factor was counted
only once per case.) The percentage was computed by taking the actual
number of cases in which a Helpful Response factor was cited, divided by
the total number of Helpful cases in that Situation, multiplied by 100.
For example, in the Situation of Death/Dying (Helpful), *took time to explain* was cited in 11 of the 38 Helpful cases, or in 29% of the Helpful
cases. Due to the fact that the total number of cases in the Situations of
Adolesence, Unmarried Mothers, Alcoholism, and Cultural Adaptation
does not exceed 20 cases, percentages cannot be considered to be statistically reliable. However, for the sake of consistency in comparison, percentages are cited throughout the tables.

Chapters 3–14 organize the statistical data presented in Tables 2.3 and
2.4 under each of the 12 Conditions/problem Situations cited by the
nurses. Each chapter is organized around one Situation and its highest
Helpful and Unhelpful Response factors are compared internally as well
as with those of other Situations. These statistics are followed by a considerable number of verbatim case accounts, which will afford the reader
first-hand reading of the raw subjective data. Further analysis of the findings is undertaken in Chapter 15, Summary of Findings.

Little more than a cursory view of this material is needed in order to be
impressed and somewhat overwhelmed by the magnitude of the various
and diverse ways in which the data might be analyzed and the potential
for generating multihypotheses that they afford. There is scarcely a
"burning issue" in nursing to which reference is not made here, each one
of which deserves to be specifically recognized and commented upon.
However, numbers of books and articles have been written in the recent
past by both nurse educators, nurse practitioners, and social scientists that
deal at least in part with many of these issues either in general terms
(Travelbee, 1971; Lambert & Lambert, 1979), specific delineation of the
psychodynamics of patient care in terms of the patient's age from infancy
to old age (Schwartz & Schwartz, 1972), or in terms of situational crises

(Hall & Weaver, 1974). The purpose of this book is not to reiterate or further expound upon these issues *as issues*. Rather the purpose is an in-depth analysis of practitioner response patterns to patients *as perceived by the practitioner* in the practitioner-patient relationship.

In some instances, where they were returned with the nurse's copy of her accounts, comments which the writer had made in her capacity of educator are included, for whatever value they may have in stimulating further thought and discussion for readers of this material. They are, however, in no way connected to the research project as such.

In terms of contributing knowledge and thereby facilitating the development of insights and skill in the crucial area of the practitioner-patient relationship, this study is offered in deep appreciation of the nurses whose thoughtful self-analyses make this casebook a unique tool for their current fellow travelers in the health professions, and for those who will follow them.

TABLE 2.3
Cross-Tabulation of Problem Situations with Helpful Response Factors: Percentages

	Pregnancy/ Birth	Adolescence[a]	Interpretation of Condition	Professional/ Personal	Psychiatric	Unmarried Mothers[a]	Convalescence[a]	Alcoholism[a]	Elderly	Colleague Relationship	Cultural Adaptation[a]	Death/ Dying
Took time to explain	70	50	58	60	37	75[b]	43	0	50	50	0	29
Was a sounding board	23	67[b]	24	40	33	50	29	0	38	39	50	53[c]
Gave moral support	67	67	62	80[b]	56	50	62	75[c]	56	61	50	66
Terms with own feelings	20	50[b]	28	33	30	50[b]	29	25	19	17	50[b]	37[c]
Initiated referral	37	33	36	40[c]	22	25	41[b]	0	25	17	0	8
Helped patient express	57	83[b]	56	33	63	75[c]	56	75[c]	69	61	25	53
Liked patient	3	0	12	7	22	25[c]	11	0	31[b]	0	25[c]	18
Not influenced	10	33[b]	4	0	11	0	21[c]	0	6	17	0	11

Nonjudgmental	37	50[c]	30	7	30	100[b]	29	50[c]	13	39	50[c]	29
Helped family members	23	0	30	40[c]	7	0	25	25	25	11	25	63[b]
Wanted to understand	50	67	54	27	44	100[b]	54	25	69[c]	56	50	32
Looked beyond behavior	33	83[b]	42	13	44	25	49	75[c]	38	28	25	26
Basis for policy change	10	0	8[c]	13[b]	4	0	3	0	0	6	0	3
Prove self to senior staff	0	0	2	0	0	0	2	0	0	6	25[b]	0
Discussed religion	0	0	0	7	4	0	3	25[b]	0	0	25[b]	0
Innovative procedure	3	33[c]	24	7	19	0	11	25	25	28[c]	75[b]	0
Physical closeness	17	33[c]	14	7	15	75[b]	3	0	13	0	25	26
Positively identified	13	33[b]	8	13	7	25	11	25	25	28	0	21
Had training in needs	0	17[b]	2	7[c]	0	0	5	0	6	6	0	3
Honest	3	0	6	7	15	0	3	25[b]	19[c]	6	0	13

[a]Indicates that total number of cases does not exceed 20; percentages shown for comparative purposes only.
[b]Indicates highest percentage of this Response factor across all Situations.
[c]Indicates second-highest percentage of this Response factor across all Situations.

33

TABLE 2.4
Cross-Tabulation of Problem Situations with Unhelpful Response Factors: Percentages

	Pregnancy/Birth	Adolescence[a]	Interpretation of Condition	Professional/Personal	Psychiatric	Unmarried Mothers[a]	Convalescence	Alcoholism[a]	Elderly	Colleague Relationship	Cultural Adaptation[a]	Death/Dying
Inadequate, hadn't resolved	38	25	28	43[c]	42	17	28	20	20	24	30	70[b]
Guilty, couldn't communicate	24	17	15	29	11	33[c]	11	0	20	32	20	53[b]
Treated condition, not patient	48	33	40	14	47	50	68[b]	60[c]	33	28	30	43
Breakdown of communication	38[b]	25	12	0	11	17	9	20	27[c]	24	10	8
Short-staffed; too little time	0	8	13[c]	14[b]	11	0	13[c]	0	7	4	0	10
Disregarded cues	33	25	25	57[c]	58[b]	33	38	20	40	24	20	30
Doing rather than coping	9	25	28	29	5	33[c]	13	0	13	8	10	38[b]
Influenced by other staff	14	17	17	14	0	0	19[c]	0	20[b]	12	0	8
Lacked training in needs	33	25	13	43[b]	26	0	13	0	7	16	30	15
Didn't want to understand	24	58[b]	33	29	32	50	40	40	53[c]	28	50	10

Afraid would cry	5	0	2	0	0	17[b]	4	0	0	0	0	8[c]
Judgmental	38	67	47	14	37	83[b]	47	80[c]	67	28	70	10
Initial negative impression	52	42	50	29	53[c]	33	58[b]	40	53[c]	44	50	10
Avoided family members	9	8	15	14	0	17[c]	15	40[b]	13	0	40[b]	40[b]
Prejudiced	9	17	13	0	16	83[b]	13	60[c]	13	8	20	10
Overidentified	0	0	2	14[b]	0	0	2	0	0	0	0	10[c]
Incapacitated by fear of death	0	0	2	0	0	0	2	0	0	16[b]	0	38[b]
Failed to seek advice	5	0	2	0	5	0	8	0	7	7	10[c]	5
Disregarded own judgment	5	8	2	0	11[c]	0	2	0	0	12[b]	0	8
Rationalized	43[b]	17	25	14	26	17	11	20	33[c]	16	20	28
Self-image threatened	38	50	35	57[c]	42	17	42	40	47	40	70[b]	40
Disliked patient	0	17	12	0	11	17	25[c]	20	40[b]	12	10	0
Lost professional role	0	0	7	14	21[b]	0	4	0	7	4	0	15[c]
Guilty, would not communicate	5	0	5	0	26[b]	0	13	20[c]	7	12	0	18

[a]Indicates that total number of cases does not exceed 20; percentage shown for comparative purposes.

[b]Indicates highest percentage of this Response factor across all Situations.

[c]Indicates second highest percentage of this Response factor across all Situations.

II/THE DATA

3

PREGNANCY/BIRTH

Of the 550 cases in the study, 9% focus on Pregnancy/Birth. Of the 51 cases that focus on Pregnancy/Birth, 59% are described as Helpful, 41% as Unhelpful.

COMPARISON WITH ALL OTHER SITUATIONS

Unhelpful Factors

Highest Rating

- Rationalized actions and thoughts.
- Breakdown of interprofessional communication/cooperation.

Helpful Factors	% of Cases in Which Cited
1. Took time to explain	70
2. Gave moral support	67
3. Helped patient express feelings	57
4. Wanted to understand how patient felt	50
5. Initiated referral to another profession/resource	37
6. Nonjudgmental	37
7. Looked beyond patient's outward response/behavior to underlying causes	33
8. Was a sounding board	23
9. Helped family members deal with the situation	23
10. Came to terms with own feelings; was able to enter into patient's problem	20

11.	Used physical closeness	17
12.	Positively identified with patient due to similar life/professional experience	13
13.	Not unduly influenced by negative opinions of other staff regarding the patient's personality	10
14.	Made this case the basis of overall policy change/improvement	10
15.	Was honest with patient/relatives	3
16.	Used innovative rehabilitative procedure	3
17.	Liked the patient	3
18.	Was trying to prove self to senior staff members	0
19.	Discussed religion with patient	0
20.	Had received training in recognizing social-emotional needs of patients	0

Unhelpful Factors		% of Cases in Which Cited
1.	Failed to look beyond initial negative impression of patient's personality	52
2.	Treated the condition, overlooking the patient	48
3.	Rationalized actions and thoughts	43
4.	Felt inadequate to enter into patient's problem because had not personally resolved the issue	38
5.	Was disapproving, judgmental	38
6.	Self-image was threatened	38
7.	Breakdown of interprofessional communication/cooperation	38
8.	Purposely disregarded significant cues in patient's statements/behavior	33
9.	Lacked training in recognizing social-emotional needs of patients	33
10.	Did not want to understand	24
11.	Felt guilty but could not communicate	24
12.	Negatively influenced by opinions of other staff members regarding personality of patient	14
13.	Felt pressured (within self) into doing things rather than coping with feeling elements (tension present)	9
14.	Avoided needs of family members	9
15.	Prejudiced toward group of which patient was a member	9
16.	Felt guilty but still would not communicate	5

17. Disregarded own judgment because wanted approval
of senior staff members   5
18. Failed to seek authoritative advice regarding innova-
tion   5
19. Short staffed; too little time to devote to the patient   0
20. Afraid would break down and cry in front of patient   0
21. Overidentified due to being similar age to patient   0
22. Incapacitated by own fear of death   0
23. Disliked patient   0
24. Lost professional role: patient became friend   0

Across all Situations, nurses describe themselves as most apt to *rationalize [their] actions and thoughts* where Pregnancy/Birth is concerned.

I was working in the obstetrical department of a large clinic. Mrs. B was expecting her third child by caesarean section. She was Roman Catholic and the doctor had recommended a tubal ligation.

Initially, Mrs. B accepted this as logical advice, but as the months passed she and her husband became more unsure and consulted their priest. She was most upset when he told her that this was entirely against church law and there was no reason for it. After many conversations with us, however, Mrs. B decided to go ahead with the ligation.

During the first few weeks after the baby was born and the ligation performed, Mrs. B became depressed and worried about whether they had done the right thing. She had been brought up in a very strict Italian home where the priest's word was law and this was an extremely difficult time for her.

I felt I was giving her sympathetic support and when she seemed to be getting too upset made arrangements for her to see the doctor. We discussed her problem and decided to advise her to consult her priest once again.

A couple of weeks later Mrs. B came in for her postpartum check. She had seen her priest and he had been very critical. This made her "so mad" that she and her husband "didn't care any more." She said, "We just aren't going to worry about it and certainly won't listen to anything *that* priest has to say!"

It was obvious to me that she hadn't resolved her problem and needed more help. But I convinced myself that this was strictly a religious problem and that I could offer nothing. The doctor felt the same way and this reinforced my thinking. Mrs. B called several times to talk about minor problems and I was well aware of her mental state. I ignored any attempts to broach the subject and talked of other things. It just wasn't my problem!

The following month Mr. B brought his wife to us in a severe depression. A usually vivacious and immaculate person, she appeared completely disheveled and very dirty and stared at us with a haunting expression. She was admitted to a psychiatric hospital that day.

This was definitely the most unnerving thing that has ever happened to me. I have worked with many psychiatric patients, but this shocked me and the memory still affects me. I couldn't blame the doctor; I spent considerable time with prenatal patients and it was his habit to let me take the lead in many of their problems. I felt directly responsible and couldn't rationalize my way out of it.

I finally had to face the fact that it was my own attitude and inability to relate to the patient that was the problem in this instance. I had felt concerned and sympathetic but the old word *empathy* hadn't meant a thing. It was too late to help Mrs. B, but this was a vivid lesson for me in the years that followed.

Yes—this was a desperate experience, though I'm sure you have made it count in the subsequent years. Many people would have rationalized it out of their minds. It is also a typical example of how patients are left to fall between professionals (the priest, you, and the doctor) with no help. It is also a very dramatic illustration of the fallacy of treating the physical in relative isolation from the emotional and spiritual. This woman's religious beliefs and her background of adherence to church authority was so central to her pattern of life that to go against them was sufficient to break her.

Would conferences with you, the doctor, the priest, and the family at several points have been to any avail?

Also, across all Situations *breakdown of interprofessional communication/cooperation* is highest in Pregnancy/Birth.

The referral requesting a home visit to the D family came from the hospital where Mrs. D had delivered a 9-pound baby boy. The form stated that the baby, suffering acute respiratory problems, had been transferred to a children's hospital right after the birth, and had subsequently died on the second day. It also showed that Mrs. D was new to the town and far removed from family and friends.

I made several unsuccessful attempts to visit her; the house appeared unoccupied with the draperies tightly drawn. However, one day as I dropped another card into the slot the door was opened by a young woman in a dressing gown.

Mrs. D: You're from the Health Department, aren't you?

Nurse: Yes. I'm Mary Day from the health unit downtown. May I come in, Mrs. D?

Mrs. D: My baby is dead . . . he died . . . so . . .

Nurse: I know—and I'm so sorry. Could we talk anyway?

Mrs. D: Come in. Please call me Iris.

The house was dimly lit. Toys were tossed about, typical of a home where young children live.

Nurse: Some like dinky toys the way my sons did!

Mrs. D: Yes. Greg—our 3-year-old. He is asleep now—thank goodness. He gets on my nerves these days. Everything does—my husband is so cross with me. He says I should stop all this crying and carrying on. The baby is dead . . . and that is that. . . . So I cry after he leaves for work . . . but I try not to let Greg see me.

Nurse: I'm sure you must feel so sad, losing your baby after carrying him for 9 months and going through a difficult labor. I would cry too, if that happened to me.

We then had some discussion of the way our society conditions men to suppress their emotions—to be embarrassed by tears. She listened intently with a sad expression on her face.

Nurse: What did your doctor tell you about your baby's death?

Mrs. D: That's part of the problem. My doctor went on vacation right after he was born. You see . . . he knew I would be due just as he was going away and so he said I should be induced. . . . I agreed because I wanted him to be with me . . . and now I know . . . I feel that . . .

Her voice trailed off as she attempted to control tears.

Nurse: Are you trying to tell me that you think the inducing process contributed to the baby's death?

She nodded in agreement, turning her face from me.

Nurse: Iris—please cry. I promise I won't be embarrassed. You'll feel better if you do. I'll feel sad with you, but I won't be embarrassed and I won't leave.

And so Iris cried and as I had predicted I felt very sad. After a few minutes she gained control of her voice.

Mrs. D: You see, I longed to see the baby after he was born. They didn't show him to me . . . they took him to another hospital . . . and whenever I think of him . . . it's awful . . .

Nurse: What is the awful part? Are you afraid he was deformed?

Mrs. D: Yes.

She began to weep again. We sat in silence—side by side.

Nurse: The referral induction form doesn't say anything like that, Iris. I feel certain that the inductions would not have contributed to his death. Give me your doctor's name and I'll find out what happened. I'll come back to see you tomorrow.

The doctor was too busy to speak to me, but his nurse told me the baby had not been deformed. There had been a long labor, caused by a shoulder presentation of the baby into the pelvis. By the time the caesarian section was performed, the baby had experienced too much distress to survive. A doctor had, in fact, tried to explain the situation to Iris, but being a new immigrant he had difficulty expressing himself in English. The office nurse made an appointment for Iris to visit her own doctor the next week.

I returned to the house the next day. Iris appeared glad to see me and listened intently to what I said. When I finished speaking she again cried for a short period of time.

Mrs. D: Every time I recall any part of the delivery I feel so terrible. I hate to think of the hospital, the doctor and nurses—even my husband—and the baby. It seems such a horrible event to remember.

Nurse: I am sorry you were not given the support you needed at the hospital. We can't change these past events, but when you think about your baby picture him as being your son. Give him the name you had chosen for him—Alan. Imagine him to have been a lovely human being who wasn't able to survive the birth process. He was not disfigured; he was conceived in love, so he was lovely.

There were more tears, but now she held her head up.

Nurse: Please open the drapes. Sunshine makes us feel "up." It sounds corny, but it's true. Take Greg out for walks and look at what springtime is doing out there. Be patient and understanding with your husband. Things are going to improve for you—I'm sure.

A week later Iris called me. Her voice sounded alive and optimistic.

Mrs. D: I think we're going to make it! Last Saturday I fixed a special dinner—even candles. When my husband wondered how I had changed my attitude I explained that I was determined that Alan's birth was going to work as a good thing for our family. He came to be because we love each other and so it can't be a *bad* thing. When I said that he cried.

She then expressed her gratitude for my concern for her and for her family, and wished me well in my studies at the university.

Analysis

From the beginning, Iris D and I experienced a good relationship. I believe this came about as a result of several factors, the most important of which was our ability to communicate effectively. As we established rapport she began to trust me. Through observation I identified her problem as her need to openly express grief. She understood the explanation of her problems and when she perceived her need, she acted out her feelings. When I sat by her in silence we conveyed our feelings through unspoken forms of communication. These attitudes she found reassuring and comforting. When she was unable to state her feelings, I verbalized them for her, indicating that I recognized her fears, that they were conceivable, even expected.

I suggested an uncomplicated plan of action to assist her to think and to act constructively. She was receptive to these suggestions because I had gained her confidence.

In my opinion Iris had been neglected (emotionally at least) while in the hospital. This fact annoyed me and increased my motivation to obtain the data that was necessary to relieve her anxiety. It was gratifying for me to see her grow strong enough to give her husband the help he needed. Our warm interaction led to effective results.

This case of *breakdown in interprofessional communication/cooperation* became the basis for in-service education.

I was working as a supervisor on an obstetrical ward. On admission, Mrs. Shane was a pleasant, 30-year-old primipara. She was relaxed and cheerful throughout her labor and delivered during the night. The baby had Down's syndrome, but the doctor saw fit not to tell the parents at that time.

When I arrived on the ward the next day the head nurse, Miss G, was upset and angry that the doctor hadn't told Mrs. Shane. I assured Miss G that he would be in later and would certainly tell her then. I left for a staff meeting before the doctor made rounds and then was off the ward for 3 days.

When I returned I found that the doctor still hadn't told Mrs. Shane and Miss G was infuriated. Apparently, Mrs. Shane was asking very direct questions that Miss G found upsetting. She closed the door on her questions by telling her she would have to ask the doctor. When I asked Miss G if she had talked to the doctor about the situation she said, ''No, I'm so mad at him I can barely speak to him.'' She felt he was shirking his duty and had no right to burden her with his unpleasant responsibility. Miss G reported that the patient was very irritable and uncooperative anyway, and she didn't have much patience with her.

Later when I visited Mrs. Shane she started in with a long list of complaints about service, various nurses, and everything in general. By being receptive and not reacting to her outburst I managed to get things down to a more rational discussion. After she had calmed down somewhat I asked her how she was getting along with the baby. It was then that she burst into tears and said she knew something was wrong but was afraid to ask the doctor. She told me her thoughts and she had guessed the truth. I told her I was fairly sure she was right but would phone the doctor immediately.

I explained to the doctor what had happened over the past few days and my conversation with Mrs. Shane. He was more than glad to be relieved of the responsibility of telling her but said he would be up right after office hours. I knew him to be a kind man and that he would be there for support as soon as he could. We were able to talk about this later and I aired my views on what his procrastination had done to our patient.

Mrs. Shane went through her ups and downs but we had established a relationship conducive to helping her. We had no social services in the hospital, but I had a social worker friend who was particularly interested in mental retardation. With the doctor's blessing I asked my friend to visit her. They seemed to relate to each other immediately and established a good relationship the first day. The social worker suggested that Mrs. Shane go home without the baby and they would continue to discuss things.

When Mr. and Mrs. Shane returned to pick up the baby they appeared confident and I felt they would be able to face the future with courage.

In talking with Miss G I was able to refer her to some appropriate reading that would help her understand her own reactions to patients. This was effective, as evident in the fact that she described this experience to the rest of the staff at an in-service education clinic. The young doctor involved helped her with a paper on communications and discussed this as a learning experience for himself.

Good—too often these experiences are not plumbed for their learning values for general staff and are simply dropped as isolated incidents—the sooner forgotten the better.

In assessing my use of self I feel I was able to guide things in a positive manner by: (1) not getting angry at Miss G for having allowed the situation to progress to such a point; (2) not reacting to the patient's or Miss G's anger and establishing rapport with them both; (3) controlling my own impatience with the doctor for his procrastination. My first thought had been to stay away from Mrs. Shane until the doctor arrived and then insist that he handle it.

The role of motherhood—welcomed or unwelcomed—is obviously one that nurses and other members of the helping team face with patients. The following accounts indicate some of the conflicts and gaps in service involved for all concerned.

Early one morning a frail-looking woman was wheeled into the delivery room. She appeared pale, tired, and very apprehensive. In a pleading voice she said, "Nurse, am I going to be all right? This is my sixth child and I hope he will be all right." I said, "Mrs. A, we will do our best for you." The doctor pointed out that Mrs. A had uterine inertia due to repeated pregnancies and faulty nutrition that resulted in poor muscle tone.

Routine care was given to Mrs. A, who was very cooperative. At intervals she spoke about her family and prayed that she would go home soon. She gave birth to an infant who appeared normal, despite prolonged labor. After care was given to both, she received the infant with expressed joy and appreciation. She then fell into a deep sleep.

When she awoke she said to me, "Nurse, the doctor advised me not to have any more babies. What can I do to prevent this?" I tried to explain the condition of her uterus and her general health. I also mentioned birth control. She listened, then said, "Nurse, all that you have said is true, but I have been married fifteen years, and my husband and I have nothing else but our children. I think I am fulfilling my role as wife and mother; that is my only contribution in life."

I was amazed to hear this woman express her role in life with so much conviction. What could I say that would make any difference in her outlook? However, I said, "Mrs. A, when you return home talk this over with your husband and ask him to go with you to your doctor for your postnatal check-up." She said, "Nurse, I know what he is going to say—he has said it many times before—but I cannot change my personality." I said, "Mrs. A, try not to worry now, your baby needs you."

Assessment

I feel I gave Mrs. A some reassurance during her delivery but I was unable to give her a satisfactory answer to her question about not having any more babies.

She had a preconceived acceptance of her role as wife and mother, and I doubt that any explanations I could give at this time would have been satisfactory. There is such a close bond between mother and child at delivery; all she wanted was to reach out and find contentment in her role as mother. Maybe nothing I could have said would have been comforting in this particular involvement.

Certainly, this was a problem that couldn't be answered within one conversation. Listening and helping her to really explore her sense of identity would be of first importance. At a later time you might have introduced the idea that her personality need not change. Obviously, it was a loving and giving one. However, there are many ways to give to one's children. What did being a good wife and mother actually mean to her—producing many children or the quality of love given to the family she now has? It would not have been good to preach to her—but to try to help her consider such a distinction, suggesting that a contribution need not necessarily be measured in numbers. Referral for on-going consideration of this problem would perhaps then have "taken."

Mrs. Otis is a 43-year-old housewife from a small town. She is a very quiet, retiring person. Her husband is a prominent businessman in the town. She has three teenaged children, and came into the hospital early in the morning in labor. She is of the Catholic faith.

I was the 4–12 nurse in maternity, and as there were no other patients in my department, I was able to spend considerable time with her.

When I arrived on duty the report stated that she was nearly ready for delivery and her condition was satisfactory. Sedation had been given.

Nurse: Hello, Mrs. Otis, how are you now?

Mrs. Otis: Hello, and don't you say I'm too old for this sort of thing.

This rather startled me as she was not the type of person to say this. I wondered what she was trying to say.

Nurse: What do you mean?

Mrs. Otis: The last nurse in here kept calling me an elderly multipara. Anyway, I hadn't planned this—it's just been terrible.

Her voice was strained. I thought 43 was rather old, too, as complications are more prevalent at this age. I also thought it unkind of the previous nurse to speak so to her.

Nurse: Perhaps I could rub your back and tidy up your bed.

Mrs. Otis: I'd like that—I'm so hot and tired.

A back rub at this time when pains are severe seems to ease the patient. You also feel you are helping her. Often a patient will talk to you when you are working around her bed. I wished to know more about her antagonistic feelings so that I might assist her with her problem.

When I examined the patient for progress, the fetal heartbeat was irregular, and I telephoned the doctor immediately. I was most anxious for the safety of the baby. However, I assumed a normal routine, hiding my real feelings of apprehension, so as not to upset the patient.

The doctor arrived and the patient was taken to the delivery room, where, under a general anesthetic, she was delivered of a stillborn female baby. I am always somewhat repelled and filled with a sense of despair when this sort of thing happens. The doctor told Mrs. Otis about the baby before we left the delivery room. Later, back in her room, Mrs. Otis turned to me.

Mrs. Otis: I'm so glad you were with me. It was a girl too. Did anyone call the priest?

I do not share her religion, but know this means a great deal to a patient to have her baby baptized. I was flattered that she wanted me with her.

Nurse: Yes.

Mrs. Otis: I can't sleep—it's all my fault.

Nurse: Do you want to talk about it? It often helps to discuss these things. I imagine you are blaming yourself.

She felt guilty and by assuring her I still cared, she began to relax. I sat down at her bedside and spoke in a friendly voice. I wanted to help her, have her feel she could confide in me and I'd understand. By my sitting down, she knew I was interested.

Mrs. Otis: Yes, I do. I didn't want to be pregnant and was annoyed with my husband and had hateful feelings toward the baby. I feel as if I'd killed her. I feel so mean.

Since I had not rejected her because of her previous conversation, she expressed her thoughts and knew I accepted her.

Mrs. Otis: Will Alex be up tonight?

Nurse: Yes. The doctor called him and he's coming.

Mrs. Otis: I'm so glad. I do feel better. It does help to bring these things into the open.

We had a mutual feeling of understanding and talked amicably until her husband and priest arrived.

I hope that Mrs. Otis was able to reveal her conflicts to her priest and be helped. Your acceptance and understanding would facilitate this, too. Actually, I think you helped her begin to resolve something that she would probably continue to think about for some time. But by not minimizing her feeling of guilt, you actually helped her along the road to eventual resolution far more so than if you had tried to "talk it down." Her guilt feelings would be very involved with her religious beliefs about birth control, love of children, etc., and she had obviously been carrying this guilt for many months—now it was climaxed—was God punishing her?

*   *   *   *

Mrs. S, 24 years old, was admitted as an outpatient for a therapeutic abortion. I first saw her after her surgery in the recovery room. I was doing a routine check on Mrs. S and she was just waking up from the anesthetic and crying. "Don't cry, Mrs. S. Your operation is over." (Still more crying.)

individually or together. There should have been some attempt to talk with them at the completion of my shift and perhaps bring them closer to this little helpless baby.

It is well known that a mother's self-accusation, hopelessness, hostility, and sense of guilt need to be expressed openly. Here was a need for strong supportive care to the parents and I failed to provide it.

Here was a perfect example of a nurse's reaction, helpless, anxious, angry, threatened and uncomfortable, leaving parents in their anxiety. It was almost with frantic relief that I received the early morning phone call, on the 4th day, that the child had died.

My failure to cope with the inevitable death of this infant and to communicate with his parents was indeed a tragic neglect on my part.

*   *   *   *

This situation involved a middle-aged mother who had been delivered of a baby with Down's syndrome. She refused to touch the child when the nurses brought "it" to her room and said that she did not intend to take "it" home when she went. The husband was more accepting of the baby, but both of them feared what the neighbors would say and what the reaction of their four teenage children would be.

Since I had experienced raising a retarded child of my own, the physician asked me if I would consider talking to this patient. I said that I would give it a try, thinking that no harm could be done by the effort.

However, as soon as I entered the room, I knew that this was a mistake. Obviously, Mrs. S had not been prepared for my visit and when I explained why I was there she immediately froze and did not utter another word. The result was a one-sided testimonial about all the community resources available to help parents of the retarded, such as schools, parent associations, and health agencies.

Mrs. S left the hospital without her baby and the child died about 3 months later for no apparent reason, except possibly the lack of mothering.

In this situation, failure was mainly due to the fact that a person with well-developed counseling skills was needed. It was an impossible task for one interview. The mother should have been asked if she wanted me to visit with her and been given the chance to refuse. I failed to show her that I was accepting of her attitudes toward the child and probably only succeeded in adding to her feelings of guilt.

Failed to look beyond initial negative impression of patient's personality is described in 52% of the Unhelpful cases. At the same time, *wanted to understand how patient felt* is described in 50% of the Helpful cases; *took time to explain* is cited in 70% of the Helpful cases; and *gave moral support* in 67% of Helpful cases. The following accounts illustrate the range of judgments involved.

On being given the night report in labor and delivery, I first learned of Mrs. M. She was 36 years old. This was her third pregnancy; she had no living children, but had had two early miscarriages. She was now only 30 weeks pregnant. She had been admitted 3 hours previously with ruptured membranes and 5-minute contractions. Her contractions were becoming bothersome and she was almost ready for a sedative.

A short personal history was also given. Mrs. M was a registered nurse with 10 years experience as a supervisor of an operating room in a large city hospital. Since her marriage to a professional man, she had done volunteer work, which included being a local Girl Scout leader.

Mrs. M was a handsome woman with a very positive manner in speaking. Her contractions were bothering her and she was sedated. With each contraction Mrs. M roused from a deep sleep, screamed, and thrashed about. I stayed with her and tried to reassure and calm her. Her only response, in a demanding voice, was "Get me a drink of water"; "Tighten the sheet"; or "Go away and leave me alone." After 4 hours of this labor she was delivered of a premature male infant. Having had an epidural anesthetic, she was awake and extremely talkative and excited following delivery. The infant was rushed to an isolette in the nursery. The obstetrician explained to Mrs. M that her son was much too small, and his chances of survival were poor. Mrs. M appeared to not even hear him and continued with her excited chatter about the baby's name and his pleased grandparents.

The infant lived only about 12 hours and died of prematurity. Mrs. M, due to her grief, was an impossible postpartum patient. She had student nurses in tears and graduate nurses close to them, because of her sarcastic remarks. She was discharged on her seventh day, much to everyone's relief.

Assessment

I was sorry that I was unable to help Mrs. M. I rationalized that perhaps if I had been on duty when she was admitted and had had a chance to establish rapport before sedation was necessary, our relationship would have been better. Her authoritative manner of speaking antagonized me. It made me feel that she, as a former nursing supervisor, resented being taken care of by a mere general duty nurse. On reviewing the situation, I can see now that this was a defense mechanism on her part. It was there because she being a nurse knew that a 30-week infant might not live. She wouldn't admit it to herself in labor and in the delivery room.

Mrs. M may have had a self-image of being able to do everything very competently. Not being able to produce a living child, after three attempts, besides her normal grief, must have frustrated her. Her behavior in labor, making such a big fuss with each contraction, indicated to me that she was not functioning normally. A nurse usually has sufficient knowledge of anatomy and the labor process to cooperate and be interested in her progress. Her response to me, when I tried to help her, indicated that she was rejecting her premature labor and me.

Her elation on the birth of her son was her refusal to admit that he might not survive. Her bad manners on the postpartum floor was her expression of grief and frustration at fate, rather than at the nursing care. At the time I felt that none of the nursing staff could help her because she needed more help than any of us were qualified to give. However, if I had understood then as much as I do now, I could have gone to her after the baby died. Instead of showing resentment to all her defense mechanisms I could have shown compassion, sympathy, and understanding. I am sure she would have responded.

This case history has a happy ending for the patient. Ten months later Mrs. M, after a short labor, was delivered of twins, a male and a female, weighing about 5 pounds each. This time she was a model patient, charming and cooperative. This immediate pregnancy verified for me her determination to produce a living child. But if Mrs. M is ever again in an unhappy situation, I hope she will have a nurse caring for her with more understanding than I had that night.

Below, the nurse describes her lack of communication with the patient who had had seven previous abortions. *Treated the condition, overlooking the patient* is cited in 48% of Unhelpful cases.

Mrs. Wilson was a 32-year-old woman who was very attractive and had a rather pleasing personality. Her husband was 47 years old. This couple had two children, and following the births of their two sons, she planned that she would have no more children. Her husband also agreed to this, but neither of them sought any information concerning family planning.

Instead, Mrs. Wilson paid the penalty by having seven criminal abortions. The last time she was admitted to the hospital, critically ill.

I gave her as much nursing care as I possibly could and reassured her, "You will soon be fine." Gradually, her condition improved and soon she had a dilatation and curretage. Later, she was able to go home.

When I look back, I am ashamed of my attitude toward this woman who was obviously needing me to just listen to her. I felt that she needed me to confide in, discuss family planning, or plainly, just talk. I am sure that she must have punished herself a thousand times, but I gave her the "professional" treatment by not wanting to discuss her private life. How she would have loved to have had a good cry when she experienced her depressive moods, but I allowed her to keep it all to herself. My opinion was that she must have been a masochist to go through this over and over again.

I concealed and camouflaged my true feelings by keeping our conversation as light and frivolous as possible. The reason for my behavior was to protect myself against criticism and rejection from the other members of the staff if I became too involved with the patients, and self-incrimination if I admitted how judgmental

I was about her actions. By refusing to try to understand her point of view I allowed this prejudice to block my listening.

The tragic thing is that, although the patient was calling out to me for help, I did not listen and we parted as strangers. If I had listened, I might have learned what she believed and why; what her fears, hopes and problems were; I might have gained some knowledge about her family life. By expressing her feelings and ideas, some of her emotional needs might have been met, and further problems redirected.

In this case, the nurse was similarly prepared to stereotype as neglectful parents whose six children had been made wards of the court.

My office was notified that I had a new family in my area.

Mrs. X had been discharged from the hospital the previous day with her 10-day-old baby. She had had a normal delivery and a tubal ligation performed on the fifth day.

Another member of the staff had visited her briefly on the previous afternoon, and had stated that Mrs. X was hopeless: she had previously had six children who were now wards of the court, but she couldn't remember how to prepare formulas or care for a baby.

I am very fond of children and my first thought was that if this woman was neglecting the baby she should not be allowed to keep it. Having heard my mother often say, "Soap, water, and love are cheap, so there is no excuse for negligence," this was deeply imbedded in my mind. With my preconceived ideas, I arrived at the home.

The apartment was above a store. Mrs. X, a woman of 38 years of age, invited me in. She was in a great state of anxiety and distraught. I observed that the apartment was poorly furnished, untidy, and cluttered. The air was heavy with cigarette smoke. Mr. X was sitting smoking; he looked rather ill, white and drawn, with beads of perspiration on his brow.

In the midst of this confusion a sweet baby lay on the davenport (there was no crib), contented, neat, and clean. In one glance I realized the baby was neither dirty nor unloved. I turned my full attention to the parents.

Mrs. X related her story: this was her second marriage, of 6 months' duration. Her first husband had committed suicide while she was in the hospital with rheumatic fever. Her six children were taken from her by the court because she was unable to provide for them on account of ill health, and they were made wards. Now she feared this baby would be taken too, if she didn't learn how to take care of it.

Mrs. X had had shock treatments in her eighth month of pregnancy, and was presently taking medication to prevent epileptic fits. She said she wasn't able to cope with everything; the home was untidy because she didn't feel strong enough to do the housework plus care for the baby. She was very fearful of losing her husband, stating he was ill.

Mr. X, an alcoholic controlled by medication for 1 year, had 18 months previously tried to commit suicide by hanging himself while depressed in jail. Three weeks prior to my visit he had had a car accident and lost his nerve for driving, and so had lost his truck driving job. He now appeared in a state of anxiety and depression.

They needed a family physician, home help, and financial assistance. I felt extremely compassionate toward them in their great need. I realized that they badly needed a parental figure at this period, and I would have to assume this role and let them be dependent upon me. By listening and quietly reassuring them, we planned and I advised. I was able to contact the Social Services Department and get promises of help. I also contacted a nearby doctor who promised to see Mr. X that afternoon. Then I began to decrease my role and to get the parents to accept some responsibility.

Rapport was established. All advice for improvement in the home and baby care was accepted. Mrs. X was much calmer and reassured. Mr. X promised to see the doctor in the afternoon; this was a great achievement because he hadn't left the house for several days because of fear.

Summary

Any feelings of prejudice were quickly forgotten in the realization of the family's needs. I recognized their cry for help, knew the role to play, and when to change that role.

I was rewarded by the parents' sincere desire to improve their situation, and to give the child a happy home, for they both loved her. They proved their sincerity by cooperation and adherence to suggestions in the many visits that followed. The confusion disappeared. The home became clean and tidy, and both learned how to care for their baby.

The patient who constantly screams during the process of childbirth has become almost a stereotype. Here the nurse faces this stereotype and deals with it.

It was very busy in the delivery room; six patients were in active labor. The staff consisted of a student and myself.

Mrs. Miller, aged 35 years, Roman Catholic, gravida 5, para 4, had a history of prolonged, painful labors, terminating in forceps extractions. She was in labor for 16 hours and had made no progress for the past 4 hours. She blamed her husband for this pregnancy and did not wish to see him. She was labelled difficult and uncooperative and I soon saw why. She screamed incessantly.

I went to see her. Her hair was matted, her face flushed, her lips were cracked, and eyes bloodshot. She was the picture of dejection and defeat. Listlessly she said, "There is nothing anyone can do. They are all tired of me." I took her hand in mine. I sympathized with her and recognized how very tired, frightened, and lonely she must be feeling. With her experience of past labors, she could not face the painful hours that stretched ahead.

Quickly I decided she needed to have her confidence restored, to know that we cared. She needed to be involved in her own labor. Realizing that she was terrified of being alone, I moved her bed next to the office. I told her, "You are not a bother to anyone. You are not alone. We are here to help you and we will do everything we can to help you," and added "You and your baby are fine."

A very nice combination of physically and verbally demonstrating your understanding.

After finishing my rounds I returned to Mrs. Miller: I bathed her and made her bed with fresh linen. I made her as comfortable as I possibly could but she still screamed and worried that she was a disgrace.

I sat by her bed and carefully explained that it was not a disgrace to scream, but that it would hinder her labor. I placed my hand on her abdomen and taught her how to relax during a contraction by controlled breathing. We practiced by doing the exercises together a few times. Gradually she grasped the idea. She faltered now and then but really began trying in earnest. I had to leave, but as I gave her the bell I repeated, "If there is anything you wish, anything at all that we can do for you, please don't hesitate to ring." I added, "Would you like me to call your husband?" She smiled and nodded.

Although I could not stay with her, I came to see her as often as I could, to stay with her during a contraction, to rub her back after one, to give her ice to suck. She was quieter and dozed between contractions. After a time I examined her and was glad to tell her that labor was progressing. She went on to have for the first time a normal delivery.

4

ADOLESCENCE

Of the 550 cases in the study, 3% focus on Adolescence. Of the 18 cases that focus on Adolescence, 6 are described as Helpful, 12 as Unhelpful. Percentages shown for comparison only (see Tables 2.3, 2.4; pp. 32–35).

COMPARISON WITH ALL OTHER SITUATIONS

Helpful Factors

Highest Rating

- Was a sounding board.
- Overcame own feelings to enter into patient's problem (same rating as Cultural Adaptation and Unmarried Mothers).
- Helped patient express feelings.
- Not unduly influenced by negative opinions of other staff regarding the patient's personality.
- Looked beyond patient's outward response/behavior to underlying causes.
- Positively identified with patient due to similar life/professional experience.
- Had received training in recognizing social-emotional needs of patients.

Unhelpful Factors

Highest Rating

- Did not want to understand.

Helpful Factors	% of Cases in Which Cited
1. Looked beyond patient's outward response/behavior to underlying causes	83
2. Helped patient express feelings	83
3. Gave moral support	67
4. Was a sounding board	67
5. Wanted to understand how patient felt	67
6. Nonjudgmental	50
7. Took time to explain	50
8. Came to terms with own feelings; was able to enter into patient's problem	50
9. Initiated referral to another profession/resource	33
10. Not unduly influenced by negative opinions of other staff regarding the patient's personality	50
11. Used innovative rehabilitative procedure	33
12. Used physical closeness	33
13. Positively identified with patient due to similar life/ professional experience	33
14. Had received training in recognizing social-emotional needs of patients	17
15. Was honest with patient/relatives	0
16. Made this case the basis for overall policy change/ improvement	0
17. Was trying to prove self to senior staff members	0
18. Discussed religion with patient	0
19. Helped family members deal with the situation	0
20. Liked the patient	0

Unhelpful Factors	% of Cases in Which Cited
1. Was disapproving, judgmental	67
2. Did not want to understand	58
3. Self-image was threatened	50
4. Failed to look beyond initial negative impression of patient's personality	42
5. Treated the condition, overlooking the patient	33
6. Felt inadequate to enter into patient's problem because had not personally resolved the issue	25
7. Breakdown of interprofessional communication/ cooperation	25

8.	Purposely disregarded significant cues in patient's statements/behavior	25
9.	Felt pressured (within self) into doing things rather than coping with feeling elements (tension present)	25
10.	Lacked training in recognizing social-emotional needs of patients	25
11.	Felt guilty but could not communicate	17
12.	Negatively influenced by opinions of other staff members regarding personality of the patient	17
13.	Prejudiced toward group of which patient was a member	17
14.	Rationalized thoughts and actions	17
15.	Disliked patient	17
16.	Short-staffed; too little time to devote to the patient	8
17.	Avoided needs of family members	8
18.	Disregarded own judgment because wanted approval of senior staff members	8
19.	Afraid would break down and cry in front of patient	0
20.	Overidentified due to being similar age to patient	0
21.	Incapacitated by own fear of death	0
22.	Failed to seek authoritative advice regarding innovation	0
23.	Lost professional role: patient became friend	0
24.	Felt guilty but still would not communicate	0

As noted, Adolescence scored highly with regard to *came to terms with own feelings; was able to enter into patient's problem* and *looked beyond patient's outward response/behavior to underlying causes.* The following case was surely the ultimate test of these responses for the nurse.

I was working in the capacity of a child-care worker in a group home for teen-age boys. To my horror one day, I found out that one of the boys had been bribing my 3-year-old to perform sexual acts for him. My initial gut level reaction was "KILL"; then I thought about sending him to a training school. Instead, I sent him to his room to think about it, while I got myself together enough to think out a rational course of action.

I decided that I must push my feelings about the boy in this situation aside, so that I could work the problem through with him therapeutically without further harming his own self-concept!

He was to spend all of his time after school at home in his room, and read a book for boys about sex, and discuss each chapter with me after it was completed.

One day I went to his room to check his progress and found him lying on his bed with a knife in his hand.

I said: You're really feeling bad about all this, aren't you?

He said: Yes, I want to die, I'm so ashamed.

I said: Really, Alex!

I was thinking, Gee, I'm really concerned, as I know shame can be a very destructive force.

He said: From reading the last chapter in this book I found out that what I did to Jerry could really have harmed him.

I thought, Wow, he really has taken this hard! I felt such empathy.

I said: Are you feeling that you are no longer capable of a good relationship with us as a family because of what happened?

I quietly took away the knife from his hand. I had just checked out my assumptions about how he was feeling with my direct question.

He said: Yes, I feel terrible!

I thought, I must help him to feel better about himself. Perhaps by discussing the book we'll get something to come out.

I said: Did you understand the parts of the book you've already read?

He said: I understand some of the book.

I said: Well, let me help you a little.

We had a brief explanation of the beginning of puberty and the games boys play, and why they shouldn't be played with youngsters. I paused, stumped.

I said: Would you help me out? I'd like you to take Jerry off my hands each day after school for an hour while I get supper. OK?

I thought, I'll try to show him I still trust him.

He said: You mean you forgive me?

I said: Well, I'm sure you are paying 10 times over for what you did. But, I still want you to finish the book and discuss each chapter with me. OK?

I was checking out and reinstating our original plan of action.

He said: Sure, I'll do that.

Then he carried on reading.

Alex was ashamed. Shame is the personal, private judgment of failure, passed on self by self. It is a merciless judgment. To have one's shame seen by others only reverberates and amplifies its awareness.

Poor Alex; although I had certainly been through my own personal turmoil, I felt empathy for him. I knew that if this whole issue was approached the wrong way, this lad could be messed up for life with guilt. This was using my knowledge of adolescent growth and development and sexuality.

I felt responsible for seeing this problem through, without my own personal needs interfering with rational thought, while still expressing my true feelings. Being aware of my own feelings and those of Alex produced a closeness, which helped communicate a sense of trust between us. I kept in tune with Alex's feelings through active listening.

By not overreacting to the knife he held, or to the incident itself, and by not letting my own personal biases get in the way, I was able to help Alex work through his guilt feelings.

The intervention in the conversation to explain the chapters in the book that he had just read was successful in increasing his knowledge of the sometimes overwhelming sexual feelings in adolescence, thus alleviating some of his guilt by making him feel more at ease with the problem. Continued conferences over subsequent chapters of the book were to serve a twofold purpose: to increase our closeness and to increase his knowledge of sex by talking it over with someone.

By trusting Alex to look after Jerry, I felt he would then understand that he was still worthwhile and that I still respected and trusted him.

At first, I had hated the boy for what he had done but by working it all through with him, we became close and both learned by the situation. When we left the home a year later, Al stayed with us for a few months as a foster boy, until he eventually returned home. So, although we grew close, Al never became overdependent; he progressed slowly away from us.

The response *did not want to understand* is highest where adolescents are concerned. Here the nurse points to her antagonistic attitude toward her own parents as the underlying reason for the way she handled the situation.

This situation occurred when I was working in a small northern town. There was one teen brought to the clinic by her parents with the complaint of having a seizure. I checked her over physically and could find no signs that there was any problem. The next day when the doctors arrived I asked them to see the girl. Nothing was found. We told the parents this and I added that if it happened again to call me and I would go and see the girl. This did happen the same night, but she was not having a true seizure.

I told the parents that it was not a true seizure and that she may have been upset and was having a tantrum. They said nothing and I told them to treat her as if she was having a tantrum. By the end of the next week there were another five children behaving similarly, all of whom had no real seizures. Their parents came to me and said that the children were sick and they did not know what they were doing. Such incidences increased over the next weeks, until I had about 25 of these children doing the same thing. They had all been checked by doctors and were cleared physically. I was being called all hours of the day and night. I felt angry at the parents for believing the children and at the children for not stopping after I had talked with them and their parents. Before the doctors had seen the children I had given a history of the occurrences and they had also talked with the parents in the presence of the children and told them that there was nothing wrong.

Every time the situation arose I found myself getting more upset at the child and parents for bothering me. I, at that time, felt that I had done all that I could and the children knew what they were doing and by doing it they were getting their own way. I felt that the parents deserved the upset because they refused to believe what I told them was true. Then the parents stopped bringing them to the clinic and teachers started to get the same situations of hysterical seizures during class. The teachers were getting upset by the disturbances in class and were asking me what to do about it. By this time I was not at the stage where I could cope with the situation and the other nurse was leaving for good and wanted nothing to do with problems. I felt very defensive and inadequate and unable to cope with the problem. I knew that I had to do something because the entire town was upset and wanted all those with the problem admitted to the hospital; I could not warrant this, since it was not a medical problem. Every time I had to deal with the families I did not listen to them any more.

Finally, I talked with one of the doctors who had had some experience with teens and was a good listener. I went to a nearby city and took a 4-day course on counseling the adolescent and other problems. At the time I still did not see where this would help and I blocked out that I was very much at the base of some of the difficulty. When I went back I talked to the principal and he and I worked out a plan to follow for the problems in the class. By his attitude I came to realize that I was doing more harm than good.

The problem still exists and I will be going back to it. By reading some professional literature, such as *Transparent Self* [Jourard, 1964] and *The Allied Health Professional and the Patient* [Purtilo, 1973], I am coming to a better realization of a problem that is more mine than the children's. I can see now that the way in which I talked to the children and the parents and not what I said had a definite effect on the behavior of both parties. From my background I have a very antagonistic attitude toward my parents and I feel that this was conveyed to the parents unknowingly in the way in which I approached them. I think now that the way I talked to the teens was supportive. Even though I was saying the opposite in words I was really giving them the message that I was in favor of what they were doing. Thus, I blocked the lines of communication and effective interaction for those parties involved. At present there is going to be a counseling program set up in conjunction with the adolescent clinic in the referring hospital and there will be follow-up conferences with the doctor from that clinic, whom I will be able to use as a resource person.

I will have to be more aware of the way in which I am getting my feelings across to those I am talking to and recognize when I am getting too involved or my personal feelings are hindering the situation.

I did not realize a great deal of how I felt until I did this paper and have found it to be a very practical help.

Again, in the following case, the nurse points to her need to side with the patient against parents. She describes her movement and professional growth through nursing a girl just 4 years younger than herself.

"In order to help our patients, must we involve ourselves to the point of becoming lost?" Nurses in my present position are constantly asking themselves this question. During my employment as a nurse I encountered a young 19-year-old girl who postoperatively developed complications that resulted in partial paralysis of her left leg, stiffness in her left arm, and loss of bowel and bladder control. Initially, I subjectively felt pity for Bette, yet objectively realized that I must assist her in adjusting to and accepting her disability. She had definite feelings of resentment (as I did) in that she was forced to accept her disability before rehabilitation had commenced. Bette identified with me since I was only 4 years older than she was. I realized her needs—for personal identity; for female and male companionship; for independence; for self-esteem; for pride and expression of self. I disputed Bette's mother's overprotective nature, which only made Bette more dependent and more aware of her physical and social limitations. So I served as a sounding board for Bette only.

In retrospect, I realize that I took her mother's role, one which I had disputed. I realized that Bette needed to establish an identity and feel needed, and I alone tried to satisfy these needs. Feeling quite emotionally drained after each visit, I could see that I was Bette's primary source of satisfaction. Gradually I came to understand that I was indeed breaking down Bette's relationship with her parents in order to satisfy my own need for security and recognition. And so, as the rehabilitation program progressed, I began to include the family. They, in turn, began to realize that Bette's demanding, irritable, supersensitive, and sometimes unbearable nature was a result of the situation they had created initially. In effect, we had been supporting her aggressive behavior and weakening her relationships.

It was a very difficult task to establish a meaningful balanced relationship between Bette and her family. I found I needed to have a great deal of patience, determination, fortitude, and self-understanding in order to offer adequate counseling. Her parents harbored feelings of guilt because of their previous lack of understanding, which I had made them realize. By encouraging them to take an active role in Bette's rehabilitation, I was hoping to relieve some of their tension and anxiety, as well as my own. I worked diligently to give support and a feeling of accomplishment to Bette's parents, realizing I had forgotten their feelings and had sided with Bette. Through mutual realistic goal-setting techniques, further frustrations were avoided as we were able to grow together and develop an understanding of each other's potentials, expectations, needs, and feelings.

In order to cope more effectively with the situation in which I was the in-between, when Bette and her family were rehabilitated sufficiently, I arranged meetings with successfully rehabilitated persons at the rehabilitation center. As I predicted, this served as an added inspiration to independence and a motivating factor.

I found I became confident in the situation as Bette increased her socialization with others and her motivation level in general. Although I had become very close to Bette, I was more and more able—through the use of self-examination—to redirect my personal feelings objectively into constructive development of the family relationship.

I know that I interfered with Bette's independence as a young adult. At times, I overidentified with her, and I was unable to objectively view potentially constructive family relationships. I was involved to the point of becoming lost in family problems, and should have discussed the program with a consulting nurse and with the family as a unit at an earlier time. Instead of realizing only Bette's reactions to stress in her emotionally aggressive outbursts, I should have examined my personal feelings in conjunction with those of the family. In similar situations since this case, I have been able to objectively analyze each member of the family and to apply this analysis in offering total family care. It really is far more satisfying than clinging to the patient.

In two-thirds of the Unhelpful cases, the nurse describes herself as being *disapproving, judgmental.*

One evening while working at a community health center I answered a knock at the door. There were two girls about 13 years old. One said that she had a dental appointment and asked whether they could come inside to wait. Just as I was questioning the absence of her name in the appointment book, another knock came to the door. Two boys about the same age were there, and one shouted, "That girl in there's a liar—she doesn't have to come! And if they can come in, so can we!" They pushed their way by me, ran and jumped on the couch, and began hassling over comics. These little people just wanted to stay to read, but all were aware of the rule that they could not come without an appointment. (Previous experience had taught us that to allow one to stay soon meant bedlam over the whole house!)

As I reminded them of the rules, they went from asking to stay, to pleading, to impudence. I told them that the clinic was for unwell people who need help, and tried to make them understand that we were not being mean—there was a justifiable reason. But to no avail. The whole incident turned into a kind of game. I became angry with their insolence and ended the episode, with the help of a medical student, by bodily evicting them and locking the door.

Although it was only a minor incident, I felt troubled about it. Sure, "kids will be kids," but I was upset with myself for losing patience with them. I was working at this community center because I was trying to help, and learn from, the people of a generally lower-class area. Although the situations that some of these people live in were depressing and seemingly unchangeable, I felt that by reaching the children of these people and educating them that there was hope of a way out. And one step was to help these children realize that people who represent authority—whether they be teachers, policemen, whatever—were not there only to dictate, push, and shove them into categorized roles. This was a common attitude of such people, resulting in mistrust and rebellion. Only through our efforts could we hope to represent friendship, guidance, and inspiration. I felt badly that by rejecting them because they would not listen, I had perhaps added to four children's already adverse feelings toward authority.

Upon looking back, I realize that I would not have listened to me, either. I had not talked with them, I had preached at them. Perhaps my attitude and intentions were too grandiose pertaining to other areas as well—too much of "Since *I* came here to help you, you'd better listen!" How could I help someone to help himself unless he became part of planning the solution?

Even though I was dealing with young adolescents in this case, had we looked at the problem together, and had they been given a chance to air their opinions and offer solutions, the situation could have turned out differently.

Fully one-half of the Unhelpful cases point to the fact that the nurse's *self-image was threatened.*

This situation occurred with an adolescent patient in the psychiatric department. The girl was in her room, sitting on the bed with her boyfriend. I went in to the room to encourage them to come out into the lounge. She told me she wasn't interested and pulled the curtain around her bed. I immediately pulled the curtain back, and she in turn pulled it closed again, resulting in my rather angry departure from the room.

I realize now that I was absolutely no help in this situation. To begin with, I was not very fond of this particular patient, and found it extremely difficult to relate to her. I obviously showed my mistrust of her by pulling back the curtain, and also my anger. I felt that I was not going to let her manipulate me, and I was the authority in the situation. I also wanted to let her know that I wasn't going to let her get away with anything. I felt that if I had let her do that, I would appear to her as ineffectual, and somewhat of a pushover. I was also no help to the rest of the staff, as they had all been trying to work with this one particular patient, who seemed to be the leader among our adolescent patients. After my display of temper she felt she had a legitimate reason for being angry with us all, and therefore, for some time, tried to refuse any suggestions we had to offer her.

I feel now, on looking back at the situation, this girl obviously wanted me to react in some way to her drawing the curtain—probably the way in which I did react. However, I would have been more help if I had ignored the pulled curtain and left the room, perhaps encouraging one of the other staff members, who related to this girl in a better way, to go in.

*　　*　　*　　*

Being a nurse at a private children's camp for 150 boys and girls aged 6 to 16 and a staff of 50 can give one many varied experiences.

It was 6:30 P.M. I thought I would relax in the back room; tonight was the staff barbecue and I wanted to attend. No interruptions tonight, please!

Suddenly the door slammed, and I could hear two girls giggling. One said, "Where is that nurse? She is never here when you want her." The door slammed as they went out. I knew the speaker was Diane.

I stayed in the back room because I was very angry. What did she mean! Why I'm always in camp and I just wanted to relax for 30 minutes. Slowly I got up, trying to compensate for her remark. Why, I had only been out of camp for 6 hours in 6 weeks. These kids!

Ten minutes later the door opened again. It was Diane. She explained she had a terrible headache and had been suffering with it since the car accident Saturday night; this was Tuesday.

I knew about the car accident. It had taken place with five other teenagers from the camp staff and some of the boys had been drinking. Only the driver remained at the scene. The other five walked back to camp. I also knew that the driver had falsely reported to the police and to the camp director. I certainly wasn't going to become involved with all these problems. What if there were legal complications and I was involved?

As these thoughts flashed through my mind Diane looked rather anxious. She didn't know how much I knew about the accident, if anything. I replied, "What car accident? It certainly hasn't been disturbing your performance on the playing field. Are you planning to attend the staff party tonight? I'll give you something for your headache but don't tell me about any car accident that happened Saturday. You go to your cabin and rest!"

Needless to say she stormed out in tears; yes, the door slammed again. I realized that what Diane needed was a sounding board. She was an exuberant, excitable girl and was really under great stress because of her association with the car accident. This tension she was bottling up was causing her headache and a little time to talk to someone at this time of stress was what she needed. I should not have been so disturbed because I was interrupted and because I might have missed the staff party.

Also, I should not have been influenced by her frivolous way with her camp duties and around the boys. Because of her family background she was insecure and this was part of the reason why she acted this way.

I should not have been concerned with legal complications because really, what could happen to me?

I lacked greatly in comprehending her immediate problem because I was concerned with myself. I attempted to rectify the increased tension I had caused by sending a senior staff member to visit her.

I have given a great deal of thought to my shortcomings in this particular situation and realize that I must not give myself an out due to my fear of becoming involved.

Treated the condition, overlooking the patient is described in one-third of the Unhelpful cases. The following case typifies the pressures that build up for both nurse and patient.

I was charge nurse on evenings on a medical pediatric floor. It was really busy and it was dinner time as well. A student nurse approached me stating that she had been unable to get a 12-year-old to take her pills. This particular patient was asthmatic as well as emotionally disturbed. I said I would give them, so off I stormed leaving what I was doing: I was annoyed at being interrupted so often as I felt the pressure of my work. I rushed into the asthmatic unit and asked the patient to please take her pills, but all she could do was scream and yell at me. I was so furious with her behavior that I lost all self-control. I did not give her a chance to reconsider taking them, nor did I give her a chance to say why she was refusing them. As well, I forgot about her emotional problem. Orders had been left to force the pills into her, so with help from the others, we restrained her and managed to get them into her in this fashion.

Afterwards, I felt so terrible and so cruel and so inhuman for what had happened, and saw where I had gone wrong. I realized that I should have got control of myself before I attempted to give her the pills. I should have finished what I was doing and that would have given both of us a chance to cool down. I was thinking only of myself and my needs. I was just so preoccupied with getting the pills into her and getting back to my work that I forgot about her. I gave her no chance to explain why she would not take them properly before we used force. I should have approached her in a calm, cool manner and spent some time trying to reason with her and talk to her, instead of accepting defeat right off the bat.

As I think you imply, both *you and your patient were reacting to pressures, though it was felt in different forms. This is a good illustration to help one truly empathize. Patients' feelings are not so different from nurses' feelings!*

*   *   *   *

I am not a city person, so yesterday I went to a park to study. I was duly impressed and began to compare the bluffs with life. Both have high, almost unaccessible peaks, smoother valleys, hidden dangers with seemingly easy ways out, just to be met with a large, dangerous overhang. There is a challenge of adventure to both. Many boys had the same feeling, and crossed the barriers to explore. Some knew the paths, venturing out boldly with no fears. Others went out carefully, stumbling forwards, clutching for help, which was not always available. It came to me that this was what the use of self was all about. It was the helping hand, sometimes needed and sometimes proffered and refused.

This was the way it was with Pete. I offered self, and was refused. Being a teenager is hard at best, but when the odds are stacked against you, well. . . . This was Pete's plight.

Pete at 17 was a gangly, withdrawn teenager, with severe adolescent acne. He had a girl friend, but was unsure of her mutual response, so he stayed by her almost constantly. They arrived at the school nurse's office just before the morning bell. Pete handed me a sealed note from his doctor, commenting that after he walked Susie to class he would return and discuss it with me. From past experience I felt that he used "discuss" in its broadest terms. I'd be lucky to get 10 words out of him.

While aware of his condition, Pete was not aware of the exact content of the note, so he peered over my shoulder as I read it. In essence it stated that he had a heart murmur of undiagnosed origin, he was not to participate in phys. ed. until he had further tests, returned to his doctor, and was referred to a specialist if necessary. When he heard about the phys. ed. exemption he became very agitated and kept murmuring, "It isn't so. It isn't so," then explosively said, "What about my basketball—the playoffs start a week from Tuesday?" Then he returned to his litany, "It isn't so." I felt so sorry for him. I too like sports and would not like to be deprived of them.

Fortunately, I knew his background history. He was an only child. His sister had died when she was 4 years old, following surgery for a congenital heart defect. Just 3 weeks previous to this incident, his father had died suddenly from a massive coronary attack. You could see unadulterated fear in his eyes, and imagine him thinking, "Heart murmur . . . undiagnosed origin. I'll be dead next." His mother, always a demanding woman, now in her grief was expecting even more from her son. He and his dad had had a close relationship; they were buddies, so his death was a major loss to Pete. But he was not allowed to mourn; his mother felt that as the wife she alone had the privilege of mourning in the family. Pete was not academically inclined, school was a bore, his girl friend had a wandering eye, and basketball was his only achievement. He surely didn't have much going for him. And now . . . his dad was dead, his basketball was on the verge of going, and if it did, Susie would likely go too—who goes steady with a loser? All told, it was a bleak hour for him.

With great difficulty I got through to him that permanent sports exemption was not yet an accomplished fact. He still had the tests and then the specialist's decision. He still should have hope. I knew that this particular doctor was very reluctant to completely rule out sports, but if this particular case merited this decision I could not raise Pete's hopes too high. It was a slim thread of offered help, but, I felt, better than none. Together we explained the medical problem to the coach, all of the time Pete soft-pedalling my explanation, "I'll be OK, sir." I could tell that he was trying to convince himself as well.

Pete would not agree to me calling his mother; he did not want to worry her he said (get a blast is what he really meant). I felt so useless; I wasn't meeting his need, neither was I meeting my own to feel helpful. My one small move could hardly be called an advancement, it was really just a stall. I tried to get Pete to talk about his dad, his home situation, his feelings, but to no avail. I was becoming frustrated and exasperated. Why could I not get through to him?

In his book, *The Transparent Self,* Sidney M. Jourard [1971] discusses self-disclosure. "Every maladjusted person is a person who has not made himself known to another human being, and in consequence does not know himself. . . . More than that, he struggles actively to avoid being known by another human being" [pp. 32–33]. It was easy to see Pete in this description. He surely did not believe in self-disclosure.

I tried a new tactic, my self-disclosure. I told him that my mother died when I was 8 years old. He still did not respond verbally, but in his expression I read that mothers were hardly on the same level as fathers. So—still not much success in communicating. At that point I dreaded the results of the tests almost as much as he did.

Friday came, and with it the results of the tests: still no Phys. Ed. until he saw the specialist. His family doctor phoned to make me aware that Pete had defied him, saying he would play ball anyway, and that I was to stop him. He also called Pete's mother, who in turn called me. She too told me to stop him. (In my inner thoughts I felt they were surely passing the buck and I was not sure that I wanted to catch it, or *How.*) I was surely in a bind. To start with I was already on very shaky ground. Until this point I was the person in whom he still had some faith. I also knew that this faith was so minimal that—poof—and it would be gone. The situation at hand could put the faith that would move mountains to the test of fire.

But I had to try. I called him out of class—I knew no other way. Even in retrospect I can think of no other way. I laid my cards on the table. He did not pick them up. I got the full blast of his agony and his anger. He was trapped—I did it—and he hated me. In vain I tried to explain the situation, my words pounding against unhearing ears. He had to get away, to be by himself. This I could comprehend, even though I was anxious about him in his present state.

He had preceded me into the room, and because of a very narrow entrance way, in which I by chance was standing, he was literally trapped this time. I foolishly again tried to reason with him. His only way of escape was to push me aside. This he proceeded to do, all the while screaming, "I don't care, I'll play, you can't stop me!" The coach unfortunately happened to be passing, heard the commotion and came into the room. This only made matters worse, as now he too had to be pushed out of the way. He was not as understanding as I thought I was. He rushed up to the principal to demand that Pete be suspended for assaulting us. After my explanation of Pete's inner turmoil, and my request on this basis to ignore the incident and also not to let Pete know this result of his outburst, the principal, an understanding man, agreed. To my surprise the coach became beligerent, but I had won my point. Pete stayed.

I felt that I had done my best all along the way, and so did the principal—but Pete—well, he did not. He refused to have anything to do with me at all. Just before the last game I received word that his exemption was lifted. I called him to my office to tell him the good news, but he refused to come, and I had to relay the message through the coach. The coach welcomed him back with open arms: he was a great guy; "Boy, he stood up for me," Pete said. In my heart, knowing the full story, I resented this, two-faced man that he was. . . .

This incident happened 2 years ago. I feel that while I failed at the time, Pete must have thought things through a bit, because now, if he can not avoid it, he will say hello to me.

I think if at the time of his dad's death all the involved staff had taken a good look at Pete and all the trauma he was facing, we could have made our efforts far more cooperative and of far more fundamental help to his basic self-image.

Here, the nurse describes herself as *not unduly influenced by negative opinions of other staff regarding the patient's personality* as the key factor in reaching out, *helping patient express feelings*. Both of these Responses score the highest ratio where Adolescence is concerned.

Linda was 13 years old and came to the hospital with the diagnosis of blastomycosis, a very severe and sometimes incurable fungus disease. Since she was from a small town, Linda left behind her maternal and family ties, as it would have been too far and too expensive for her parents to come and visit. This deprivation, along with the strange and painful treatments, confronted Linda unprepared. As a result she became very withdrawn and depressed and unfortunately she went unnoticed by the staff.

Other children on the ward came in and went out, but Linda always stayed, and consequently the nurses took her for granted and treated her almost as part of the surroundings. With all the physical care that had to be given to the other patients, the nurses never seemed to have the time to spend with her and really deal with her problems: she evidenced silence and withdrawal.

One evening, while I was in charge, the security guard came to me and stated that he had seen a patient standing at the landing of the stairwell at the end of the hall. She was hovered over the windowsill and was apparently crying. Other staff nurses on the floor with me said that it was Linda, but to just leave her, that she wanted to be left alone and was probably in one of her moods again. In spite of their protests I felt that something should really be done with her now as she was obviously upset and needed help.

I walked down the hall and out to the stairs. There was poor Linda sobbing as if her heart would burst. On approaching her I received a very weary, "Leave me alone, I don't want to talk to anyone!" For the first time it occurred to me that this isolated behavior was Linda's way of really asking for help. She needed someone to look beyond her overt personality and care enough to find out what was actually bothering her.

I sat on the stairs and remained silent, hopefully showing her that I was not going to be satisfied with her unconvincing reply. She continued to cry, so I went over to her and to my surprise she threw her arms around me and really let herself go. She blurted out all her feelings about being away from her family for so long, about her medications, about the tedious long days in and out of X ray, but most significantly her lack of any close friends while she was in hospital. After talking to her for about 20 minutes I felt a great guilt for not responding sooner.

In analyzing this situation I cannot help but recognize the needs of each individual patient and the way in which each projects them. Because Linda was an older girl and seemed to cope, although passively, with her hospitalization, she went ignored as far as any special attention was concerned. The staff were preoccupied with the toddlers and preschoolers, as younger children seemed to require more attention. Along with that the staff tended to spend time with the aggressive or hostile patients as their needs are much more obvious and often more immediate.

The outcome of my experience with Linda resulted in a favorable change in her behavior. She became more outgoing, although it did take a little more support on my behalf. I arranged for a day to take her downtown for a break in her day-to-day routine in the hospital. We became good friends and I am sure that she appreciated the hand that was held out to her.

While in the following case the nurse helped this teenager to express some of her feelings, their connection to the girl's resentment of her family, and in fact the pattern of her whole existence, appears not to have been treated.

The situation in which I feel I was helpful involved myself and a 15-year-old girl, whom I will refer to as Sarah. During the past 1½ years Sarah had been coming to my public health office for monthly prophylactic injections against rheumatic heart disease. At first she was resistant to coming, but after many low-keyed home visits about her condition we built up a working relationship. She came in very regularly for her injections and she usually talked about some of her concerns about her home situation and herself while I listened and gave her support. She was the oldest of four children, had quit school and spent her days baby-sitting for her younger siblings. Her parents were heavy drinkers and she seemed to resent having to baby-sit day and night while they got drunk. She often complained that her parents did not let her go out with friends and on occasion she ran away from home. Six months earlier she took an overdose of digoxin in reaction to her unhappy home situation.

One day Sarah came into the office for her Bicillin injection, appearing downcast and sad, contrary to her usual perky self. The following interaction occurred.

Nurse: How are you doing today, Sarah?

She looked very sad—I wondered what had happened.

Sarah: I'm OK.

She looked sadder and avoided usual eye contact.

Nurse: What sorts of things have you been doing lately?

I wanted to see if she could tell me on her own—it sometimes took a while. I knew she did not like the needle and usually felt more relaxed after it. I really felt concerned about her.

Sarah: Not much.
Nurse: Would you like the needle now and if you wish we can talk after it?

I was letting her know that I would like to talk with her, and also that she had the choice to do so.

Sarah: OK.

The needle was given. She was not usually this sullen—she was not smiling in her spontaneous way. I thought she was trying to give me the message that there was something bothering her.

Nurse: You look very sad to me, Sarah. Is there something bothering you?
Sarah: Yes, I do feel sad.
Nurse: Can you tell me about what is making you sad?

I hoped she could talk about it—I had not seen her this despondent since she took the digoxin overdose, but I did not want to push her. She smiled a little.

Sarah: I don't feel like talking about it now.

I felt a little uneasy—I wanted her to talk but I could not push her. I wondered what to say. I tried to empathize a little.

Nurse: I can understand that it is a difficult thing to talk about something that is bothering you. . . . Sometimes it can help to talk about it and get it off your chest.

I spoke in a deliberately calm and soft voice. She did not respond; she just kept looking at the floor. I wanted to let her know that I accepted "where she was at"—I would not reject her because she did not want to talk; I would sit with her. After a few minutes I began again.

Nurse: I am really concerned about you, Sarah. It must be something pretty important to make you feel this sad.

She nodded her head and started to cry. I put my arm around her.

Nurse: You know, Sarah, sometimes it helps to have a good cry.

I wanted to let her feel free to cry. I felt relieved that there was now an emotional response. After a few minutes she stopped crying on her own. I sat quietly with her for a few seconds after she had stopped crying.

Nurse: Do you think you can talk about it now? I think it might help you feel less sad.
Sarah: Yes, I do.

Sarah stated that she was afraid she was pregnant, and that her mother had told her a long time ago that if she ever got pregnant it would kill her because of her heart condition. It seems that Sarah had sex for the first time in November, but had no more relations since then (this was mid-January). She had an early period in December and was now a week overdue. I could understand the great fear she must have had. I wanted to decrease quickly her fear and anxiety. I felt quite sure she was not pregnant after having a period in December.

I told Sarah that I was fairly sure that she was not pregnant and that if she were, the doctor would thoroughly check her over and make sure that her heart was all right. She seemed a little relieved. I then explained the menstrual cycle to her, with the use of diagrams. This information seemed to be new to her; however, it appeared that she comprehended it. I also emphasized the effect of one's emotions on the cycle and told her that this irregularity had happened to me several times when I had been upset or worried. This also seemed to relieve her. I asked Sarah to come back to see me within a week and we would take the situation from there. She left looking relieved and happier. (She returned in a couple of days, stating she had her period. We discussed her sexual activity and the desirability of birth control if she chose to be sexually active, as well as a physical examination and consultation with the doctor.)

Sarah's activities may also have been an acting out of her rebellion against her parents.

I feel that I was helpful toward Sarah in that I helped her talk about what was upsetting her and hence relieved some of her fears and anxieties. Since we had a good rapport already, I was able to assess quickly that something was bothering her. I tried to accept her by not pressuring her to talk before she was ready. I showed this acceptance and my concern by comforting her and allowing her to cry.

I gave her ego support and encouragement to express her feelings when she was ready. I had recently had an experience of wanting to talk about something difficult, but was unable to until someone encouraged me to do so. I remembered the feeling and how relieved I felt after I was able to talk about what was upsetting me. I allowed Sarah to describe the situation in her own way and listened intently trying to understand the situation the way she perceived it, and trying to understand the amount of fear and anxiety she was experiencing.

I focused on the problem that was creating the greatest amount of fear and anxiety.

Temporarily—yes, and on the surface, but perhaps not fundamentally (see previous comment).

By giving her some knowledge of the menstrual cycle I reassured her that the probability of her being pregnant was very slight. I gave verbal and nonverbal reassurance that I was sure she was not pregnant. I knew I was risking her future trust in me if I were wrong but I felt she needed my reassurance and I was quite certain I was right. I also helped her deal with her feelings toward herself. I chose to deal with other issues such as her sexuality and birth control at our next meeting as I felt she would be more receptive to dealing with these issues then.

During the interaction, I tried to be aware of my own feelings. I realized I felt pressured to discover what was upsetting her in fear that she might overdose again. I also became aware of my anxiety when she was not willing to talk. I had previously resolved my own feelings toward adolescent sexuality and premarital sex, so that I was able to listen to her without being judgmental in my mind or words. By recognizing my feelings, I think I was able to prevent them from interfering with my interactions. I feel I was able to help her at her own rate to express her feelings, so that she could help herself.

Did you deal with the fact that her mother had always told her that if Sarah ever got pregnant, it would kill her because of her heart condition? This needed to be very carefully looked at with both mother and Sarah in terms of Sarah's whole future: marriage, self-image, etc. It seems that Sarah's life was pretty intolerable and she and the family needed help with a change in the whole pattern of her existence.

5

INTERPRETATION OF CONDITION

Of the 550 cases in the study, 20% focus on Interpretation of Condition. Of the 112 cases that focus on Interpretation of Condition, 45% are described as Helpful, 55% as Unhelpful.

COMPARISON WITH ALL OTHER SITUATIONS

Neither Helpful nor Unhelpful factors render highest ratings.

Helpful Factors	% of Cases in Which Cited
1. Gave moral support	62
2. Took time to explain	58
3. Helped patient express feelings	56
4. Wanted to understand how patient felt	54
5. Looked beyond patient's outward response/behavior to underlying causes	42
6. Initiated referral to another profession/resource	36
7. Nonjudgmental	30
8. Helped family members deal with the situation	30
9. Came to terms with own feelings; was able to enter into patient's problem	28
10. Was sounding board	24
11. Used innovative rehabilitative procedure	24
12. Used physical closeness	14
13. Liked the patient	12

14. Made this case the basis for overall policy change/
    improvement   8
15. Positively identified with patient due to similar life/
    professional experience   8
16. Was honest with patient/relatives   6
17. Not unduly influenced by negative opinions of other
    staff regarding the patient's personality   4
18. Had received training in recognizing social-emotional
    needs of patients   2
19. Was trying to prove self to senior staff members   2
20. Discussed religion with patient   0

Unhelpful Factors	% of Cases in Which Cited
1. Failed to look beyond initial negative impression of patient's personality	50
2. Was disapproving, judgmental	47
3. Treated the condition, overlooking the patient	40
4. Self-image was threatened	35
5. Did not want to understand	33
6. Felt pressured (within self) into doing things rather than coping with feeling elements (tension present)	28
7. Felt inadequate to enter into patient's problem because had not personally resolved the issue	28
8. Rationalized actions and thoughts	25
9. Purposely disregarded significant cues in patient's statements/behavior	25
10. Negatively influenced by opinions of other staff members regarding personality of the patient	17
11. Avoided needs of family members	15
12. Felt guilty but could not communicate	15
13. Lacked training in recognizing social-emotional needs of patients	13
14. Short-staffed; too little time to devote to the patient	13
15. Prejudiced toward group of which patient was a member	13
16. Disliked patient	12
17. Breakdown of interprofessional communication/ cooperation	12
18. Lost professional role: patient became friend	7

19. Felt guilty but still would not communicate   5
20. Disregarded own judgment because wanted approval
     of senior staff members   2
21. Failed to seek authoritative advice regarding inno-
     vation   2
22. Incapacitated by own fear of death   2
23. Overidentified due to being similar age to patient   2
24. Afraid would break down and cry in front of patient   2

It is clear that the nurse's *failure to look beyond an initial negative impression of the patient* (in 50% of the Unhelpful cases), and conversely, a willingness to *look beyond patient's outward response/behavior* (in 42% of the Helpful cases) are key factors in the balance between a Helpful and an Unhelpful relationship. The following account illustrates this dramatically.

This situation began on a Monday afternoon as I was rushing to the orthopedic ward to start work. Oh, how I hated afternoons and an entire week of it was just a dreadful thought. After report I proceeded to look over my patients' charts. I had 13 patients and 6 of them were diagnosed as lumbosacral pain, origin not known. On top of this dreadful shift, I had six patients who would be terrific complainers (as back patients usually are). You see, I had a label for people with back pain: neurotics.

So there I sat, anticipating the worst, and I had not even seen the patients yet. I was actually stewing about which patient would be the worst complainer and ruin my routine. On my tour of patients I found "the one" and did he ever give me a blast. He lashed out at me for dozens of things that were wrong. His bed sheets were wrinkled, the drinking water was warm, the room was too hot, the music from the next room was too loud, and a number of other items were not to his taste. After trying to settle Mr. J down I was positive I was in for a terrible week. My theory on undiagnosed back pain patients was correct—they were nothing but complainers.

As I was handing out the 6:00 P.M. medication, Mr. J proceeded to give me a detailed account of how this hospital did not measure up to the Eastside General in any way. This statement was the end. I thought this was a good hospital and this man had his nerve to think otherwise! By the time I left that room I was ready to say, "Okay, chum, up and off to the General!" However, I felt that this was no way for a nurse to behave and actually I feared the fact that Mr. J might report me to the head nurse.

During bedtime care, Mr. J continued to rave about the Eastside General and complain bitterly about the stupid nurses in this institution. Not one nurse had given him a decent back rub and mine certainly left much to be desired. By this time, I could not stand the criticism and felt I just had to leave the room. Thus I rationalized and nastily told Mr. J that I had 12 other sick patients who needed care also. Naturally these words made no impression; instead he just lashed out at me again. He did not care how many patients there were, he was ill and required attention. To make matters worse, I just rushed out of that room like a scared rabbit. I simply could not handle the situation so I tried to repress it by leaving.

Then in my haste I bumped into the orderly carrying a tray. Items spilled all over the floor. Since I was already angry at Mr. J and couldn't show it, it was very easy to project the anger onto the poor orderly. Later in the evening I felt sorry for losing my temper and apologized to the orderly.

Finally, after the preceding encounter I reached the desk and related my interaction with Mr. J to an older nurse. Of course, I rationalized my part, making myself out to be the angelic nurse, and Mr. J the ungrateful patient. Naturally, the other nurse agreed with me. Mr. J was a terrific complainer and a neurotic. She also advised me not to pay attention to all his demands.

Then his call light went on. Mr. J wanted a pain pill for the third time that evening. I was certain nothing could keep that man quiet—I knew the pills were not strong but I still felt that if he would settle down his pain would disappear. I still did not believe Mr. J had physical pain—he simply thought he did. By the time the shift was completed I felt exhausted. I certainly was not looking forward to the next evening.

The next day the interaction between Mr. J and myself continued to be one of conflict. If I showed my anger, he just increased his hostility and his demands. The entire evening consisted of one incident after another, leading to frustration on my part. Not once did I stop to think about the cause for Mr. J's hostility. I remained too concerned about my own feelings and just how this patient disturbed my routine.

The following afternoon I noticed Mr. J's myelogram report. To my amazement he had a protruding disc pressing on nerves, which caused him much discomfort. At that moment I felt terrible: I had completely failed to believe in my patient's pain. My first impulse was to apologize to him for acting so negatively, but I was simply too proud. I knew how upset my ego would be if the apology was refused.

That evening I tried to be considerate by listening to all Mr. J's demands and complaints without rejecting them. This was very difficult because I still felt his attitude was wrong. I even came quickly when his call light came on and paid attention to his every whim. I felt that I should do this to compensate for my previous behavior. I needed to prove to myself that I could communicate to Mr. J without further conflict. I still did not understand his hostility and his comments could still cause sparks of anger to fume within me.

The next evening I tried to remain thoughtful and considerate although Mr. J maintained his hostility. By the fifth evening I just thought of his negative reactions as part of his character and did not feel flustered when the hostility appeared. This was the time I began to notice that Mr. J did not complain as much any more. If I came soon after he called he made fewer unnecessary demands. The speeches concerning the Eastside General Hospital ceased. I felt our relationship was becoming a beneficial one. I could even sit down and answer his questions without getting upset. Then I realized that Mr. J was actually afraid of the hospital and the different tests that he was subjected to. So I explained the reasons behind the X rays and other special tests. After this he became relaxed and we could communicate. When his fears were overcome by reassurance and thoughtfulness the hostility disappeared. By this time Mr. J was interacting well with all staff members and his back pain was slowly decreasing as the disc returned into place.

In the beginning I failed Mr. J by putting my own feelings before his. I did not enjoy afternoon shifts nor did I enjoy orthopedic patients. I had managed to label them as neurotics. Then I attempted to prove this theory when they complained. Not for a single minute did I believe Mr. J had a legitimate excuse for his complaint because I had not really been concerned about him. Instead I thought of how much bother his demands caused me.

When Mr. J compared the hospital to the Eastside General I became angry. I did not enjoy accepting a viewpoint that differed from my own. I expected Mr. J to think of my hospital as the best when this fact had not been proven to him.

Now, I finally realize why I was able to help Mr. J. I had been able to show him by my action that I could accept him as a person, hostility included. It is a lot easier to read about accepting the patient as he is than to do it. I felt a certain amount of tension and anxiety before I could bring myself to truly accept this patient. After this happened within myself I could help to develop a working relationship with Mr. J. Once he felt reassured and secure there remained no reason for the hostility.

Now I can look back and realize that this experience shows definite proof of the need for accepting an individual. I just took this for granted before and never realized the significance of the word "acceptance." In the future when difficulties occur and I believe I am not using the correct approach, I shall look within to see if I am accepting this person. Until one can honestly accept a patient as a total individual any relationship will be false and accomplish very little.

It seems to me you moved from (1) needing to prove to yourself that you could communicate with Mr. J as a compensation for your erroneous labelling to (2) a patient-centered approach, where you focused on his problems and fears.

Then, rather than accepting him in spite of his hostility (which is really only a sufferance through clenched teeth!), you began accepting him with his hostility and began to diagnose and treat it from his point of need. Those are some moves!

*   *   *   *

One evening, working part-time at the Children's Hospital, I was thrown into a position of responsibility on a ward with unknown patients. I was feeling unusually harassed and anxious to see visitors leave as near the appointed time as possible. In one room a mother with a female friend was lingering, reluctant to leave her apparently sleeping child of about 6 years. Rather brusquely, I suggested she go home to rest herself and return in the morning—and she quietly complied. Only about an hour later, having seen to the more severely ill patients and while reviewing the rest, with their diagnoses, did I discover that this particular child was in the hospital for a minor problem, but was also severely mentally retarded.

Although the next hour or so was very busy, I couldn't rid myself of nagging feelings of guilt at not having offered this mother the simple assurance she so obviously needed. Finally, although it was almost 10:30 P.M., I decided to telephone her at home, in case she was worrying about anything. After explaining that I had not known her child was retarded and would not be able to express her needs adequately, I asked about any feeding, sleeping, toilet, and other habits from which she might derive comfort.

Mother, with obvious relief, answered these questions in detail, then went on to explain her feelings of unease, in spite of repeated hospitalizations, at leaving her little girl in the care of strangers who would not understand her. She cited other occasions of having been briskly dismissed by nursing staff, hence her reluctance to interrupt anyone's work to explain her child's variety of peculiarities. In closing the conversation she again expressed relief and a certainty that now she would surely get to sleep more easily.

Suddenly the things that had kept me so busy earlier seemed relatively unimportant, mere details and more institutional routine. There was suddenly time to spend with this little girl, in coaxing her to drink in the way her mother had suggested and rocking her awhile before settling her to sleep. This time thus spent was satisfying to me in itself, to the little girl in her response, and, it is hoped, to her mother's state of mind while away from her. I can only hope to always remember this situation before slipping back into the let's-get-on-with-our-work attitude unfortunately so often encountered in hospitals, forgetting that our work is people.

I find it very easy to slip at times into such involvement in doing things and in being as organized and neat as possible at the same time, that attention to the person involved, rather than just a body, falls behind. Perhaps fortunately, I'm easily stirred by others' tears or expressions of concern and usually respond compassionately and, it is hoped, reassuringly. It's situations like this, however, that serve as an important reminder that concern and apprehension are not always so obviously expressed.

A very important point.

Treated the condition, overlooking the patient is described in 40% of the Unhelpful cases.

It was 11:00 P.M. on a busy Sunday evening when I received a message that Mr. B in room 152 wanted to see the supervisor right away. When I arrived in the patient's room a few minutes later I found him extremely angry and upset. He had been in the hospital for a week for diagnostic purposes and had been on a 24-hour urine collection as part of the investigation. A nursing assistant had just thrown a specimen away, which would ruin the test! I was confronted with a myriad of questions. "Are you in charge of the hospital tonight? Is there anyone of any higher authority on the premises? What are you going to do with this stupid staff member? Do you stand for this kind of stupidity or will you relieve him of his position? Why do you employ such people to start with? How is the doctor ever going to find out what's wrong with me if a stupid so-and-so ruins the test?"

I agreed with the patient wholeheartedly that the nursing assistant had made a stupid mistake and I, too, was angry with him, because even though he was a relief staff member for that evening only, the tests were clearly marked to avoid errors. I agreed that I would most certainly talk with the person involved about the error and the consequences, and I would also inform the doctor. I felt Mr. B's present state of anxiety and complete exasperation and frustration was increasing and that it must surely be related to other negative incidences while he had been in hospital or deeper and more involved feelings and worries. I tried to receive the real message, but was unable to. I commented on the fact that he had been able to leave the hospital to have Sunday dinner with his family that day, but his only reply was that he had conscientiously voided before he left and not again until he had returned for the accuracy of the test.

Perhaps not really listening for his deeper worries, but rather attempting to vindicate the hospital?

His only consolation seemed to be that he planned to see the administrator of the hospital first thing Monday morning to report the incompetency of the staff member. I left the patient's room 40 minutes later, feeling that I had completely failed in this situation.

I had been in a supervisory position in a large city hospital for 7 years and certainly interaction with patients, families, nursing and medical staff, and all hospital staff was an integral part of my work. Situations of misunderstandings, conflicts, complaints, and so on, were not rare but common occurrences. I met Mr. B with a genuine regret that the incident had happened and a genuine concern that he was so overwrought. I felt that even though I couldn't retrieve the lost urine (Oh! how I wished that I could!) I could create a helping relationship.

However, such was not the case. Mr. B and I were not on the same wavelengths, and I was not hearing or understanding his real message. My defenses were up as well as those of the patient. I became anxious about the time and other problems yet to be solved before midnight. I concluded that because Mr. B was a chartered accountant, he was a perfectionist: his figures were always correct and in line, therefore making him intolerant of human frailties.

No doubt he was very concerned basically as to how and when (following a week's testing) his diagnostic investigation was going to add up and frustrated that the human body (his own) didn't always operate according to calculations or specifications. This fact of life was further borne out in the assistant's mistake and provided a specific act around which he could summon all his anger and anxiety.

Furthermore, his wife was an active, well-known leader in the nursing profession, and I failed to understand why I found it impossible to communicate with him, and why he had not been indoctrinated into some of the problems of nursing by his wife. This increased my frustration and annoyance. I was aware of my own feelings to a certain extent, but was unable to control or change them at the time—thus never meeting Mr. B with anything more than very cold comfort.

Here a young nurse describes the combination of administrative and self factors that prevented her from supporting this patient or his family.

I was not interested in doing intensive care nursing because I was afraid of the unit and the very close contact with patients. I also wondered if I would be able to cope and measure up to what was expected of me. I am sure that these feelings also helped me fail in dealing with Mr. R.

Half of our graduating class was chosen to do a 3-month period in the unit, and I was one of the chosen. While doing my training, I looked after Mr. R, a 24-year-old who had just been admitted a few days before as a result of a car accident. Mr. R was not married, extremely good-looking, and had a fantastic physique. He had also just returned from a vacation in Barbados with a dark tan, and had only been back a week when the accident had occurred.

Mr. R was on a Stryker frame and had tongs in his head. He was also paralyzed from vertebra one down. He had only head movement, slight sensation in his right hand, and slight movement in one shoulder. He had no sensation in any other part of his body.

During my time in intensive care, I was often assigned to Mr. R. At first Mr. R was most cheerful and looked forward to chatting with me. He had not been told the extent of his injury and I believe he was still in a state of shock. We never mentioned the accident and talked of everything else. I was relieved that the accident was never mentioned because I did not know what to say if he brought it up; rather I encouraged all other topics of conversation so that the issue would be avoided. At times we talked about the future, but very superficially, because I knew and was afraid of what the outcome would be. His parents had requested, on advice from the doctors, that Mr. R not be told that he would probably never recover, and that he might only regain very limited usage of his right hand.

At this point, I had mixed feelings. I was terrified that one slip of the tongue and I would blurt out the truth; thus my conversation was guarded. I also felt the frustration of not telling Mr. R the situation, as I thought that he had a right to know.

Each day I watched Mr. R look at his body and I wondered if he knew or suspected his condition. He often asked me if I thought that he was losing muscle tone and sometimes he told me that he could feel sensations in his feet. I felt annoyed because I knew his probable outcome; why did I have to hide this from him? I lied and said that he was doing as well as could be expected at this point, but I also felt very guilty about saying so.

I was also afraid of any mention of Mr. R's future, because of my inadequacy to offer support and comfort. Already I felt that such a tragedy was a senseless waste of a human being.

As a result, my contact with Mr. R became less than it had been. I did the necessary physical care required but never really involved emotional support. If he asked any questions, I gave brief answers because I was beginning to pity Mr. R. I was also afraid of becoming more emotionally involved with Mr. R: that is, he was coming to expect more of me as a person than as a nurse. So before more of such a relationship could develop, I backed away quickly. I couldn't cope with such a dependence. I never realized that possibly Mr. R was trying to reidentify himself as a person and was probably very concerned with his body image and trying to cope with loneliness as well.

Each time his parents came to visit, I left quickly. I couldn't face the bleakness in their faces and then the forced false cheerfulness when they saw their son. It seemed as if nothing had happened to their son. I wanted to scream at them that there was no hope of Mr. R ever regaining the use of his body. What were they hoping to gain? Not once did I try to talk to them about their son, or tell them of a little of his progress. I didn't even try to realize what his parents must have been going through. I felt inadequate and overwhelmed by the senselessness of such a tragedy. I felt, too, most selfish. What could I offer them anyway?

As time went on Mr. R became more and more aware of his situation. He began asking why he still didn't have any feeling in his legs, or regain the use of his arms. I told him that it would just take time and to have patience and that I knew how he felt. Again a useless answer! How could I possibly know how he felt! Here I was, a person who could walk and use my arms and legs, clearly showing Mr. R that he could not. I also probably increased Mr. R's anxiety level as well as my own, because I had probably led Mr. R to believe that he was undesirable and useless.

At a later date, after completing the morning bath, Mr. R asked me to leave the curtains closed for a while. He said that he would like to have a quiet period to himself to think. After a short interval I returned and asked if I could enter. A muffled voice greeted me, and I found Mr. R crying. My reactions were mixed. I thought, how could a man cry and what for? Immediately I felt helpless and uncomfortable. In our society, men were not supposed to cry, no matter how tough the going was. I asked what the matter was, but in a tone of voice that conveyed that I couldn't help him anyway. I never realized that Mr. R was crying from the sheer terror of what his life now was, and his uncertain future.

Even when Mr. R lashed out at me verbally, blaming me and those around for his present state, I took this as a personal affront to me, not realizing that frustration, fear, and helplessness led Mr. R to show denial and resentment of his condition. Also, I was most often in contact with Mr. R. I was the closest one he could express his feelings toward. I was hurt and felt Mr. R shouldn't have done this to me.

Thinking back now, I really failed that young man. How much easier it would have been for both of us to have first created a meaningful relationship—to be able to talk about the future, to talk about what was really troubling him, and to offer possibly some hope or short-term goals. I should have listened effectively and been more supportive and understanding, instead of only being concerned with myself. But because of my fear of becoming involved, I chose the easy way out. Feelings that I could not cope with, such as pity, fear, frustration, and anxiety, made me most ineffective in my dealings with Mr. R.

In 35% of the Unhelpful cases the nurse identifies the fact that her *self-image was threatened*. In the following case, the nurse also refers to her vulnerability, but moves through this to give invaluable *moral support* (62% of cases).

Working on a male surgical ward, I came in contact with a boy named Jerry. Together, we faced a situation in which I was vulnerable.

Jerry's face had been burned away following a freak accident. He was driving a truck that hit a culvert, throwing him free of the vehicle, but the motor of the truck landed on his face, completely destroying it. No brain damage resulted, and despite a religious faith that prohibited blood transfusions, Jerry lived and began a painful, slow climb back to life.

One day, he posed a question to me and I had to face reality as it was, not as I desperately wished it could be. "Margie, what does my nose look like?"

I felt the relationship we had developed to this point was being tested and only the truth could sustain this helping relationship. In order to help Jerry cope with life, develop, and improve his functioning I would have to be honest. Honest in a way that didn't observe through rose-tinted glasses; honest in a way that was caring and yet cruel. I suspected Jerry had asked others the same question and for a moment I hesitated, wondering what I should say.

I told Jerry the truth as I saw it. He had no nose, nor was there much of a face left on his head. After we had talked regarding his physical appearance, he said quietly, "Thank you for being honest, you are the first person who has been really honest with me."

At that moment, I realized I had fully accepted Jerry for himself. Despite his hideous face, I had seen beyond it to the boy named Jerry. I had met him halfway by being honest and, therefore, could use myself to help him in becoming a more complete person.

We had developed a trusting relationship on the basis of honesty. This relationship continued as I spent extra time with Jerry, learning to empathize with him and comprehend the great void there would be in his life.

Helped patient express feelings is cited in 56% of the Helpful cases.

It started out with a teacher asking me to see Melinda T regarding a rash on her arms. The teacher also asked me to chat with Melinda for a while as she often made remarks in class such as, "I hate my father because he killed my mother."

The T family had just moved into the area so I had no school health records for reference. I felt strongly though that this 9-year-old girl was asking for help with such an attention-getting statement.

Very shortly an unkempt-looking young girl was at my office door. It was Melinda, in minor distress due to the itchy nature of her rash. She was wearing a new blouse, so I presumed that a substance in the blouse was causing the skin reaction. I asked her if someone was home so that she could go home to change. She replied that her father was home. Upon further inquiry, I learned that her mother had died of cancer 10 months earlier. Very matter of factly she added that her father was also dying because he drank a bottle of rum every day and that now his liver was shot.

My concern was raised as to just what kind of a household this child was living in. (She also had a 12-year-old brother.) I thought that perhaps this lonely widower was trying to solve his problems in a bottle or that maybe Melinda was telling fibs to get attention.

That afternoon I visited the T household on the pretense of seeing how Melinda's rash was. Mr. T was sitting on the living room couch and appeared in a very debilitated state. He was impossible to talk with as his responses were inappropriate and irrelevant and he was hallucinating. Yet I did not think that he was drunk. He came with me readily to see Dr. G. The doctor admitted him directly to the hospital with a diagnosis of Korsakoff's syndrome. Two days later he was further diagnosed as having cancer of the left lung; he was dead 6 days later.

Within this short time period, I got hold of Melinda's 16-year-old sister, Joan, who was living with a young man in town. She really impressed me as a responsible, level-headed young lady, and quickly took over the care of the children. Other chores involved contacting Social Services, arranging for welfare assistance, and having Joan get all necessary papers together for the lawyers.

Feelings about their dad's impending death were sorrow, guilt, fear as to their future, and a desperate feeling of being all alone. Due to the extremely short time element between diagnosis and death they reacted with denial. I spent much time with them and gradually they passed through all the stages of mourning.

There was much ambivalence in their feelings toward their dad. He had drunk and abused the family for years. Yet he was their father and they wanted to feel that they loved him. What really tore these kids up was that they truly felt that he had killed their mother. They had been very close to their mom. Mrs. T died from a primary cancer of the breast. It seems that their doctor had told them the cancer started from a hard blow Mr. T had given her in the chest with a lamp. Mr. T had been in one of his usual drunken rages at the time. They were very open with these feelings and through many many talks I got them to see how very justified their feelings were and not to feel guilty about having them. I really think that this was a great comfort to them and that they understood themselves better.

The major problem was that there were no relatives to care for them. The possibility of becoming foster children under court custody was a very real concern. Joan wanted custody of her younger brother and sister and she and her boyfriend were planning to get married so that they would have a chance to do this. I wanted desperately for this to happen, yet I felt it unfair for Joan to have such heavy responsibilities at such a young age. I urged her to think of herself in this matter. Much counseling was done by myself and social workers. All aspects were thoroughly examined and Joan and her newly acquired husband presently have temporary custody of the children. All is going well.

For a period of several weeks, I visited the T family regularly. I became their older sister and confidant, and they felt free to discuss anything at all with me. They relied heavily on me before and until shortly after the death of their father.

They are now gaining independence and self-assurance daily. I strongly believe that my involvement with this family allowed them to remain a family unit—and a good one.

I hope the family will continue to be seen. You are right that Joan has a heavy burden—which needs on-going support. It would be easy enough to assume all will be well and later find that tensions had developed—more guilt, breakdown, etc.

Took time to explain is specifically cited in 58% of cases, indicating that this response is not considered to be automatic. Here the nurse is able to draw on the interpretations and concerns of the family, rather than explaining them away.

This situation began with a phone call from the nurse for the ENT specialist, Dr. C, who called to give me a T and A booking for one of our patients. This child, Jill H, had been seen in consultation by Dr. C because of recurring ear infections and Dr. C had advised a T and A. It was standard procedure for Dr. C's office to arrange the hospital booking and phone the information to me; I then called the family to inform them of the date and to answer any questions that they might have. I had seen the Hs many times in recent weeks so Mrs. H knew who I was when I called.

Mrs. H's Reaction

Mrs. H became alarmed that the T and A was to take place, stating that Jill was now well and that it did not seem right to take a well child to the hospital and make her "sick." I questioned her and found out that Dr. C had fully explained the operation and why it was being done. She protested that while she was happy to agree to the T and A at the time of the consultation under the pressure of Jill's illness, she now considered the risks of the operation too great to go ahead.

My Reaction

My feeling about the situation was sympathy toward her. My eldest daughter had recently undergone a T and A and I had been surprised at what a traumatic experience it had been for me. Although I was familiar with the hospital and the operative procedure, and confident in the ability of the surgeon (the same one incidently, as Jill's), I had been quite shaken by my fears and doubts. I knew my fears were unfounded but was not at ease until my daughter was safely home.

However, as I listened to Mrs. H, I detected more than the usual amount of apprehension. By listening with that third ear I interpreted her protests as indicating a troubled area that she wished to communicate without verbalizing the actual cause.

Progression of the Situation

Mrs. H further revealed that she was afraid that Dr. M, the pediatrician, would be cross at her for not following the advice of the doctor to whom Jill had been referred, and that she would be scolded if the ear infections recurred; that she would be, or be thought to be, neglectful for refusing necessary treatment.

Since Mrs. H was reluctant to speak to Dr. M herself, I suggested that I discuss it with Dr. M and with Dr. C's nurse and call her back. I hoped that if I was better informed, the problem could be overcome.

The family file provided some of the missing pieces to the puzzle. Jill was the youngest of two girls of an immigrant family. An older daughter was a patient in an institution for retarded children. Dr. M provided more information. The older child had been born normal, but had been reduced to vegetable existence by meningitis at an early age.

I spoke to Dr. C's nurse, who assured me that the T and A was advised but certainly not essential to Jill's life. Dr. M added his assurance that the choice was Mrs. H's, and would be respected whichever way she decided. Armed with this information, and choosing a quiet time of the office day, I called Mrs. H back.

How I Handled the Situation

The problem had changed from convincing Mrs. H to agree to the T and A, to assuring her that her reasons were understood and valid: that Jill's health would not be jeopardized without the operation, and that Jill's future care would be in no way influenced by her decision.

Mrs. H's reaction was one of great relief. She also seemed surprised that her feelings were really understood.

Evaluation of Myself

I feel there were several factors that helped me to help Mrs. H.

1. I had had personal experience in a similar situation and was able to recognize an appropriate reaction.
2. My reply to her was not judgmental, argumentative, or scolding.
3. Patience and a listening attitude encouraged her to enlarge on and explain her fears.
4. My sixth sense made me aware of deep feelings and fears about this child.
5. By using other sources of information that I knew to be available, it was not necessary to probe too deeply with Mrs. H.
6. I respected Mrs. H's ability to make the right decision for her own child.

By recognizing that she had made the right decision and by communicating this to her, I was able to allay her fears about future treatment. By recognizing this seemingly small incident as a major crisis in Mrs. H's life, I was motivated to give the situation my full concern and attention and to bring about a solution that was mutually satisfactory.

Excellent—you were able to lay aside any need to sell this mother on the operation and thus appear efficient. Too often our own need to succeed blocks our listening to our sixth sense and actually defeats the helping process, real efficiency, and true success.

In this case the nurse describes taking time to explain syphillis.

Recently, a field nurse and I were having our weekly conference about the district, when suddenly she complained, "I am getting nowhere with Mr. Jones. That man is supposed to be a VD contact, and so far I cannot persuade him to attend a clinic or see his family physician. He keeps saying he'll go tomorrow, and nothing happens. Will you take over the case for me?" I had a feeling this nurse was uncomfortable in this situation, and maybe had created some of her difficulties by her attitude. In the past, she had frequently grumbled about VD cases, and the "baby-sitting" we were expected to do with such cases. Having had my own problems with clients, I could sympathize with her. Although one tries to comfort oneself with the conflict of personality theory, and struggle along somehow, there are occasions when it is better to turn the case over to someone else.

After trading assignments, I decided to try to contact my new client by telephone. It seemed only fair that my visit should be at his convenience, if at all possible. Mr. Jones sounded cautious and hesitant, but agreed that I might see him the next afternoon. I was careful to check his file to get what background data I could.

It appeared that I would be dealing with a 30-year-old swinger. I began to plan my visit, confirming clinic addresses and hours and reviewing information as to the usual plan of action at each clinic.

Arriving at the agreed time, I was greeted at the door by a defensive Mr. Jones. He invited me in; I felt relieved at that. Somewhat nervously he asked me to sit down, then he sat across the room, tense and rigid in his chair.

After the usual polite preliminaries, I inquired, "The nurse who visited you previously has stated that you are a contractor, and very busy at this time of year. Do you work long hours?" Suddenly, he moved to a chair across from me, and in great detail explained how important it was for him to be at work every day. His employer really depended on him to see that everything on the construction site went like clockwork. I noticed that he was now relaxed in his chair, his voice was less tense, and he seemed at ease with me. I hoped this was the correct time. If I dragged out the visit, he might feel that I was evading the issue, and both of us would end up uncomfortable in our bogged down conversation. I decided to try.

"You know, of course, why I was so anxious to see you today, Mr. Jones. I hope I did not inconvenience you by asking to see you, on such short notice?" He leaned forward and somewhat abruptly said, "You think I have syphilis, and I must be examined. Well, I should know. I don't have it and I won't waste my time visiting doctors. I have read all about syphilis. I am certainly not stupid. I protect myself!"

I could understand his indignant remarks. He seemed so positive: was he trying to convince himself? Struggling to remain calm I managed: "People sometimes are misinformed about syphilis. You know, the symptoms vary. Our concern is that you may have been in contact with someone who now has a diagnosed disease. If you have the test it will alleviate any doubt in your mind. If you have been infected, the earlier you are treated the more advantageous it is for you. After all, you are a young man; it would be a tragedy to find in a few years that you have medical problems because you neglected to care for yourself."

I waited. Had I talked too much? I only hoped my concern was on the same wavelength as his. After a few seconds of silence, he smiled and said, "You know, I really think you care what happens to me. So I'll go to the clinic, if they will see me after 5:30 P.M. You can telephone from here, and save yourself a trip."

Quickly, arrangements were finalized and, fortunately, he kept his appointment. A week later he telephoned the office and asked for me. I was surprised to hear this cheerful voice yelling, "Hey, Nurse. I'm OK. Thanks a lot. Call me any time you think I might have a problem. OK?"

Unexpected as the call was it was reassuring to know that my attempt to help a patient had been effective. Learning not to make value judgments is difficult, but rewarding on occasion.

At the same time, there is a difference between informing a patient about a condition and understanding their more fundamental questions.

Mrs. B was admitted to the medical floor of our hospital. Her admitting diagnosis was vertigo, unspecified cause. Mrs. B was a very attractive, sophisticated woman of about 40. She was accompanied by her husband, who seemed genuinely concerned. The Bs had no children and were a career couple.

The neurologist, on examination, felt that Mrs. B had been having mild epileptic seizures. However, any suggestion of this was met with denial and indignation. The neurologist's questioning had been most tactful. Mrs. B stated that she would occasionally have dizzy spells and fall down. These she had been having since approximately the age of 20, and it was their increase in frequency that finally urged her to seek medical attention.

The neurologist still felt that she had been having convulsions, however mild, and stated this to the nurse. I couldn't believe that a seemingly mature, intelligent woman could be so opposed to even the possibility that she might have had a convulsion. I decided to see if I could build some sort of a relationship with this woman, where we could talk about her illness comfortably. This was my challenge.

Mrs. B was very easy to talk to on almost any topic except her illness. I was quite discouraged, as whenever I tried to approach the subject Mrs. B would change it. Finally, one day she asked, "What is a convulsion like?" I was really excited at this first sign of interest from Mrs. B. However, I tried not to convey this feeling and tried to answer her in a sincere and interested manner. It seemed that Mrs. B had been quite embarrassed by her fainting spells and concerned about them for some time. In spite of her beginning interest Mrs. B still maintained that she couldn't possibly have a convulsion. There had been no history of epilepsy in her family and she would be a disgrace to her family if this were so in her case. I explained that there were many epileptics holding down good jobs and that she might even know one; with the proper medication and doctor's care she could lead a very normal and productive life. With this type of care she would be able to go about her business without the constant fear of having one of these fainting spells.

The tests that had been ordered by the doctor were confirming his diagnosis. Mrs. B phoned her sister and told her that she was under treatment, but couldn't tell her exactly why, as it was a shameful disease.

Mrs. B's treatment was begun and in due time she was discharged. The success of this challenge was not complete by any means, but I suppose one step was taken in the right direction when she consented to the medical staff that Yes, these spells could possibly be mild convulsions. However, there was still shame and doubt about her condition, as far as her family and friends were concerned.

I feel that my role was that of an informer about her condition at a time when she was receptive. I realized her feelings about the disease and tried to be supportive. Although Mrs. B was still denying to a point, I feel she had taken the first step in accepting her condition.

Did you simply inform her of the positives regarding job, medication, etc., or did you also explore with her the misconceptions about people who have "something wrong with their heads?" She needed to come to terms with the latter before she could accept the former.

Was *disapproving, judgmental* or *nonjudgmental* are indeed major factors in Interpretation of Condition. These responses are cited in 47% of the Unhelpful cases and 30% of the Helpful cases, respectively.

This situation occurred when I was working in the capacity of a public health nurse in the health department of a large city.

My district, and the schools I visited, were located in an old section of the city known for its high incidence of multiproblem families. I had excluded from school the member of one such family. The five or six children from that family were examined and found to have pediculasis (head lice). An official form from the health department, signed by myself, and endorsed by the principal, was sent home with the youngsters requesting treatment and a return to school as soon as possible.

When the children failed to turn up at school within the week, I decided (mainly due to the principal's insistence) to drop around to the home. I had known from previous nursing records this was a multiproblem family, well known to the health department, and various social agencies as well, but I was quite unprepared for the sight that greeted me!

The house was badly in need of repair, steps were missing, screens half off; the house was dirty, squalid, unkempt, full of flies, and an unwashed odor prevailed.

I know I wasn't able to hide the feelings of disgust and indignation I felt, and the fact that I was 3 months pregnant, and fighting back a wave of nausea, didn't help the situation any.

I inquired as to why the children hadn't returned to school. Their mother explained with a series of weak excuses. I couldn't have cared less about establishing rapport at this point, and I assumed my authoritarian role; armed with the knowledge that public health regulations backed me up, I informed her she must have the children's heads cleared up and them in school without delay! And as an extra reinforcement, I reminded her that if the children weren't attending school regularly, she could lose her public assistance check! (This was the principal's suggestion.)

I was successful in that the children were back to school very promptly, and in satisfactory condition, but I was never able to go back into the home and establish any kind of a working relationship.

I failed to put myself in the patient's position. I considered her a stupid, ignorant, sloppy woman, and I made no attempt to approach her intelligently, or to consider her feelings and her frustrations from years of living in these depressing surroundings. I allowed my own feelings of disgust and indignation, the fact that I wasn't feeling well, and my annoyance at the principal for foisting off part of his job onto me (it was an attendance problem as well as a health problem) to contribute to my improper handling of the situation.

*   *   *   *

Mrs. Z was admitted to the intensive care unit for investigation of gastric hemorrhage, which occurred several times at home prior to her hospitalization. She was a new citizen from Latvia, aged 45 years, married to a technician; the couple had no children. Mrs. Z was a private patient since her husband had very good health insurance. She spoke English well enough to make herself understood and in turn was able to understand when spoken to slowly.

Monday morning, following a weekend off, I came on duty and in the course of the night-nurse's report I learned about Mrs. Z's condition, her doctor's orders, and her present behavior in the unit. I was told that she was a difficult and demanding patient but not in any apparent physical distress. As was my custom, following the report I went on rounds and chatted with every patient for a while to find out more about their current health problems.

I came to Mrs. Z and asked her how she was, to which she replied angrily, "What do you mean how I am! How could I be in this terrible public ward where men and women are together? I want you to phone my doctor right away to get me out of here. My husband is paying for a private accommodation and I demand a decent room." I felt anger swelling in me at this rude tirade and trying hard to be calm I replied, "This is not a public ward, Mrs. Z, and many patients would be very grateful to be here. This is the intensive care unit where the hospital provides the best available care, which your husband could not buy for you unless he was a millionaire." Without saying anything else I walked away thinking, silly woman.

I completed my rounds with the rest of the patients and had returned to the desk, when Mrs. Z beckoned me. She had had clear fluids for breakfast because of her history of hemoptysis and intended investigations. When I arrived she pushed her tray away and said to me, "I am not going to eat this, so take it away because I think you made a mistake in the first place giving it to me." Woman, I thought, you have no manners, you are rude and should be put in your place! Thus I said to her, "You are not going to be operated on today or tomorrow since the doctors have to investigate first what causes your bleeding. I did not make any mistake and next time when you have any complaints about your food, would you please tell your nurse instead of calling me. I can assure you that if there is anything that I should know, your nurse will report it to me." "Honey," said Mrs. Z, "You do not understand, I have to have an operation because that is what my doctor told me." What could you tell someone like that, I thought, when she does not want to believe you anyway. To Mrs. Z I replied, "I will speak to your doctor and he will explain to you your treatment."

When the surgeon and medical consultant arrived in the unit, I explained to both that Mrs. Z did not understand why she was in the unit and insisted that she would be operated on that day. The doctors agreed to speak to her and went with me to her bedside. I introduced them to Mrs. Z, saying that she would be able now to find out anything she would like to know about her treatment. To my surprise, instead of asking any questions pertaining to her condition, Mrs. Z proceeded to tell them about her eating patterns at home, that she ate very little but good food because of a rather delicate constitution, and called both gentlemen repeatedly honey and darling, which needless to say sounded completely out of place. She smiled coquettishly at both of them and interrupted constantly whatever they were saying. They looked at me and I blushed for Mrs. Z's childish display. When we left her bedside the two gentlemen expressed a unanimous opinion that she was a silly woman. I felt embarrassed, for I felt that Mrs. Z, being a European, might have created an unfavorable impression of European women (with whom I too may be identified). I resented her even more now than I did following our initial meeting. My attitude, I am sure, must have been conveyed to the rest of the staff, since everybody had something unpleasant to say about her. In short, in my own mind I had labelled her a silly, uncooperative patient and that label stuck extremely well, as reflected in the staff's attitude towards her.

The next few days went on very much the same without change. I avoided Mrs. Z as much as I could and she grew progressively more demanding and rude toward the staff. I am ashamed to admit that I was totally blind to this patient's needs until an event occurred that shook me out of my selfish callousness.

One afternoon one of the nurses whom I assigned to nurse Mrs. Z came to me with a kidney-basin full of clotted blood and said, ''She just vomited this, would you please have a look at her?'' I went to Mrs. Z's bedside and suddenly when I looked at her pale face I saw for the first time what I should have seen from the beginning, a helpless, extremely frightened fellow creature in dire need of understanding and sympathy. I took her cold hand with both my hands and said, ''Would you like me to call your husband to come and see you?'' She nodded yes, and tears began to stream down her pale cheeks. I added that I would also place a call for one of her doctors and she said, ''Call my own doctor please.'' ''You mean your family doctor?'' I asked. Again she nodded and I said, ''Is he your countryman?'' She said, ''Yes, but it is she not he,'' and smiling faintly at me she said apologetically, ''I hope you don't mind.'' I realized that she was trying hard to communicate with me but was afraid that she might offend me again and I would brush her off as I had done until now. Her anxious expression seemed to say, ''Don't close your heart and your mind to me, I need you.'' She put her other hand on mine and said simply, ''Stay with me for a while.''

I learned a great deal about her and myself in the following few minutes that I spent with her. She certainly was not a silly woman or rude as I had imagined before. She did not measure up to the stereotype role of a good patient because she herself had not been in a hospital before and this was her first admission, although she had visited some of her friends, who had private and semiprivate accommodations. Thus, instead of giving a proper explanation of the unit to her, I had been offended by her seemingly unreasonable demand and did not fulfill my role as a nurse. She challenged my authority and status as a head nurse. I thought she doubted my knowledge and prestige, whereas she simply wanted to know what was going to happen to her due to conflicting information she received from her family doctor on the one hand and the hospital personnel on the other. Naturally she trusted her family doctor, who spoke her own language and who had known her for a long time. Thus if I had not projected my own pride on her, but found out earlier more about her family doctor and elicited the proper information of her illness and the explanation she received, I could have been of help to her and her hospital medical attendants. The family doctor had referred her to the two specialists but they had not secured enough information from her doctor regarding Mrs. Z to be able to understand her behavior in the hospital. They treated an extremely interesting and puzzling case of a disease, but not Mrs. Z. I was too preoccupied with fears for my own self-image to be of assistance to the patient and to them. I should have tried to find out why Mrs. Z did not ask questions pertinent to her condition but spoke to the doctors about her eating habits. The whole pattern stretched clearly before my eyes and I began to try to change the communication from incongruent to congruent.

Mrs. Z's unexpressed fear of cancer was the underlying reason why she did not ask the specialist anything about her condition. She did not want her fear to be confirmed; it was safer to avoid the dangerous question and cling to her family doctor's reassuring statement that it is most likely a peptic ulcer, which the surgeon could remove in a relatively simple operation. The medical terminology frightened her even more, and thus she regressed in her behavior towards the doctors and adopted the pleading attitude of a child to a father figure. She was surrounded by a strange environment and hostility, which she could not understand, and thus reacted aggressively in order to protect herself and her human rights.

When her family physician arrived, I had a long talk with her and showed her all the results from the various tests we received, imparting to her all I knew about Mrs. Z's treatment. I asked her, in turn, to explain the treatments to her patient, which she did gladly. I spoke to her hospital specialists and imparted to them all I knew about Mrs. Z's fears about cancer. They too in simple language reassured her that she did not have a cancer but a benign tumor, which would be easy to remove by a surgical procedure. She responded with a quiet smile and handshake with both of them.

Now able to be a European rather than continuing to court the doctors in what she considered to be an acceptable North American approach.

The nursing staff and I had a conference where I admitted to them that it was me, not the patient who had created the misunderstanding and difficulty.

Good for you! Probably one of the most valuable learning experiences you could ever give to your staff.

We discussed a plan of care for her and with her, which consisted of moral support in the form of explanations of everything we had to do.

Her only family was her husband, with whom she had a very good relationship, but who was unable to visit her during regular visiting hours. I gave him special permission to visit her at his convenience. He gave us more information about his wife, namely, that she was a very independent woman, a good housekeeper and cook. She did not make friends easily but once befriended was a good and loyal friend.

Mrs. Z's tumor was removed and her recovery in the unit proceeded quietly and uneventfully. She cooperated very willingly in her postoperative treatment and on the 5th day we were able to transfer her into an ordinary surgical semiprivate accommodation. On the day of her transfer from the unit I came to say goodbye to her. She thanked me for her care in the unit, and suddenly picking up my hand, she pressed it to her lips and said with feeling, "You are an angel and I could never forget your kindness."

"Mrs. Z," I replied sadly, "Not an angel but a very inadequate human being, who needs to stand on guard constantly against her own judgments of others and emotions toward them, in order to be humane."

Was disapproving, judgmental or *nonjudgmental* can be closely related to *did not want to understand* or *wanted to understand how patient felt.* Of the Helpful cases 33% describe wanting to understand, while 54% of the Unhelpful cases point to not wanting to understand.

The incident in which I feel I was not helpful is one which will take me a long time to forget. It concerns a chronic peritoneal-dialysis patient, an older man whose wife had left him. He was really a very lonely man and complained quite often. As a result, many of the nurses found it very difficult to be pleasant to him. He became progressively more ill and more lonely. I distinctly remember hollering at him one day to hurry with his dressing and go home. I remember being very tense that day and instead of letting him take his time and perhaps sitting down with him and asking what was on his mind, I resorted to my nonprofessional habit of yelling to get action. He died a week later. He overate one day and admitted himself to the hospital. He knew he should not have eaten foods not included in his renal diet. He had a cardiac arrest in the middle of the night, probably due to a severely high serum potassium level.

The guilt I felt at the time was quite strong. Could this have been prevented if I had tried to convey some understanding to him that day? I knew he was always being rejected and yet I still rejected him myself.

In a very real sense these rejections probably had a direct association with his wife leaving him and his feeling about himself as an unlikeable person. Perhaps this related to his need to compensate by overeating—also a cry for help.

I let my own problems take precedence over his. I fulfilled my own needs at that time instead of trying to fulfill his. Every action of his that day had been a plea for acceptance and understanding (groaning, complaining) and yet I consciously ignored this because I had a deadline to meet and work to get done.

I feel that another reason for my unprofessional behavior was perhaps the fact that I had felt I would have no control over the situation if I let him go on moaning.

This is very often one's fear. Related to this is "What will others think?"

I also failed to recognize priorities. Mrs. X's bath really could have waited 10 more minutes. A chat with Mr. B would have postponed my work, but then again, it all depends on how one defines work.

In the following cases, failure to recognize the need for referral for mental health counseling was critical.

A young woman came into the emergency department early one evening when the benches were full of people waiting to see the doctor. She had cuts and bruises that looked more sore than dangerous and soon left us all in no doubt as to how she had acquired them by asking us to look at what her husband had done to her. She then said, "What would you do, nurse, if your husband came home from work, flung you on the bed and tried to make love to you, even before supper?" This brought forth several comments from some of the men concerning her husband's stamina, so without any thought at all I answered, "Leave him," and promptly escaped into the treatment room.

Later I found out that we already had a card for her because she had been beaten up several times previously by her husband. From the card I also found out that this man was not her legal husband, who at that time was serving a prison term.

While I carried out her care she talked freely, mostly about the beating, saying several times that she had done nothing to upset her husband as she had been innocently watching TV all afternoon and was just going to get supper. I pointed out that she had no legal obligation to the man and asked her why she stayed with him. She replied, "What can I do nurse—I haven't any job." I reminded her that she was young and as she had no children to care for she should have no problem finding work, and surely anything was better than being beaten up all the time, even if it meant scrubbing floors. She thanked me and we both knew that she would continue to live with the man and in all probability would be beaten up again.

On looking back on this, I realize that besides letting several opportunities slip by when I might have been of some help to this girl, my biggest mistake was in viewing this episode from my own middle-class point of view—particularly biased because I have rather strong views on the rights of women. I was shocked when she made a public disclosure about such an intimate aspect of her life, especially when she involved me in it as well, so I dissociated myself from her pretty quickly and made sure that those who were listening knew that I would never allow myself to be treated like that.

I think now that she wanted support for the fact that she had refused this man's request, some boost to justify her own behavior because she had a sense of guilt. I wonder now what understanding there might have been between them that was implicit in this couple's relationship? He supported her in return for what? Sexual satisfaction and other creature comforts? She obviously hadn't started to get any supper ready, and one would wonder about her housekeeping, as she looked pretty bedraggled herself and by her own admission had been watching TV all afternoon. I should have worked with what she already had, namely the partnership she had established with her common-law husband. Perhaps she could have been helped to see what initiated his bad temper and so seen where it could have been circumvented. Perhaps she could have been helped to think about her legal husband's release from jail and what plans she would need to make, and she could have been given the name of the organizations that exist to help prisoners and their families.

Yes, she needed (and in many ways was really acting out her need for) professional counseling.

Instead I assumed that she held the same attitudes as myself. I forgot that she probably saw nothing wrong in being bossed and ordered around by a man. I assumed that she wanted to be self-reliant and ignored all the evidence to the contrary. Even though she had virtually told me that she had no skills, I gave her no indication that I appreciated her difficult problems and airily told her that she would have no difficulty finding a job. No wonder I was so little help to her.

In this case the nurse points to purposely cutting off the cues that the mother gave her.

Mr. and Mrs. P and their four children lived in an apartment, a public housing development. Mr. P gambled at the race track and lost what little money they had. The boys (aged 6 years, 4 years, 11 months, and 7 days old) would have been a handful for any mother. But for Mrs. P the problem was compounded by the fact that David, aged 11 months, had a congenital measles syndrome. He was blind, deaf, retarded, and had some obvious physical deformities. Shortly after David was born the doctor told Mr. and Mrs. P to place him in an institution. Mr.

P refused. This forced Mrs. P to care for the child at home. Mrs. P soon became pregnant for the fourth time. Mr. P refused any discussion of David and his gambling increased.

When the baby, Peter, was born, David was admitted to the hospital for tests and surgery. When Mrs. P and the baby arrived home the rent was almost due, the baby needed special attention, the older children had to be cared for, and David was to be discharged from the hospital any day.

A nurse had been visiting regularly since David's birth. From her notes I knew most of the basic information, though I didn't know about Mr. P's gambling. I also didn't realize until the day before my visit that Mrs. P had already had the baby. I felt very rusty on postnatal care and this concerned me.

When I entered Mrs. P was almost immediately cool and remote. Any attempt to open the subject of David met with resistance. As we spoke Mrs. P's composure and manner completely unnerved me. She spoke without feeling and her thoughts wandered. I didn't understand this and I didn't know how to take it. Finally she concluded aloud, "I don't need help now as much as I did before." "You mean the crisis has past and things seem better now?" I asked.

Her response was immediate and unexpected. She began quietly, "Yes, before I could not talk about David. I would just turn around and cry if anybody mentioned him to me. But now it is different. I am not the only mother who has had a baby like this one. I am thinking about David now." As she spoke she appeared to forget her composure for the first time and anger showed in her voice as she continued: "Someone is going to have to talk to my husband, though; someone with more knowledge than I have. I don't know if I can keep David when he is discharged and if I can't someone will have to talk to my husband. He won't give him up."

I listened. It was the first meaningful thing she had said but my immediate reaction was to change the topic and regrettably I did. "How are the other children?" I asked. Mrs. P returned stoically to her "cool." She wanted and needed to talk about David. By changing the topic, cutting her off in effect, I failed to help her.

I lacked self-insight. Though I would not have admitted it to even myself then, I just could not accept Mrs. P's rejection of David. Without realizing it I made this judgment. I knew it was wrong to judge so I could not bring myself to think that I had done this. To myself, then, I denied it. Hence, I was tense and uncomfortable with myself; this was reflected in my behavior. Mrs. P picked this up. She was on guard and my changing the topic left no room for doubt. My rejection of any further discussion of the topic spoke for itself.

I feel that I have learned from this experience but it has had a lasting effect on my relationship with Mrs. P. I have found it difficult to resolve my feelings and though I have more insight into her behavior and mine now, the mistakes that I made during and prior to my first visit have made it very difficult to rebuild any sort of a trusting, open, helping relationship.

Do you still feel that placing David in an institution constitutes rejection? What has been done about Mrs. P's plea that someone talk to her husband? Have you explored your need for consultation on this family and their need for in-depth counseling? There is no need for you to "go it alone."

Here sexuality, role conflict, and self-image are discussed as the chief problems for both patient and nurse. The nurse describes her movement through the entire range of Responses cited most often in Interpretation of Condition.

Joe Smith was a 32-year-old male, admitted into a four-bed semiprivate room with the diagnosis of left-sided epididymitis. There was no formal history written for his chart. Therefore, all information regarding his condition was obtained through conversation with Mrs. Smith, Joe, and the doctor.

Joe was born in Maine and started school there. When his family moved to Vermont, he completed his elementary education in Warren. He attended trade school occasionally. Joe said he was now a mechanic or television repair man, but presently was driving a bus. The story varied with each telling.

Important early cue to problem regarding self-image.

He said he was buying a home in the suburbs and enjoyed doing his own home repairs and gardening. Mrs. Smith was shy and friendly. She appeared to be younger than Joe by several years. They had two children, a boy of 3 and a girl of 6.

Several weeks previous to hospital admission, Joe had had a left vasectomy in the outpatient department. This procedure had failed to relieve the infection and the doctor was unable to determine the cause of it. Joe was admitted for X rays, evaluation, and possible surgery.

I discovered that Joe had a good understanding of his condition. He realized that without treatment his present discomfort would continue and possibly lead to sterility. He also knew that the surgery involved might also render him sterile.

My first contact with Joe and his roommates was during bathing and bed-making Monday morning. The three other patients were older than Joe by 20 to 30 years. The older men asked me the usual questions: "Are you married? How long? Where did you train? Where do you live?" I was very pleased to be able to talk so easily with them and readily told them I had trained in this hospital and lived on Parkside Drive. Like anyone else, I was happy to be able to talk about myself and was even more pleased to discover that these three patients had also lived in my area most of their lives. Although I turned the conversation over to them, I was glad to have found common interests for talking to them. I noticed that Joe did not join in their discussions of the good old days or present politics.

In fact, if we talked for too long (20 minutes) Joe would interrupt with an off-color joke or some reference to his sexual activities prior to his marriage or how lucky his wife was to trap him into marriage. Joe became increasingly rowdy and his use of foul language more the rule than the exception.

At first I attempted to ignore Joe. I felt his jokes were in very poor taste and his bragging made me uncomfortable. He reminded me of an adolescent. I failed to realize this was his way of expressing concern over his possible sterility. I wanted Joe to be quiet and cooperative instead of disturbing the whole room.

Joe made a point of disregarding his doctor's orders to drink extra fluids and remain in bed, wearing a scrotal support. He frequently got out of bed and took off his support with the explanation that the hospital did not have one large enough to fit him.

At first I patiently explained to Joe why he should follow the doctor's orders but when I realized that Joe was fully aware of the reason for the support and bed rest, I lost my temper. I felt Joe should have accepted the responsibility for helping himself. I never stopped to consider that maybe Joe felt inadequate to help himself.

My behavior probably seemed inconsistent to Joe. One time I was telling him to act adult and be responsible for his own actions and the next time I would expect him to accept my authority and wisdom as a nurse.

I really thought that Joe was trying to prove himself to me as a female instead of simply seeking recognition from another human being.

Joe had to be the center of attention. He would not allow me to prepare the other patients for surgery the following day. I felt that, since Joe was not even booked for surgery, he could wait his turn. I was the nurse and I wanted to set the teaching program my own way. Looking back, I can see that Joe was undermining my authority and prestige, or so I thought.

Joe bragged about his role as head of his own home. He talked a great deal about a woman's place in the home: bearing children and waiting on her husband. He strongly asserted that housework was fine for a woman but only a man could handle a job outside the home.

Very concerned at the fact that his wife might now appear to be the strong one and desperately trying to figure out the whole sick role and especially his adequacy in the male role.

I honestly felt Joe was directing this at me and snapped at him, "Who would look after you four if I stayed home?" Joe looked blank for a few seconds and said, "Oh, nurses are different."

Unfortunately, Joe had touched one of my sensitive points. The weekend previous to this I had been forced to attend an old-fashioned Irish wake for one of my in-laws and there I had been subjected to several lectures on this same subject. Also at this time I was making plans to attend a university in September, much to the horror of my own relatives. Needless to say, I had already heard enough about the role of women. It was much easier to strike out at Joe than my own family.

There was also something much deeper here. My eldest and favorite sister felt that child bearing was a woman's only role in life. Against her doctor's advice, she had a large family and spent much time in psychiatric hospitals after the births of the last two children. At first it was considered to be only postpartum depression, but they now feel she is a schizophrenic and have little hope that she will ever be completely normal again. I have always felt that a nurse must not allow her personal feelings to interfere with the care of her patients and I am ashamed that I lost control of them in this case.

Joe had other habits that came to the notice of the other staff members. I was feeling rather pleased that we all agreed that he was a pest and nuisance until one nurse told me what she had said to him. Joe mocked all religious belief.

The man in the bed opposite Joe was a quiet, elderly lay preacher who spent most of his time reading the Bible and church publications. Joe mocked and ridiculed the man and increased swearing in his presence. Nurse A said she lectured Joe on being a nice Christian like Mr. Green. It was this that made me realize that I was as wrong as A in failing to accept Joe as he was and meeting his unspoken needs.

After giving the whole situation much thought, I approached that room with some hesitation but much determination. At the first opportunity I told the patients of my background. I corrected their mistaken impression that I lived in a swanky house on Parkside, and described our tiny apartment. I made certain that Joe heard this. Then the conversation moved to the outdoor life, fishing and hunting. Joe was not only joining the talk but the men were listening attentively to what he was saying. When Joe did revert to crude jokes or bad language, I listened politely instead of reproving him.

I attempted to repair the damage I had done by belittling Joe with a sharp word or glance. I felt Joe could not identify me as someone who could understand him, as our backgrounds and education were so far apart. By giving Joe a more accurate sketch of my past I was hoping that he would see I was not so far removed from his way of speaking and thinking.

To do any health teaching, I used the method of group discussion. By starting with Joe's questions and problems and then proceeding to those of the other patients I was attempting to reduce the tension caused by leaving Joe until the last. I recognized that Joe needed to be the center of attention and wanted to have the others look up to him. Quite often Joe would repeat the same question several times and the last time he would answer his own question. This also gave Joe the required outlet to express his fears.

To increase Joe's sense of importance, I asked him to be responsible for calling me when the postoperative patients needed anything. Joe took his responsibility so seriously he almost drove me wild by checking the levels in the intravenous bottles every 10 minutes! By answering the bell promptly and accepting Joe's estimation of the situation (within reason), I increased his own sense of worth and reassured him of the importance of his opinion. This was not a dangerous practice as I was in the room every few minutes even if Joe did not ring the bell.

I had noticed that Mrs. Smith appeared embarrassed by Joe's loud and sometimes foul language. She did not seem to say much except to attempt to quiet him. This had the same effect as my own attempts: his rowdiness increased. I stopped Mrs. Smith and sat down with her at the nursing station. At first, I talked in general terms about men being afraid and how they reveal their fear. I stressed Joe's actions were typical and normal. Mrs. Smith was so relieved, I thought she was going to cry. She said Joe was being a big baby and making too much out of this. She did not want more children and did not care if Joe were sterile. I asked her if she could talk to Joe and tell him this. She said she would try. Until now, she had been too worried about Joe bothering the patients and staff to think about Joe himself. That cut me quite deeply! I wondered if she knew that I had done the same thing.

Later Joe thanked me for talking to his wife. He said they had been unable to talk about it before. They both had felt these were things you did not discuss.

Joe and I became friends. I never knew when one of his simple questions would lead to a crude remark but I accepted these as part of Joe and he was aware of this. Working with Joe was not easy. It was very difficult for me to give up my role of total authority. Gradually, Joe divided the area of authority between us. I was responsible for interpreting medical orders and nothing else. Joe was able to accept me as a nurse whom he could trust, regardless of my behavior in the first 2 days of hospitalization.

Joe would need continuing verbalized help (from everyone) concerning his maleness. His wife, who, following his hospitalization, might well become the focus for Joe's identity problems, would also need support.

Short-staffed; too little time to devote to the patient is not a major factor in any of the 12 Situations. It is cited in 13% of the Unhelpful cases of Interpretation of Condition. Here, a nurse—a student at the time—recalls her attempt to meet this problem as well as some of her own status needs.

The setting is a busy surgical floor of a large general hospital. My assignment, as a student nurse, was to physically prepare two middle-aged women for major surgery on the following day. Rather than shave and give enemas to the women in their rooms with the other two patients, I took them individually into two separate rooms and initially questioned them as to what their doctors had told them and their interpretation of this information about surgery and specifically their type of surgery. During the actual physical preparation, I explained the surgical procedure to them in detail. As well, I told them exactly what to expect postoperatively, e.g., pain, and what would be expected of them, e.g., early ambulation. I showed the apparatus with which they would return from the recovery room, e.g., intravenous, and demonstrated to each of them the equipment that they would be using to speed up their recovery, e.g., aerosol therapy. Both of the ladies practiced using this equipment. Also, I reinforced what their doctors had told them and corrected and interpreted any misconceptions.

Both women progressed so rapidly following the surgical procedure they were discharged 3 and 5 days prior to the average length of stay for this type of surgery.

Before analyzing my actions in this situation, there are several factors to be considered. First, as previously stated, the setting was a large general hospital. In a hospital of this size and caliber, generally speaking, the emphasis preoperatively is placed on the physical rather than the emotional preparation of the patients. Surgery is not seen as a traumatic experience, or if a few of the staff do consider the emotional trauma involved, the common complaint of the lack of time to do preoperative teaching is heard.

Another factor to consider is that in a teaching hospital, there is a definite stigma attached to student nurses. This comment is based on personal experience. Generally, student nurses are treated in such a way as to make them feel inferior.

Last, but in all probability the most important factor that influenced my actions was the fact that I had just completed a 3-month psychiatric affiliation. Still fresh in my mind was the fact that surgery is indeed a very traumatic experience.

Also, I feel my actions were a type of experiment to see if the complaint of the lack of time really was valid or if it was an excuse for laziness or lack of knowledge on the part of the nursing staff. As can be seen, the extra 15 minutes saved 3 and 5 days, so this completely nullifies the time element involved.

I think that I impressed on the graduate staff that my actions made me a little more than useless. This feeling only shows that I was indeed suffering from an inferiority complex because it was an attempt to prove my own worth to them.

I proved to myself that if my knowledge was beneficial to these patients that I was correct in assuming that the lack of preoperative teaching was an excuse to hide some other factor and that this type of teaching would be helpful to other patients.

Have you since explored what these "other factor(s)" are and how nursing may deal with them?

In the following case the nurse was determined to pursue her conviction that beyond surface gains, no basic change would occur unless she could help the child's mother to interpret the meaning of fundamental family problems. The time and sensitivity required to get through the barrier is clearly demanding.

I had been asked to make a home visit by the school authorities as the result of a nurse-teacher conference concerning Jill, a 7-year-old girl.

Jill, they said, was a disruptive influence in class, smoked at recess, and was suspected of having mental problems. Apparently she came from an excellent home, had well-educated parents, and had brothers and sisters who had attended that school and were good students with no behavioral problems. Theirs was a beautiful home, set on two acres of orchards, and my first visit was a pleasant one, in a formal way, since Mrs. P did not really relax with me. Jill had been difficult since she was born, she said, and I got the impression that she would really rather not talk about it.

In the weeks that followed, the more I thought about this case, the more it seemed like a jigsaw puzzle, with too many missing pieces to be able to recognize the picture. I had built up a good rapport with Mrs. P and with Jill but I was very conscious of the tension between them when we visited together. Jill was quite a tomboy and wanted a horse very badly and with her parents' permission, between us we managed to motivate her to working toward and saving for a horse by picking apples and later taking a paper route. Her behavior improved and she appeared to be less frustrated, but her remark to me one day that her mother hated her and the mother's obvious tension in her presence caused me to continue my visits.

By visiting on a regular basis, ostensibly on Jill's behalf, I managed, eventually to get through to Mrs. P, and one day she told me the whole story. She and her husband, both only children, had been married straight out of college. She had a degree in home economics and he in agriculture. They had had the family almost immediately and they were fairly close. They were happy with each other and with the family until he was transfered to an isolated area and she refused to join him. There was a period of estrangement, another woman, and later a would-be lover for her whom she was unable to accept because of her rigid upbringing. A year or so later, they were reunited and almost immediately she became pregnant. The pregnancy brought renewed fears of losing her husband again and she tried to have an abortion, but it was before the days of easy abortions and she failed. She had feelings of guilt and hated every minute of her pregnancy, resenting the child who was making things so difficult for her. Although Mrs. P was a very efficient homemaker and mother, she felt insecure and inadequate as a person. She felt trapped and wanted to prove herself as a person and as a wage earner, and she doubted if she could survive on her own should her husband leave. She appeared to have so much and yet she felt deprived as she never had any money to call her own unless she asked her husband for it.

Since they had a huge undeveloped basement and so much space outside, and there was a real need in that community for a nursery school, I suggested that she study for her certificate and set up a nursery school in her home. In that way, she would still be in the home with her preschooler, but would have a goal for personal development and the potential wage earning she was so concerned about. I was surprised how quickly she achieved her goal. By involving her husband, who was very clever with his hands and had all the equipment necessary, she soon had small tables, chairs, and all the paraphernalia pertaining to the world of young folks, and the show was underway. I discovered that he had felt shut out, since she had been almost wholly involved with the young since their marriage began. He became involved with the project with tremendous enthusiasm and energy and together with the help of the children, who painted, collected old tricycles, and such, they produced the most successful nursery school in the city.

Some time later, when I then became involved as a nurse visiting this nursery school in my area, it never ceased to amaze me how much had been achieved with so little effort on my part. Here was a family who were working together, using their combined skills, to give the community a service that was required badly. It would have been so easy for me to have stopped visiting when Jill's immediate problem appeared to have been solved and things had quieted down at school, but as a nurse, I had recognized the underlying needs and turmoil of the mother. By being a good listener, and showing my concern as a woman, I had acted as a potentiator and catalyst to bring together Mrs. P's latent self-motivation, Mr. P's skills and need to be involved and the children's several needs and skills, so that their joint project brought them together as a family and solved many of their problems while meeting the needs of the community.

Now 10 years later, the P's eldest daughter is married, has a 3-year-old son, and runs their venture as a nursery school very successfully.

Professional closeness is possible, when one can recognize the need, has the skills to interpret and motivate, and the maturity to realize that only in pooling joint skills of the professional and patient can one hope to achieve the ultimate goal of optimum health for both.

6

PROFESSIONAL/ PERSONAL RELATIONSHIP

Of the 550 cases in the study, 4% focus on the Professional/Personal Relationship. Of the 22 cases that focus on the Professional/Personal Relationship, 68% are described as Helpful, 32% as Unhelpful.

COMPARISON WITH ALL OTHER SITUATIONS

Helpful Factors

Highest Rating

- Gave moral support.
- Made this case the basis for overall policy change/improvement.

Unhelpful Factors

Highest Rating

- Lacked training in recognizing social-emotional needs of patients.
- Short-staffed; too little time to devote to the patient.
- Overidentified due to being similar age to patient.

Helpful Factors	% of Cases in Which Cited
1. Gave moral support	80
2. Took time to explain	60

110

3. Was a sounding board	40
4. Initiated referral to another profession/resource	40
5. Helped family members deal with the situation	40
6. Came to terms with own feelings; was able to enter into patient's problem	33
7. Helped patient express feelings	33
8. Wanted to understand how patient felt	27
9. Looked beyond patient's outward response/behavior to underlying causes	13
10. Made this case the basis for overall policy change/improvement	13
11. Positively identified with patient due to similar life/professional experience	13
12. Liked the patient	7
13. Nonjudgmental	7
14. Discussed religion with patient	7
15. Used innovative rehabilitative procedure	7
16. Used physical closeness	7
17. Had received training in recognizing social-emotional needs of patients	7
18. Was honest with patient/relatives	7
19. Was trying to prove self to senior staff members	0
20. Not unduly influenced by negative opinions of other staff regarding the patient's personality	0

Unhelpful Factors	% of Cases in Which Cited
1. Purposely disregarded significant cues in patient's statements/behavior	57
2. Self-image was threatened	57
3. Felt inadequate to enter into patient's problem because had not personally resolved the issue	43
4. Lacked training in recognizing social-emotional needs of patients	43
5. Felt guilty but could not communicate	29
6. Felt pressured (within self) into doing things rather than coping with feeling elements (tension present)	29
7. Failed to look beyond initial negative impression of patient's personality	29
8. Did not want to understand	29
9. Treated the condition, overlooking the patient	14
10. Short-staffed; too little time to devote to the patient	14

11. Negatively influenced by opinions of other staff
    members regarding personality of the patient   14
12. Was disapproving, judgmental   14
13. Avoided needs of family members   14
14. Overidentified due to being similar age to patient   14
15. Rationalized actions and thoughts   14
16. Lost professional role: patient became friend   14
17. Breakdown of interprofessional communication/
    cooperation   0
18. Afraid would break down and cry in front of patient   0
19. Prejudiced toward group of which patient was a
    member   0
20. Incapacitated by own fear of death   0
21. Failed to seek authoritative advice regarding
    innovation   0
22. Disregarded own judgment because wanted approval
    of senior staff members   0
23. Disliked patient   0
24. Felt guilty, but still would not communicate   0

In 43% of cases the nurse *felt inadequate to enter into patient's problem because she had not personally resolved the issue.* In 57% of cases her *self-image was threatened.* The following cases illustrate these Responses.

J was 8 days postoperative. He had recovered well, but was undergoing further tests for gastric pain. His medication included small amounts of Librium. He had been a laborer in my husband's firm and I hadn't seen him for about 7 years. He told me that he had hurt his back and was now employed with another firm in the city. I had returned to nursing, and was doing part-time general duty. My children were in school and I had been separated from my husband for 2 years at this time.

One of the rooms to which I had been assigned was the four-bed ward in which J was a patient. Here was someone I had known, who might probe and uncover some nameless horror because my marriage had failed! All the emotions of guilt, rejection, hostility, and self-pity that I thought I had rationalized were let loose. I was reduced to a quivering bit of vulnerability and was so preoccupied with myself that I didn't realize until later that J couldn't have cared less about my shabby secrets. He had his own problems! I pulled myself together enough to ask him about himself. He told me that his mother had died with cancer a year ago. The doctors were trying to find out what was the matter with him, but he knew it was no use, for he was sure that he had cancer himself. Then I remembered that he had taken Communion that morning in his room. He was a very frightened, dejected man. He needed reassurance and I, an old acquaintance, was the person he turned to at that time.

Here was a strength he was calling upon that you might have followed up with J's clergyman, enlisting his help as a member of your team.

I wasn't much help to him. I said the usual things about his doctor being the best in the city, and I was sure that he would be all right. Later in the day, after reading his history, I returned to try and reassure him that nothing had been found, and that the tests would soon be finished, but he was obviously unconvinced.

I could have been some help to him in the morning if I had been capable of really listening to him, but the time in which I could have been of some support to him had passed. J relegated me to the "they" who, he thought, really knew that his case was hopeless.

* * * *

When I was at Brookside hospital, the grandmother of a very good friend was admitted to the ward where I was working. Her diagnosis was pneumonia. She was approximately 70 years old, a diabetic, and had been a cardiac invalid for many years. Her daughter, Mrs. L, had postponed her admission for over 2 weeks, as she felt she could look after her mother much better at home. As a result, Mrs. D (the grandmother), was in critical condition on admission to hospital. She had improved quite nicely when she suffered a stroke, causing her to fall out of bed and fracture her hip. Naturally, with these complications her condition deteriorated rapidly. She was unconscious, and probably had extensive brain damage. The doctors considered her inoperable and terminal.

Ever since her mother's admission, Mrs. L had been complaining to her daughter about the nursing care her mother was receiving. In fact, she had been quite demonstrative about it during visiting hours, in that she always set about immediately to wash, turn, and generally fuss about her mother, who, according to her nurse's estimation, was in a comfortable state.

I was very fond of Mrs. L, but I found it difficult to accept her behavior, and I was angry with her for having delayed her mother's admission. I knew she was unhappy with the nursing care, and I felt that if she saw me on the ward she would equate me with this so-called poor care, even though I had never looked after her mother. I therefore made myself quite scarce during visiting hours.

Of course, the inevitable happened—she approached me in the nursing station, and the following conversation ensued.

Nurse: Yes, Mrs. L?

Mrs. L: Would you tell me please why my mother isn't being looked after properly?

Nurse: I don't understand, Mrs. L.

Mrs. L: Well, I never see any nurses when I come in, and my mother is always in a mess. She needs to be turned every 15 minutes, you know.

Nurse: Do you think she is uncomfortable now? The nurse was just in there changing her.

Mrs. L: Well, I've just had to wash her and turn her myself. She is moaning all the time. She must be in terrible pain, and nobody seems to care.

Nurse: Your mother is unconscious. She doesn't feel any pain.

Mrs. L: That certainly can't be true if she is moaning all the time. Why won't they operate on her?

Nurse: The doctors think she is a poor risk for surgery, Mrs. L. Her pneumonia is so bad right now, she probably wouldn't survive an anesthetic.

Mrs. L: You mean she is going to die, so they just don't want to bother.

Nurse: That's not what they mean at all, Mrs. L. They will operate on her as soon as her condition improves.

Mrs. L: And why did they take away the oxygen tent?

Nurse: The doctors didn't feel it was helping her. Not everyone with pneumonia needs an oxygen tent.

Mrs. L: I know exactly why there is no oxygen tent, and no medicine for pain, and no operation—it's exactly what they do when you are going to die—stop treatment.

Nurse: Oh, Mrs. L, you've been watching too much television.

Mrs. L: I'm really disappointed in you; you're just a typical nurse; you don't really care.

Influence of the Self Factor

The situation was too personal for me. I was unable to function as a nurse, as I had always, in the past, gone to Mrs. L for help myself. I could not see her in the "need" role, nor myself in the "help" role.

My own personal needs were involved. I was concerned with my professional status, which would be diminished if she associated me at all with her mother's nursing care. I was not especially anxious to have the staff sitting at the desk know that I was a friend of this so-called neurotic woman. I was embarrassed by the lack of privacy, and by her behavior.

I was suffering from guilt pangs about the delayed hospitalization myself, as I knew Mrs. D had been ill and had really done nothing concrete in trying to persuade Mrs. L to have her hospitalized. I think in trying to relieve my own guilt, I was trying to make Mrs. L more guilty.

I think I had made up my mind not to be helpful at all. Mrs. L was threatening me with her accusations of poor nursing care, thus displacing her guilt on me, and trying to prove through her attentions to her mother that she was good, and the nurses were bad, and I was not going to let her do it. I think I wanted her to suffer her guilt, and not displace it on me, the nurses, or the hospital. I would say that I lacked ethical motivation; I was trying to make her look foolish. I wanted her to be grateful for the nursing care her mother was receiving from the staff.

I was misinterpreting the situation perhaps. There may have been more than displacement of guilt involved in her actions and words. She may have been afraid of death itself, and worried about what she would do with herself if her mother died. What would she do to fill her time?

I wasn't sure of what she expected of me, and I was seeking her approval. I wasn't being myself; I was trying to play a role. I obviously lacked maturity, and was greatly influenced by social pressure.

Perhaps Mrs. L delayed her mother's hospitalization for one of several reasons: (1) she felt guilty that she had "allowed" her mother to contract pneumonia (often lay people think pneumonia is regarded by the medical profession as symptomatic of negligence) and therefore had to prove her devotion both to herself and others; (2) either Mrs. L or her mother had fought against putting the elderly lady in an institution with all the rejecting overtones this can carry in the minds of either or both (irrational perhaps, but nonetheless real). As you say, the patient had been an invalid for some years. Exploration of these various dimensions would have given you a clue to Mrs. L's real doubts and fears and would have allowed both you and her to be real with each other, and you to be both friend and professional.

Being in the same group and *overidentifying due to being similar age to patient* can compound the *threat of self-image*, as illustrated below.

Jackie and Dave—teachers—were having problems, and now they wanted me to help. This was just too much to ask: didn't I have enough work to do without trying to straighten out a troubled marriage with the Smiths?

Dave was 32 and this was his second marriage. He drank a little too much and appeared to be the strong, silent type. Jackie was 25. She had left home at the age of 16 because she and her parents just couldn't get along. At the age of 17 she was unmarried and pregnant; when the baby was born she gave it up for adoption. At 19 she married and had another child, which she still has. At 21 she was divorced and then remarried at 23 to Dave. Now she and Dave were expecting their first child and they didn't want it. Jackie also admitted to drinking more than was good for her, but at night it was the only way she could get to sleep—a few stiff belts and a couple of sleeping pills. What could I do? I ignored the problem; didn't even try to pick up the feelers Jackie put out. If I didn't know what was happening, how could I help? It was great for a while, sneaking away from the responsibility.

Then all hell broke loose: Jackie had what appeared to be an agitated manic depressive breakdown. So what did I do? I shipped her out to the nearest hospital to see a psychiatrist, and advised her husband to go with her, and for both of them to seek help in trying to work out their problems. Again I succeeded in shrugging off the responsibility. The sun shone again.

Three days later both were back, with a letter from a GP and the psychiatrist, and they wanted me to do all the follow-up. Fantastic. Just what I wanted: back to square one.

What was I going to do now? It was as if the weight of the world was on my shoulders. I did very little. I made sure Jackie had her routine prenatal checks and that she took the medication prescribed by the psychiatrist, but I appeared very busy whenever she was around. I also informed her that I didn't feel competent to deal with her and Dave's problem and advised them to go out to the hospital for counseling (not very realistic on my part). I even offered to supply free transportation—very good of me, wasn't it?

Now looking back on the situation I can see I could have been of help by just listening, by being there when they needed me, and by trying to help them think through their problem to find a workable conclusion. If I hadn't been so wrapped up in the feeling of "poor me," I probably could have done more.

Dave and Jackie also presented another problem for me—there are few whites in my area and we tend to stick together as a group. We all get together for parties, suppers, and other small social gatherings—we're all drinking buddies. I found it impossible to divide the friend-patient relationship and to be objective. If they had had a medical problem I could have coped with the situation, but presented with a very personal problem, marital difficulties and an unwanted pregnancy, I felt as if they might suck me dry of emotions and I wanted to run away from the whole thing. This assignment has made me much more aware of my performance as an individual and as a nurse.

You were quite justified in feeling you needed help with the counseling—particularly in view of the personal relationships you shared with Dave and Jackie. Perhaps you could have combined what you suggest, with consulting help from the psychiatrist.

*   *   *   *

In this case, the nurse recounts the responsibility she feels toward her friends concerning taking drugs. She describes her conflict about imposing her own values on her friends, about interfering, about doubting herself as a truly accepting person, and about her concern and guilt in being a helping person.

A situation in which I feel very uncomfortable as a nurse is one in which I expect myself to give a professional opinion to acquaintances with whom I'm trying to become friends about the nonmedical use of narcotics. I find I have conflicting ideas between the moral and the physiological aspects of drug use.

I know that the use of narcotics can be both physically and mentally dangerous; however, I feel that in giving an opinion relative to my feelings I would be placing the friendship at jeopardy.

I realize that one of the reasons for my failure is that I identify with my friends and feel that I might be in the same position had I not the fears of endangering my license, becoming addicted, or being ostracized by other friends and family. I know the pressures of the group and of university society, so am further hesitant to lecture, as I escape from those same pressures in other ways.

Another reason for my failure is an ignorance of the immediate effect of drugs from personal experience. I know this point should not trouble me as I can advise a peptic ulcer patient to avoid irritating foods or an emaciated person on nutrition, neither condition of which I have personally experienced, but these are straightforward matters and not ones involving moral values.

It upsets me when I realize that if these people are really my friends I should be doing all possible to protect them. My fear is that I will lose them as friends: my rationalization is that then I'll be unable to help them in other matters (e.g., sickness or physical injury).

Perhaps the basis for my lack of confidence is that I have difficulty accepting the people without accepting their actions.

In order to deal with my inadequacies in handling the drug situation, I will have to study why people turn to drugs and try to help them from that standpoint. To cope with my fears of loss of friendships I'll have to analyze what a friendship means to me. If I deal with a problem in a professional manner can I still be a friend?

Based on this nurse's experience, she suggests a concept that has become a policy in several centers, particularly with respect to dying patients and their families. In fact, making an *individual case the basis for overall policy change/improvement* rates highest across all Situations in the Professional/Personal Relationship. It would appear that as the practitioner is involved as a friend, she may have more conviction about the need for basic changes.

This situation occurred while I was working in emergency. I was working part-time, but a brief encounter one evening led to the extensive use of self for the following year. I noticed a woman, whose face was familiar, standing in the corridor with a young boy at her side. I approached her and we quickly identified our common denominator. Our teenage daughters were friends. I queried, "What brings you to the hospital at this late hour with your son?" Her reply came like a bolt of thunder, "Two months ago he was diagnosed as having acute leukemia." The last few words were broken with sobs. I stood there in shocked disbelief, reacting to my innermost thoughts. Why was I so blunt with my question? What should I say now? The automatic response of "I'm sorry, so sorry" was elicited. Since I was working only on a part-time basis, I was not sufficiently in control to suggest that we go to a quiet corner where my friend could regain her composure in dignity, away from the masses that spill out of every cubicle in an emergency setting.

While listening to details of her son Michael's past admission I sensed the need for this mother to have someone to relate to that was affiliated with the hospital. I made it very clear that I would be willing to discuss with her any problems, whenever she cared to call. On that particular evening the parents had been unable to contact their family doctor to consult about their son's epistaxis. They had registered in emergency, where his past record of admission was on file. Previous and initial contacts made with medical personnel at this center had been good.

Two weeks later my friend called to say that Michael was attending school daily but that his appetite was declining and she was wearying of the demanding schedule that involved taxiing him to school each day. In that message I saw a young woman burdened with care, sensing some of the inevitable uncertainty, exhaustion, and despair that were in store for her in the months that lay ahead. I saw the need for some companionship and diversion. I suggested that she accompany me to some ceramic classes. This seemed to be of interest and she appeared to enjoy both the hobby and the fellowship of the other women. While traveling back from the class she again expressed real concern for her son's lack of interest in food. I thought, how futile it was to push food in the face of a terminally ill person. My response was, "A certain loss of appetite is to be expected, as frustrating as it may be."

At this early stage I was questioning myself as to how supportive I could be in the terminal stages. I had nursed an adult dying with cancer and found it very depressing. Why must a child be struck with a fatal illness? Although I recognized the threat of working with the family of a dying child, I felt a strong sense of personal commitment to the helping relationship.

I was informed by my daughter of each hospital admission, and visited my friend and her son in his room each Wednesday before going on duty. I was always warmly received and given reports of various blood testings and forms of treatment. All of these indicated a steady decline. I vividly remember walking down the corridor of the leukemia section one afternoon and being acutely aware of how easily our roles could be reversed, as I also have a son. A very handsome 10-year-old boy was rapidly dying as indicated by loss of weight, hair, and variations in skin tone. I said a silent prayer each time I entered his room: God, give me the courage to be of some support.

Close to Christmas, Michael reached a crisis stage and was transfused. When I made a delivery to the house at that time I found the pathos of the tree in the living room evoking a tear.

My friend discussed with ease results of recent blood work, doctors' reports, and nursing care. She also referred to her husband's difficulty in accepting the inevitable and his unwillingness to discuss it. (I now see the need to do some reading in the area of the dying patient and grief. By enriching my own understanding I could have felt less threatened and could have been more helpful in the use of self. I did not attempt discussing her husband's needs with my friend.)

Michael was home for Christmas and the day was uneventful, but a sudden onset of hematemesis necessitated an emergency readmission. The next time I visited them Michael had been transferred to a single room at the end of the hall. As I walked the corridor I found myself identifying with his mother. She met me at the door and ushered me into the death chamber. There before my eyes was the white, flaccid, skeletonlike remains of a handsome 10-year-old male. I played the role of the active listener as my friend recounted the details of many nightly vigils. The need for the next of kin to communicate at this time is great. All too frequently the nurses working with these patients are very reluctant to give of themselves. Is it due to a lack of preparation or a refusal to get involved emotionally, or both? I think it is essential for nurses working in these areas to have classes in psychosocial medicine.

For Michael, it was obvious that death was imminent. He had rallied, following a cardiac arrest, and one of the doctors suggested that formal treatment should be discontinued.

My friend told me of her inner struggle with this issue. She was clinging to all measures that would prolong life. I felt it was not within my right to suggest that it might be more fair to her son to discontinue treatment, as I have not walked in her shoes. My own spiritual background accounts for my feeling that this is a very personal decision. Therefore, in all honesty I could only say to the mother, "I am sure it is an extremely difficult decision." A week later when I attended Michael's funeral my eyes were brimming as I touched that mourning mother's arm, but I had kept my commitment to myself to use the strongest possible self to the bitter end.

I was aware that there are many feelings tied up in a grief reaction. I made a point of drawing alongside my friend for the following few months by inviting her to my home or swimming club. In this period of time she expressed her disbelief that God could allow this fate to fall on a child. Since I share this premise, I could simply offer support by listening. There was a clergyman visiting periodically, so I encouraged her to discuss this issue with him. A year later I received a phone call that imparted a great deal of deferred gratification. My friend said she had purposely delayed the call, as she was aware that the content of the message would evoke an emotional reaction. She said she honestly felt that without the sustenance from the likes of myself she could not have coped during that stressful period.

That is the major reason for my assessment of having been helpful. It represents to me the continuous and comprehensive use of self over a period of a year. Although I entered this relationship on a professional basis, much of it was practiced at the level of a paraprofessional. I see great possibilities for trained paraprofessionals to be involved in helping relationships. A local mental health clinic could provide the training and placement could be arranged by clinic referrals.

In the following case, the nurse points out that due to *lack of training in recognizing social-emotional needs,* she failed to be helpful (43% of cases).

This situation deals with a friend who, unexpectedly, telephoned me late on a Sunday afternoon to ask if I would be home in the evening because she wanted to come for a visit. This was unusual because she had three young children who normally went to bed quite early in the evening, and my friend lived in a distant city, about 2 hours' drive away. This friend had a mental illness about 3 years ago and was hospitalized for about 3 weeks. Her condition was diagnosed as paranoid schizophrenia.

When she and her family arrived she seemed very agitated and complained about being overworked and that her husband never took her out. I attempted to carry on light conversation but was not successful. She became increasingly agitated and appeared to be annoyed at whatever I talked about. I had purchased a blouse for her daughter, who had a birthday a few weeks previously. I gave it to her, and my friend looked at it and said that it was too big and that it had to be exchanged. I suggested that the little girl try it on because I wanted to see how it fit and also asked the mother if she preferred another color. The girl's mother shouted, "Don't you believe me? I know when it is too big." Later, when talking about the children's pet turtle, my husband remarked on the huge paws for its size. My friend immediately burst out saying who did my husband think he was trying to make her believe a wild tale like that. She took exception to everything that was said, especially by her husband. I suggested that she quiet down, but this only seemed to aggravate her. The men then went downstairs to the recreation room, and she and I remained upstairs. While we were talking I was busy folding clothes and she said that if she had known that I had work to do she would not have come. I probably was occupying myself folding clothes because I was ill at ease.

She told me that she had an appointment with her doctor the next day, and I strongly encouraged her to keep her appointment.

After the short visit was over, I felt I had inadequately helped my friend. In analyzing the situation I realize that I had placed her in the position of having to make a decision about the blouse, which probably at that time she was not capable of making. I also realized that I should have given her my complete attention and should not have folded clothes. Also, I should not have told her to quiet down. I felt I assisted her when I encouraged her to see her doctor, but I should have also suggested that she contact a social worker or a public health nurse in her city for assistance. Because of my many responsibilities (going to school, looking after my family and home), I probably felt that I could not become involved in someone else's problems at that time. Probably, my friend was looking for some help from me, because as a friend and a nurse I should have been able to assist her. I feel that I did not have the knowledge and felt inadequate in being able to help her. I felt that I had not been much help to her as a friend or as a nurse.

Of the Helpful cases, 80% cite *gave moral support.* This is the highest rating in relation to any Condition.

Henri was a crew member of an oil tanker on the Great Lakes. While in the process of assisting to tie up the ship, he had fallen on the slippery deck, thus bruising his back and buttocks, although not severely. He was brought to hospital by taxi: his ship continued on to its winter berth, where he would rejoin it later and stay on board alone as watchman for the winter.

It was Christmas Day when I returned to work after some days off and met Henri. My role at that time was staff nurse on a male surgical floor of a suburban general hospital. The floor was almost empty of patients, as elective surgery had been canceled for the holidays. Therefore, there was a surplus of time to spend with the remaining patients—to communicate and to enjoy the relaxed, festive atmosphere.

When I entered Henri's room on that fateful morning, I was met by a short, smiling, nervous bachelor of about 45 years. He was up, dressed, had made his bed (better than most nurses would do, I remember), and was in the process of sorting through a coin collection he had brought with him. He immediately stood up to introduce himself and to proudly display the cigarette lighter and electric razor he had received as Christmas presents. He would not accept a back wash or rub, but obviously was happy to talk.

It was later at coffee with the head nurse that I learned the truth about the presents. On December 23, Henri had given her money to make these purchases for him and at the same time, he had given her money for herself to buy French perfume. Obviously he had a great need to receive a Christmas gift from someone and to give one in return.

During the next 4 days I learned more about this kind, sensitive man. Our common interest in numismatics helped break the ice, although communication came easily and spontaneously, as if we had known each other for years. We had time to play cards and he enjoyed helping about the floor with tidying up and handing out meal trays. He was really enjoying his stay in hospital!

Henri grew up in Spain, but ran away at age 14 after his father had been shot, because he felt he was a burden on his mother, the sole supporter of the family of five boys, three younger and one older than himself. He obtained a job as a deckhand on a freighter that sailed the South Pacific and in all those years had returned home only once, when he received word that his mother was ill and was to undergo major surgery. His brothers had done well, were married with families, and he felt like the black sheep of the family. His older brother sent news and photographs regularly via the shipping company, but Henri would not answer. He just could not bring himself to do so, although he wanted to. It was a very painful conflict. His brothers encouraged him to come home to see their mother and their children—it was obvious they cared.

In 1962, Henri arrived in Buffalo in a severe state of depression. He quit his job and stayed at a mariner's residence for 2 years, his first time on shore for any length of time since he had left Spain. During that time he spent his savings on alcohol, gambling, and gifts to acquaintances, which only lowered further his feelings of worth and self-esteem. He tried to buy friendship and was only hurt further in the process. It was at this time that he contemplated suicide. Fortunately, the captain of a Great Lakes oil tanker recognized his despair and persuaded him to go aboard and try his present job. For the last few years, with the help of this very perceptive, humane captain, Henri had pulled himself out of his depressed mental state. In the course of conversation, I learned that this captain was retiring that year and that Henri felt this upcoming loss very deeply. There seemed to be nobody else.

Looking back, perhaps that is why I gave Henri my address and telephone number when he was discharged from hospital. It was the first time I had ever done so for any patient. I had misgivings about this at the time (due to learned role definition) but felt compelled to do so anyway. Perhaps subconsciously at the time I knew that there was an unspoken need of another person. I was married with two preschool children and realized the complications that might ensue (husband's attitude, my own needs, etc.). I, in return, made a note of his address.

I feel I helped this man, not so much as a nurse, but as another human being who cared and who recognized signs and symptoms of a very great need. Nursing training might have made the recognition possible.

Six years have passed now, and, looking back, I see indications of progress having been made. That first winter, as a family, we went to visit Henri, who was alone on board that eerie, empty, creaking ship for 3 months. The realization of his loneliness and fortitude was overwhelming. He could not contain his emotion when we arrived unexpectedly and could not do enough to make us comfortable. He took our 4-year-old son on a tour of the ship and enjoyed bouncing and holding our year-old daughter, wet diapers and all.

That was the beginning of a lasting friendship. Since then, we have corresponded by letter and have visited personally at our home and at various ports. At the beginning, Henri showered us with expensive gifts. It was difficult to refuse his well-meant gestures, realizing his need, but I felt it was of more benefit to him to realize that we cared for him as a person, that we valued his friendship, that gifts were not necessary. This realization on his part had some effect, although he found it difficult to refrain from gift-giving altogether. It was at this point that he admitted the truth about the Christmas presents and how badly and childish he felt about it. I felt this was a big step forward, facing reality and toward growth.

Four years ago, on New Year's Eve, after much encouragement (and a few drinks), I helped Henri write a letter to his older brother and mother. It was a very trying, anxiety-producing ordeal for him to write that letter, but he did it. Once he began writing, words and emotion flowed freely. Twenty-three pages later, on into the early hours of the morning, after much sweat and many tears, the letter was finished and we both sat there crying tears of relief, then went right out and mailed it. It was obvious that Henri's self-esteem had risen to a point where he felt of some worth and value and he communicated this to his family. I felt that I, and my family, had helped him to arrive at this point by giving freely of ourselves, our time, and our love and by accepting his in return.

A few months after this great event, I received a letter from Henri, announcing his plans to go to Spain for a holiday to visit his family. After they had received his letter, nearly every relative had written in reply, encouraging him to return home. His mother was old and ill and desired to see him. This was the end result I had hoped for, a reunion with the family he loved but had been too proud and fearful to get involved with again because of the intense amount of feeling and vulnerability involved.

I feel that I helped him recognize how he had hidden away on ships behind his facade of pride. He admitted that he felt it was unmasculine or a sign of weakness to want to establish a relationship with his brothers after all these years; he just did not know how to go about doing it. I think I helped show him the way by helping to build up his sense of worth, helping him to see himself as an asset to his family, not a hindrance. Our family had become Henri's substitute family and had filled a very great need on his part, to be with children and to have a home to go to when he was in the vicinity. We still keep in touch to this day, although not as regularly as before.

Henri is still on board the same ship, traveling between the Great Lakes and the East Coast. Each winter now, rather than staying on board alone as watchman, he returns to Spain for those 3 months. His letters indicate he is happy and much more optimistic about life in general. He writes enthusiastically about his family, about all his nieces and nephews and what they are doing and what his plans are for the next holiday. It is amazing to see the many changes and to realize that this progress took so many years. The main thing is, however, that change and progress have taken place. It is difficult to evaluate one's use of self intellectually in such a situation, but it is one I feel right about, not knowing exactly how it all came about but realizing that somehow, someone was understood, cared for, and helped by a friend.

You moved from what had essentially been a professional relationship to take on what you felt he most needed—a personal friendship. You were right in questioning what the complications could have been, which is perhaps why the transition worked so positively for everyone concerned.

7

PSYCHIATRIC

Of the 550 cases in the study, 8% focus on the Psychiatric patient. Of the 46 cases that focus on the Psychiatric patient, 59% are described as Helpful, 41% as Unhelpful.

COMPARISON WITH ALL OTHER SITUATIONS

Unhelpful Factors

Highest Rating

- Purposely disregarded significant cues in patient's statements/behavior.
- Lost professional role: patient became friend.
- Felt guilty but still would not communicate.

Helpful Factors	% of Cases in Which Cited
1. Helped patient express feelings	63
2. Gave moral support	56
3. Wanted to understand how patient felt	44
4. Looked beyond patient's outward response/behavior to underlying causes	44
5. Took time to explain	37
6. Was a sounding board	33
7. Came to terms with own feelings; was able to enter into patient's problem	30

8.	Nonjudgmental	30
9.	Initiated referral to another profession/resource	22
10.	Liked the patient	22
11.	Used innovative rehabilitative procedure	19
12.	Used physical closeness	15
13.	Was honest with patient/relatives	15
14.	Not unduly influenced by negative opinions of other staff regarding the patient's personality	11
15.	Helped family members deal with the situation	7
16.	Positively identified with patient due to similar life/professional experience	7
17.	Made this case the basis for overall policy change/improvement	4
18.	Discussed religion with patient	4
19.	Was trying to prove self to senior staff members	0
20.	Had received training in recognizing social-emotional needs of patients	0

Unhelpful Factors		% of Cases in Which Cited
1.	Purposely disregarded significant cues in patient's statements/behavior	58
2.	Failed to look beyond initial negative impression of patient's personality	53
3.	Treated the condition, overlooking the patient	47
4.	Felt inadequate to enter into patient's problem because had not personally resolved the issue	42
5.	Self-image was threatened	42
6.	Was disapproving, judgmental	37
7.	Did not want to understand	32
8.	Felt guilty but still would not communicate	26
9.	Lacked training in recognizing social-emotional needs of patients	26
10.	Rationalized actions and thoughts	26
11.	Lost professional role: patient became friend	21
12.	Prejudiced toward group of which patient was member	16
13.	Felt guilty but could not communicate	11
14.	Breakdown of interprofessional communication/cooperation	11
15.	Short-staffed; too little time to devote to the patient	11

16. Disregarded own judgment because wanted approval of senior staff members — 11
17. Disliked patient — 11
18. Felt pressured (within self) into doing things rather than coping with feeling elements (tension present) — 5
19. Failed to seek authoritative advice regarding innovation — 5
20. Negatively influenced by opinions of other staff members regarding personality of the patient — 0
21. Afraid would break down and cry in front of patient — 0
22. Avoided needs of family members — 0
23. Overidentified due to being similar age to patient — 0
24. Incapacitated by own fear of death — 0

As noted, *helped patient express feelings* is the factor that nurses cite most often (in 63% of cases) in being Helpful to Psychiatric patients.

My positive use of self concerns a 19-year-old boy, whom I nursed in the hospital on a psychiatric floor. Mike was a strong, healthy, but very depressed boy. Prior to admission Mike had been mixed up in the drug scene for a period of 2 years. He had been in the hospital 4 months before I was assigned to be his nurse. The only facts I knew about Mike were that he had taken large doses of amphetamines prior to admission and, most important, that he had not spoken a word to anyone since admission. His parents had disowned him and also had forbidden his two younger brothers to visit. Before I met Mike I felt much pity for him. It must be terrible to be so alone, and not to have anyone close to turn to and lean on when you need them the most.

The first day I met Mike there was no need for an introduction. He was sitting in the lounge looking at the floor with his hands on his lap. His face was filled with sadness. When I said, "Hello, Mike," he slowly glanced at me but said nothing. There wasn't any expression in his eyes at all. I knew then the loneliness he was experiencing must have been very deep. Mike was not my only patient, but I felt sympathy toward him, probably because there was no verbal communication.

The next 4 weeks were a strain on me, because I never really knew what Mike was thinking. I admit that there were times when I felt like giving up, but I realized that if I had built up any trust, I couldn't take the chance on losing it. My positive use of self was to communicate just by caring. When we were in group therapy, or in the lounge, I would make a point of sitting beside him or across from him. At recreation, there was always something to comment on without asking too many questions. It would have been so easy to forget this quiet boy in the corner. At mealtimes I would make some comment about coming to the cafeteria. ("Are you ready for lunch, Mike?") My only visible accomplishment after 4 weeks was that he was now eating regular meals.

One day after group therapy Mike sat alone after the others had left. I returned and sat beside him in silence. In previous weeks I had asked if he wanted to talk about anything, but got no response. This day I chose not to say anything. After a few moments he turned his face and looked at me for the longest time.

"My father hates me," he said, with tears in his eyes. At that moment I felt sorrow for Mike but at the same time excitement, joy, and happiness. I took his hand and he continued to talk. It was the beginning for Mike. I offered him the understanding and sympathy that he needed so desperately. In the weeks to follow Mike was a different boy. It made me feel good to see him laughing and talking with other patients.

In the preceding case, the process of building sufficient trust for verbal communication took a period of some weeks. In the following example, a specific crisis helped to precipitate expression of feelings. Just as the nurse is about to leave—after a 2-hour interview—the basic problem is blurted out.

On a routine visit to one of my schools I was hastily summoned to the vice-principal's office. On arriving there he informed me that he had received a telephone call from the leader of a Scout troop to the effect that Sally Black had attempted suicide the previous evening while attending a meeting. I discussed the situation with the vice-principal, checked Sally's school record, and discovered she had only arrived in the area 3 weeks ago. She had also presented several problems at her last school. She had a terrible home life; her father and mother were always quarreling and were now together again after several separations. Sally was the eldest of three children (all girls) and was expected to shoulder a lot of responsibilities, e.g., getting her sisters dressed for school and giving them breakfast, with the result that she was always late for school. Sally was 10 years old.

I also discovered that the family had been recommended for psychiatric services and for this reason left the previous area where they had been living. This was Sally's second attempt to commit suicide.

It was evident that something had to be done and done quickly, too. I had permission to contact her Scout leader, which I did. I had an interview with the class teacher, who confirmed what Sally's Scout leader had told me: Sally was an introvert, did not participate in any play or activity with the other children, and thought, actually said, that no one liked her. I spoke to Sally for a short time. She was smartly dressed, well spoken, and talked about her sisters and an aunt who was living with them, but I had to ask direct questions concerning her mother and father. She told me she had been to the Scout meeting the previous evening, but did not mention anything about attempting to commit suicide. She looked pale and withdrawn. Incidentally, Sally had an IQ of 130.

At the end of this interview the principal came to see me and requested a home visit. Mrs. Black lived a few blocks from the school, so I decided to walk, hoping this would give me time to put my thoughts together as to a line of approach. I realized this was going to be a difficult visit from several points of view.

1. The family was new in the area.
2. Their history showed they resented and had refused professional help.
3. Mrs. Black had previously refused to admit that Sally had a problem and was a disturbed child.
4. There were marital problems that Mrs. Black might resent discussing with someone she had neither seen nor heard of before.

In fact, there was nothing in my favor.

I arrived at the home and introduced myself. Mrs. Black was very apprehensive, pale, and even resentful. Before I could state the reason for my visit she blurted out, "There is nothing wrong with Sally. My God, I wish I were dead," and then burst into tears. I took her by the hand and told her to sit down and I did likewise. I waited patiently and silently while Mrs. Black cried.

Finally, she stopped and apologized for her behavior, but I reassured her that a good cry was often the best thing that could happen. I said, "Mrs. Black, if you feel you can talk about it, I am here to listen and to offer any help I can if you desire to accept it. I know you do not know me, but the situation is such an important one we cannot afford to lose too much time."

She told me her problems, at the same time blaming her husband, who she claimed was a shifter. Most important, she admitted Sally had a problem and that she needed help immediately. Could I help her? Being new in the area she did not have a family doctor. She then remembered that 5 years earlier she had lived in a neighboring area and had had a family doctor whom she liked and who also knew all her problems. She telephoned and after discussing the situation, the doctor, realizing the urgency, was able to make an appointment for her and Sally to attend the mental health clinic that very afternoon. After spending approximately 2 hours there and as I was about to leave, Mrs. Black said, "Nurse, I have been very hard on Sally. Maybe it's because she was born out of wedlock that I resent her so much. I feel she is the cause of all my problems." She had married Sally's father a year after Sally was born and since then her husband had repeatedly disowned paternity of the child. This he had told Sally and all their quarrels centered around that fact: hence, the reason for Sally feeling unwanted.

This was a situation in which I felt I was helpful. Because of the rapport I was able to establish with Mrs. Black she was able to talk about her problems and analyze them, as well as try to do something about solving them. My approach was accepting and nonjudgmental. I was patient and a good listener. By being able to talk about her marital problems she was able to see that Sally had become the family scapegoat. The family is still being treated at the clinic.

"What is normal? Who am I?" The following case involves a university student in acute depression.

Sheldon G was a 19-year-old university student, admitted to our floor with a diagnosis of acute depression. For the first few days of his hospitalization he remained completely immobile and withdrawn. I was in his room at regular intervals. I worked quietly and efficiently and kept stimuli to a minimum.

The admission note revealed that Sheldon was a second-year university student at the top of his physics and chemistry classes. His parents had had the tendency to overprotect him in childhood; Sheldon showed no liking for sports and had formed few relationships outside the home. Prior to admission Sheldon had apparently lost interest in school and schoolwork had lapsed in this period of severe depression.

A few days after admission Sheldon started to rouse. During this time I spoke to him slowly in short sentences and said, "I am your nurse, Miss Butler. What you are going through is pretty rough. I want you to know that if things get too bad or if you need someone I would like to help."

I stayed with him as much as I could and slowly he came around. Understandably, this was a slow process. Sheldon revealed that as a child he had no friends. At the university he had got to know a few of his classmates, but these relationships generally upset Sheldon because of his classmates' apparent preoccupation with girls and sex. He was confused by their cool, aloof attitude to the opposite sex in contrast to his father's teaching that love and respect were of prime importance. The conflict Sheldon had in trying to see this matter in its proper perspective led to intense feelings of self-doubt, doubt about the value of a brilliant mind when athletic prowess and personality appeared more important to social acceptance. Sheldon was really just beginning a stage of growth that his classmates had been experiencing since high school—that of discovering who you are and what you are while (it is hoped) having the support and mutual interests of other members of the peer group, who are also trying out different roles to establish an identity.

As we developed a relationship of trust I discussed with him his goals as he saw them: (1) to get his Ph.D.; (2) to meet a girl with an outlook on life similar to his own, someone who would not mind that his only experience had been with bunsen burners.

He realized that he would probably experience no difficulty achieving his first goal. But unfortunately from his exposure to girls at the university he had convinced himself that nice, moral girls just weren't around.

Through our discussions he seemed able to see that his girl would not be the easiest to find. She would have to be fairly refined and possess a genuine liking for him as a person. I assured him that there would probably be many times when he would envy his classmates for their knack with girls but that at the same time he would be envied for his academic ability.

In time he seemed able to distinguish himself as an individual with likable qualities worthy of self-esteem. He accepted himself with his limitations and capabilities quite well. He realized the need for independence from his parents and expected that it would be awhile before he met the girl who could replace them. He was able to perceive that his new acceptance of himself would enable others to accept him—perhaps members of his class with similar academic interests.

Why I Feel I Was Helpful in This Situation

1. I was able to establish an atmosphere of trust.
2. I was able to understand Sheldon's concerns as he saw them and show a genuine liking for him just as he was.

As noted, of the Unhelpful Responses to psychiatric patients, *purposely disregarded significant cues in patient's statements/behavior* is cited most often (in 58% of the cases). This is also the highest rating of this response among all 12 Conditions. *Lost professional role: patient became friend* is also more prevalent with Psychiatric patients than with any other group.

In the following cases, the nurses relate these responses to their *threatened self-image:* their need to be acceptable to the patient and thereby prove their competence to co-workers.

I was working as a nurse in a psychiatric setting as a student, far from my friends, family, and boyfriend. I was lonely. I knew very little of the therapeutic helping relationship. I feel I grew close to one of my patients, Martin, and in this manner, did not come near the goal of helping him to develop and become responsible for his actions.

A particular interview went something like this:

Martin: I hate this place, and I don't belong in it!

I thought, he'll like me better if I go along with what he says.

I said: I know you don't belong here, Martin. You and I get along fine, so you must be OK!

Martin: Sure we do, Susan, so let's go for a walk.

That sounded like fun; no harm in that! I said OK, laughing, and jokingly hooked my arm in his. I thought, gee, this is a close relationship!

Martin: Would you go out with me if I ever get out of here?

Oh, dear. I should have listened to the warnings of my instructors. What do I say now?

I said: Well, I don't know about that!

In this short part of a typical encounter I see many things I did wrong. This was not the type of patient with whom to let down the air of professionalism at all! This was not a helping relationship but instead a flippant boy-girl social visit.

I did not listen to the true feelings Martin was trying to express, about being normal and not needing "this place." I was too caught up in my own little ego trip, in my need to be liked. This produced a detrimental dependence on the part of both of us. Acknowledging the fact that he didn't need to be in hospital certainly did not help him toward gaining his health!

I used his first name and let him use mine, which in this particular case was not a good idea, as he was already a dependent type of personality who would read me wrong, producing more dependency. Martin was clinging to anyone who would pay attention to him, and I let myself become caught in a bind—sopping up all the attention myself also!

In my taking his arm I was not acting appropriately in this instance. I was joking, but again Martin was the type of patient of whose feelings one must be careful, as he was a dependent type of person. He misinterpreted my touch with something else.

When he asked if I'd ever go out with him, through my insecurity my answer was quite inadequate. I should have explained why I did not feel this would be appropriate. I was unable to handle the sexual component in our relationship; it was not of my doing (or was it?). I came on as a social partner, not a nurse. I answered in a confusing manner as I did not know how to handle what I had got myself into. I did not have the perception to recognize that he may have been asking just for verification that he was still desirable. My seemingly turning down his offer of a date only proved to him that his experiences with rejection were well founded, as once more he was being rejected.

This relationship carried on and was very difficult to terminate, as I had not been personal, but intimate. I had not helped Martin assume responsibility for himself, but instead had fostered dependence. My own needs for feeling worthwhile, my lack of knowledge of the therapeutic relationship, and my need to succeed as a student had tremendously interfered with the needs of the patient. I was of no help to him at all; instead I was a destructive influence in his recovery.

*   *   *   *

Miss J had been a psychiatric patient, and had been diagnosed as schizophrenic; she had been in the psychiatric hospital for a period of a year, and had been discharged about 18 months earlier. Miss J had her own home and a female friend boarded with her. Miss J was visited monthly by a nurse as well as a social worker, who visited periodically. The hospital had hoped to turn this lady over to local facilities; as the district health nurse, I was contacted. I was to visit in order to assess if Miss J was slipping again, and to notify the hospital if necessary, in order to avoid another hospital admission. I was to check on her personal hygiene, as she tended to let this slip when ill, and I was to see that she was socializing, taking her medications, and keeping house properly.

According to the history, it was advised that the nurse make the first visit with the social worker, as the patient's behavior was unpredictable. I decided that I wouldn't be afraid of her; after all, I had some experience in psychiatric nursing. Therefore I chose not to call the social worker for the first visit, and contacted him later.

Miss J was pleasant on the first visit, but did look "spooky." Conversation centered on the weather and I said I would return for another social visit. After all, I didn't want her to reject me, or to make her angry, so I couldn't get to the point yet! And what would the nurse or social worker think if I blew it!

Even after establishing the fact that she liked my visits, I just couldn't tell Miss J her appearance was really poor.

Would this have been necessary?

I tried to tell myself that I was starting out being too critical of her. I asked all the questions about pills and her social life and she just said yes. Now where to go! I just couldn't bring myself to tell her about her appearance. Maybe she would get mad because she thought these were social visits. My visits became less frequent. I was very busy doing other things!

Then I heard from the psychiatric nurse, who said she thought Miss J had slipped and hadn't I noticed! Besides that, the nurse told Miss J exactly why I was visiting! The next two visits I didn't find Miss J at home; more fear for me. When I did find her at home, she was very nice, to my surprise, but would you believe it, I still evaded the issue!

Perhaps I did *not* take the social worker because I wanted to forget that this was a psychiatric patient. I didn't really know how to handle this case, but refused to admit it. My social-visit approach avoided irritating Miss J, and I really was afraid! I didn't want this patient to reject me, and this was important to me because the other workers had established a relationship with her. Also, I knew I wasn't too busy to make visits, because I passed her house regularly. Most of all, I just could not bring myself to criticize another openly.

You may want to consider why you see criticism as an inevitable part of working with Miss J.

What I should have done in the first place was to swallow my pride and make the first visit with the social worker and have things straight from the start. By doing this, I would have received some guidelines as to how to work out my problems. I have since made arrangements to visit the hospital with the supervisor of psychiatric social workers (I gathered up the courage to admit to her that I really had goofed!) and discuss this case with the people involved and then go back to discuss things with Miss J.

Great!

Forty-four percent of Helpful cases describe *looked beyond patient's outward response/behavior to underlying causes.* The following cases describe how this can lead to innovation and change in hospital programming.

Last year I was working in a male residential ward at a psychiatric hospital. The hospital was in the process of integrating the male and female areas and I was one of the first nurses to be sent to the male side. The ward was staffed by one male nursing supervisor and an attendant staff. There were 60 male patients ranging in age from 30 to 90. Their diagnoses were mostly senile psychosis, but we had some suffering from mental retardation and brain damage.

Many of them exhibited bizarre behavior and were quite suspicious of a woman on the ward. No one ever had much time or inclination to talk with these people and I tried to talk to them all about three times a day, when I made rounds. It was amazing how quickly they responded and it took a very short time for them to accept me. I was genuinely fond of all of them and they seemed to sense it. In time they were overprotecting me. No one swore in my presence and if anyone ever tried to be aggressive toward me, the others were all ready to do battle with the aggressor.

In the spring a psychologist was added to the unit staff and we decided to set up a program to reactivate as many of these people as we could. An arts and crafts program was launched as our first project. We had no supplies, no money, and no trained occupational therapy staff. These things did come later. We begged, borrowed, and almost stole supplies. We chose 20 patients to participate and they were simply delighted to be doing something useful again. We reinforced them positively with loud and long verbal praise, tailor-made cigarettes, and candy. The hospital had a bazaar in the summer and we sold $89 worth of crafts. (I have used the word *we* a great deal instead of *I* because this really had to be a multidiscipline team effort.)

In terms of myself, this was one of the most rewarding and challenging experiences of my life. I seemed to be able to accept their bizarre behavior most matter of factly. I thought their plight in life was simply appalling and I tried to help modify it. They knew this and appreciated it. For the first time in years they were doing something useful and interesting. But most important of all, I cared, and they knew it.

The following also describes the initiation of a new area of programming for patients. It is the mutual support factor between nurse and patient that is described as the catalyst. Given much *moral support* by the nurse, the patient reciprocates by giving the nurse the confidence to become involved in an area that heretofore she has been unable to discuss with patients.

I started working with Miss X 4 ½ years ago as a patient in our psychiatric day care program. She was very shy, timid, and withdrawn. Her weight was 88 pounds after losing 50 pounds in one month. She was never a person who smoked but now she chain-smoked.

After 3 months with Miss X, I felt we were making slow progress. We would sit for hours involved in some kind of an activity or just sitting and talking, but our conversation would be superficial. I knew she could not be rushed. I knew she wanted help, because she came every day. I wanted to help but felt helpless because I did not know her needs.

She was afraid and angry, but also afraid to expose herself. When we sat in group therapy she would save me a seat; I felt I was building trust and should not give up. The other members of the team felt she was playing games with me and I should confront her; I knew she was too fragile for that approach.

I suggested that, because she was underweight, I would exchange my extra pounds for her thinness. She looked me in the face and for the first time smiled. I knew I had broken the barrier. I was excited and yet afraid she would freeze up again, so I told her she made me feel comfortable when she smiled and she smiled and touched my hand.

I was anxious to know why she was losing weight. With my fingers crossed I ventured in: I asked her how she was able to lose weight and I could not. With head downcast and tears rolling down her face she said, ''Get fired when you are on vacation.'' I was glad to see her cry I forgot we were in a public park. Her voice was stronger but she was angry and frightened. I put my hand on her shoulder and told her to keep on crying if she wanted to, I was there to listen to her.

Through her sobs and tears she told me her boyfriend was laid off, so they decided to go home on her vacation to meet her parents. She said her boyfriend had never traveled and they enjoyed themselves so much. She returned to be told she was fired, but they called it a layoff. She said she lived with her aunt, but could not bring herself to tell her aunt, or her boyfriend, that she was not working. She felt her aunt would not understand and it would depress her boyfriend.

She left home every morning for work and sat in libraries and parks. She was not eating or sleeping. She did not even tell her aunt she was attending the center or taking medication. I asked her why, and she told me her aunt would say that she just had to be tough, fight it, speak up, and forget the pills. She said she tried that for 8 weeks and got more depressed.

I was so intent on listening to her that we forgot the time, until she told me we had been out for 2 hours (and I had not even checked my watch once). ''Thanks for listening,'' she said.

After a couple of days I asked her what her aunt thought of her weight loss. She said her aunt thought she was homesick, but she had been away from home for 8 years.

After she began socializing with others and not relating only to me, I asked her how she felt within herself, and she said that she felt less depressed but not better. I asked in what way she would like to feel better, and with sadness in her eyes she said, ''No one can help in this area.''

I told her she had made great progress and she should give it a try. But she looked reluctant, so I told her to think about it. I knew she could not be pushed. As I was walking away, she said it had to be a female whom she would turn to; when I asked her why she acted surprised and said she was just thinking aloud.

I thought about what she had said—''It must be female''—and I thought this must be very personal. Every day I spent half an hour with her, teaching her how to breathe and relax properly. I introduced the subject of nutrition, and asked her to get a little book or diary and write down some of the things she thought she needed help with and we could discuss them. She agreed, but after 2 weeks of not having discussed it with me, I asked her about it. She took out of her purse an up-to-date diary. She had gained 20 pounds, but she looked a bit embarrassed, so I asked her to let me hear the list. She seemed relieved that I did not read her diary. The list went as follows:

1. Express myself to say what I am really feeling.
2. Get a job working with people in trouble.
3. Feel comfortable with people.
4. Get over my fear—speak with confidence.
5. Sex and marriage.

As we went over the list, I felt I could help her with most of them, but not sex and marriage! I started my own battle with myself. I was never married. Sure, I had seen my parents', relatives', and my friends' marriages—some good, some bad—but who was I to speak of marriage?

Sex was really personal! Sure, I could talk to my friends, but to a patient, I wondered, can I be expressive enough as a person that she will understand what I am communicating? I could have found an easy way out; I could have refered her to a social worker, but I would have failed myself and her. I felt she would perceive me as not dependable or consistent if I said she should see someone else. How much of her freedom should I interfere with, or should I impose my ideas and beliefs on this person, or will she be able to choose her own freedom? These were the questions that plagued my mind.

After speaking with her doctor, she advised me to go ahead, because Miss X trusted me and opened up more to me than she ever had done to her in the 5 years she had known her. This reassured me a little, but did not help much with the inner me.

I decided to be honest with Miss X and let her know my feelings. She could not believe that nurses did not know everything and that I had fears and doubts as she did. I thought, here goes honesty, but she responded by patting me on the shoulder and saying, "The doctors and ministers are terrible at explaining sex and marriage to you. It takes a sensitive person to work with people with bad nerves." At that moment I saw her strength and knew that she knew what she was shopping for and I could use those strengths.

We did work through these areas together and she helped me to set up a workshop for the other patients. In talking about sexual problems, she selected films and collected them for me; she was also sharing this knowledge with her fiance.

Our meetings together became less frequent. She had too many other things with which she was involved: she was active in voice and drama at the YMCA, cooking and sewing at night school, and working with a skid row project. Having previously put off her wedding five times by being sick and depressed, she was now making her wedding dress. It took the best of 4 years of this lady to reach this stage of development in her life, and it was the start for me of teaching sexuality to male and female patients in my job.

I chose this case because, after it, I felt I really became a true nurse.

1. In helping the patient grow, I was growing too.
2. I had to abandon the rigid interpersonal armour that I had worn as a nurse when working with patients and in doing so I became more emotionally involved.
3. I found out that not only the patient gets stuck in stages of development, but the nurse does also.

I let the patient know the real me, and it was frightening. I had exposed myself as not knowing everything, but was willing to learn. The patient identified with me—no one can know everything. My colleagues said I would be sorry in the end because she was manipulating me for attention, but I saw a person in need. Moreover, I learned to really listen and observe, and not to look at my watch, because the patient is also observing.

Failed to look beyond initial negative impression of patient's personality (53% of cases) and *was disapproving, judgmental* (37% of cases) are aptly illustrated in the following accounts—the first two involving suicide attempts.

It was an extremely busy evening in the emergency department when a semi-comatose woman was wheeled in on the ambulance stretcher. She had taken an overdose of pills and although busy with two car-accident victims, we had to work quickly before any more of the pills were absorbed into her bloodstream and she became more deeply comatose. We worked earnestly for about 1 ½ hours, during which a policeman came in to say that the patient was Miss C, a 45-year-old who had tried this same thing four times in the past 6 months and was under the care of a psychiatrist.

She started to awaken and 3 hours after admission she was conscious and talking. Meanwhile, in the next room was a 40-year-old man with a serious head injury who was unconscious; in the opposite room was a hit-and-run car accident victim, a 17-year-old boy who was bleeding extensively from abdominal injuries and had many fractures. We were short-staffed and I resented having to spend my time with this overdose patient.

Then Miss C became extremely restless, started swearing and tried to climb out of bed. We restrained her and she soon calmed down. She wanted to know what had happened and I told her. I asked her why she had taken the pills and she replied, "I felt like it." I was becoming angrier by the minute and showed it with stern words and orders of what she could and could not do. I did not explore her thoughts or feelings any further, blocking all communication and tending only to her physical needs. I was glad when she was ready to leave the department.

I partially resented having to spend my time with this woman who had willfully tried to kill herself when in the next two rooms were people fighting for their lives who had not caused or asked for their conditions. When I did try to communicate with her and she was offhand, my anger was increased and I became more impatient. Actually, there were many problems under her flippant surface but I was too angry to try to explore them.

In this case the nurse describes a wall between herself and her patient.

Marion was a sad, pathetic girl who was well known on the psychiatric ward. She was transferred from a respiratory unit to the observation ward on which I worked.

The history left me with disgust: sixth attempt at suicide. This incident had been planned and was to be discovered before death ensued; however, her roommates didn't arrive home as expected and the attempt was almost fatal. Marion quick-wittedly called the telephone company to inform them of her mistake.

For the 4 days Marion was on the ward, she became more alert and orientated. I cared for her physical needs, but was unable to give of myself in order to help her psychologically. Marion, for me, stopped at the words "sixth suicidal attempt." In the back of my mind were all the pat phrases: "suicide is a plea for help," "form of attention seeking," and so on; but in Marion's case, they were hollow words. I felt like taking that girl and shaking some sense into her head.

My inability to comprehend the desire to self-destruct left me with the inability to accept Marion for herself with all the facets of her personality. Perhaps, because I have never tasted from the bitter cup of despair, I shall never fully empathize with people who have.

Marion had positive aspects that I was unable to bring to the fore, because I saw her as hopeless. Attention-seeking by attempted suicide, however sick a method, was working for her. The hospital reinforced her pattern. Thus, Marion never learned a more socially acceptable method.

As a result of this hopeless feeling, I was frustrated in my attempt to support Marion. Reviewing my feelings toward this girl, I realize I did not function to my full potential because I did not communicate. I built a wall between us that I expected Marion to surmount because the hospitalization was her problem, not mine. In actual fact, it was my problem. I failed to have basic human compassion for Marion, because I saw a symptom and not the individual. I failed to remind myself, "There, but for the grace of God, go I."

Actually, in a sense both you and Marion had each built walls of despair. Perhaps this insight into your feelings of despair and hopelessness will help you to more fully understand this emotion in others.

The fear and stigmatization of the psychiatric patient is described below both as it affected the nurse and the community.

The area where I work is isolated in the north of Canada and the people are Cree Indian. They originally belonged to a village 12 miles up the river but split away due to religious problems between the Anglicans and Roman Catholics. This occurred approximately 20 to 25 years ago and the feud is still alive. The chief presides over both villages. In spite of their common religious ground, the village I am in is very disjointed in villagers' concern for each other. The only time they seem to get together is when someone from the other village creates a problem and then there is a village meeting. If there is trouble at one home very few if any go to help the person, even if they are relatives. At first I found this very hard to accept and found myself getting angry when something happened to someone that could have been avoided. I have been in this area for 10 months now and am slowly learning not to ask too much about the circumstances surrounding some injuries.

The following situation involved a former psychiatric patient. Joseph was hospitalized for schizophrenia until he was under control with medication. He then required mostly custodial care at home. His mother had another child permanently in the hospital with mental illness, but seemed to be able to handle Joseph. The other nurse and I took turns making weekly visits to the home to make sure Joseph was taking his medication and to see how the mother was coping. She told us that he was taking medication and was doing well.

Just a week before Christmas, the other nurse and I were called and told that Joseph was upset and wouldn't settle down. We went together to his home because he does not like women and is 5 feet 7 inches tall and weighs 350 pounds. We spoke to his mother and the other members of the family and they told us he was getting more upset and no one could sleep in the house because they were afraid of him. That night we gave him sedation by injection since he refused pills; I was to check on him the next day. Upon checking, I found he had settled down and was sleeping; his mother said he would be better now.

The third day I checked him he was pacing and no one could go near him. He refused both injections and pills. I was afraid of him myself and found it very difficult to talk to him. I was told he was unpredictable and the other nurse did not want to look after him, so I was on my own.

Joseph had gone into his room and I didn't want to be alone with him in his small room. I decided to talk to the mother and try to figure out what I could do. I found out he had not taken any medication since the last spring and I realized that there was a problem in the way we had approached or talked with the mother. She had not realized that his medication was necessary to control him. I felt that to say anything now would only make her feel responsible for the situation and she would not talk at all.

From his record I knew he was on a high maintenance dose of sedative and it would take a fair amount to calm him down now that he had reached the state he was in. I tried to explain what needed to be done immediately and how we could work together to calm him down—that he would have to go back to the hospital to be put on another regime to control him. His family was very willing to talk and explain his behavior and I felt my fears of being hit or hurt might not be as realistic as I had felt.

I had let my own personal fears interfere too much and I had to reassess my approach to him. I realized that I had to be the first to talk to him without running when he started to move. I think when I finally realized this and did not show my apprehension as much as I had earlier, Joseph picked up this change in my attitude.

During my next conversation with him he continued to just say "Leave me alone" and pace around the house, but I did not leave him and did explain that he needed something to help him feel not so upset inside. I felt that I could not rush him into anything. But it came to the point that we would have to hold him down to give him enough sedation to get him on a plane. I then talked to one man in town that I knew Joseph was comfortable talking to and he was able to get some men in town together to hold him so I could get him sedated. The first time I tried, the men ran out of the house when he started to move around and would not touch him. The next day I had to talk with the men and explain that it was up to them to help Joseph since he couldn't help himself and unless he was sedated the pilots wouldn't fly him south.

Since I or anyone else could remember, the men had never been able to work together to do anything like this. I did not know until I went back to the house with the sedation whether or not they would stay with him until I could give him the needles. When the time came, the men were there and Joseph was just about ready to run out of the house. But the men did get him and hold him and even stayed with him until the medication took effect. I felt it was very important that the men had stayed together and helped and I thanked them and told them that it was very much appreciated.

The parents were still a little upset about him having to go to the hospital. They wanted him to look proper, so we changed his clothes and they bought him a new coat, etc. They accompanied him to the plane and they talked with him for a few minutes before the plane took off. The people in this culture are afraid of any form of mental illness and I felt that it was commendable that they were able to stay with him. I talked with the parents about the hospital and what would be done for Joseph, and told them that we would let them know what was going on with Joseph and that they could write him whenever they wanted. Contact was kept with the hospital and the parents and they are visiting the nurses' station more frequently than they used to.

I feel that if I had just insisted that Joseph be held and then sent him out in the plane the parents and others in the community would have been even more upset and their beliefs about mental illness would have been even more confirmed.

Future situations could be avoided by more open communication and me trying to understand their feelings and to cope with mine so that we can work together for the betterment of the individuals involved.

The next two cases concern the discharge of patients from a psychiatric ward. They are concerned with the effect of hospital procedures on the therapeutic environment, and the nurse's analysis of *treated the condition, overlooking the patient* (47% of Unhelpful cases).

This episode took place on a psychiatric ward. Mary, a confirmed manic depressive for the past 15 years, would suffer for many weeks in a deep depression before she finally responded to treatment. Her usual pattern of improvement was to suddenly become slightly euphoric overnight, and in a day or two, her mood would stabilize. At that point she would be given a trial weekend leave to see if she could cope in the community. Her psychiatrist, Dr. Brown, recognized Mary's need to be independent when possible; consequently, she was allowed to go home by herself on the public transportation system for her short leave. Since no one in Mary's family had a car, it was a very long trip for anyone who might have to pick her up and thus two needs were met by this arrangement.

Unfortunately, during one of her many admissions, Mary became ready for her weekend at home when Dr. Brown was off duty. Dr. Smith, the unit director, took over her caseload; she was more authoritarian in her management of patients and rescinded the standing order allowing Mary to go home by herself. Thus, Mary had to ask her sister to come to the hospital to take her home.

What a blow that was to Mary's pride, confidence, and esteem. She felt very bitter against Dr. Smith because she had to inconvenience her sister. Resentment, hostility, and frustration immediately replaced the anticipated joy of the two-day leave. She picked up her suitcase and threatened, in a loud voice, that she would go home alone and not return on Sunday evening.

Knowing that Dr. Brown would have been more democratic regarding Mary's responsibility to manage alone, I sympathized with her, but I still had to remain loyal to Dr. Smith and her ward policy. I invited Mary into our small office and encouraged her to express her feelings. Her frustration level was continuing to rise because the sister who had promised to call for her was overdue. I suggested that she phone to see if there had been a sudden change in plans; when her sister didn't answer the call, it seemed logical to assume that she was already on her way. Mary accepted that, but kept repeating, "It just isn't fair; Dr. Brown always lets me go home alone, why can't Dr. Smith?"

I agreed with her readily, but pointed out that it was Mary herself, not Dr. Smith, who would suffer any setback if we couldn't work this disappointment out. I asked her, "If you can't control yourself because of a change in routine, perhaps you aren't as ready for your weekend as you think?" We talked in this vein for several more minutes and her tension lessened somewhat. At this point I could explain that Dr. Smith was not familiar with Dr. Brown's treatment for Mary. As head of the department, Dr. Smith had one broad policy for the ward and often it did not suit one individual, as Mary had just experienced.

She responded to my sympathetic reception and was even able to acknowledge a slight legitimacy for Dr. Smith's action in canceling her privilege.

Thus, by according her the dignity a responsible adult deserves, she eventually calmed down without requiring medication. Her resentment of Dr. Smith had not dissipated, but I felt that we successfully had weathered this crisis together. She did return at the proper time on Sunday and was discharged early in the week as usual.

$$* \quad * \quad * \quad *$$

This case occurred on a psychiatric ward with someone who was not mentally ill. A young girl, in her mid-20s, had given a party in her apartment the night before. Late in the evening, she had left her party for a few quick moments and walked to a nearby park. Presumably she had had a few alcoholic drinks that made her sleepy and she fell asleep on the ground. On a routine check of the area, the police discovered her, but on questioning her they drew a blank for co-operation. Not wanting to arrest her as a vagrant and give her a record, they decided to have her admitted overnight to our psychiatric hospital and have things sort themselves out in the morning. During the admitting process she ran around the halls like a frightened, wild creature, and the 15-minute procedure lasted for over an hour.

When I came on duty the next morning, after a few days off, there was very little information in the files about the docile-looking girl in bed 10. I identified myself to her and inquired how she felt this morning. Since she was a night admission, she had not been shown around the ward. This I did immediately, and also introduced her to another young girl with whom she could sit for breakfast.

Later, when our routine morning work was finished, I sat down to talk in an attempt to find out something about her. However, Sally was preoccupied and revealed no information about herself except that she had no business being in the hospital.

She inquired as to when the doctor would make rounds. This was the weekend our ward was covered by a duty doctor, who only came when we called for him. Although he would have seen her at admission time, her request to see him now seemed reasonable. Thus, I put in a call for him, but when he learned why we wanted him, he refused to come to our ward. He said, "Anyone who acted on admission as Sally did needs the hospital confinement for at least the weekend and on Monday her fate can be decided." That was setback number one for her. Number two came when I asked her to take the prescribed tranquilizer, which she obviously needed. She refused, and as reasoning with her was not going to change her mind, I bartered with her. If she would take her pill she could use the office phone. The bribe was accepted.

However, tension continued to mount in her, even after the phone call. She expressed how wrong it was that the police had brought her here. I tried to imagine how mistreated and frightened she must feel; after all, she had only intended to leave her party for a few minutes and instead had been admitted to a psychiatric ward. What a catastrophe had befallen this young girl.

With a feeling of empathy, I tried to reason with her because she was not out of touch with reality. If the circumstances were as she described them, she would certainly be discharged the next day. Could she not get through this one, long day? "Nonsense," she said, "I want out today—now!"

Since that approach failed I tried reality therapy: "Regardless of how unfair and cruel you think that you have been treated, you are here; we can't do a thing about it because the doctor will not see you. Try to make the best of a bad experience." This technique also was rejected.

Frustration and tension were obviously building in Sally, and we wondered how we could help her to control them. Sympathy, reasoning, and reality had not worked. What was our next move to be? As we wondered how we could help her to contain her emotions, the nursing office informed us that Sally had given her roommate's name on the admitting record. No wonder that the poor girl's anxiety level was high; not only was she in a hospital where she knew she didn't belong, but she had involved an innocent person who trusted her.

When asked to confirm this, Sally's endurance for her nightmare ended and she "blew her cool." Running to the bedroom area, she smashed several windows, using the footstool, and so released her overflowing tension.

Unfortunately, this is a relationship in which I could not be helpful. And, yes, Sally was discharged the next day.

A nurse's struggle with the seeming futility of long-term outpatient care of the chronic psychiatric patient, inadequate support services, and personal feelings of inadequacy and guilt are vividly described in the following account.

I wish you to consider the case of CM, a young man, 22 years of age, of Indian origin, who returned to a particular Indian reservation at a time when I had just about managed to build up some agreeable form of relationship with the community. This is quite a process, as Indians rarely fully accept an outsider. Depending on a person's attitude toward them some do, after a considerable time, accept or at least tolerate the outsider. I should state here and now that I never saw an American Indian before 1971, except in western films, which usually depicted the savage Indian versus the white hero. Therefore, I do not claim to be an authority, and my statements are based on personal experiences and assumptions I made during my brief contact with them.

CM had, like many others, a chronic bilateral otitis media since infancy; this resulted in deafness and a deformed external left ear due to poor surgical techniques following two mastoidectomys. Also, as a lad of 13 years of age he had had investigations for pulmonary tuberculosis because of frequent chest infections. However, he had never been diagnosed as such. His appearance was tall, very slim, anemic-looking, and definitely undernourished.

Eleven years ago, he had been admitted to the mental hospital following several episodes of antisocial behavior at a residential school and diagnosed as an undifferentiated schizophrenic. He had been hospitalized intermittently for 9 years, sometimes discharging himself, other times being discharged to continue as an outpatient. But there had never been a successful follow-up throughout the years. Several social workers had probably been involved in attempts to rehabilitate; however, there seemed to be no continuity, probably because CM had no fixed abode.

His mother, brothers and sisters, living in the city, had rejected him completely. The parents were separated and, although the father seemed to have some affection for his son, he too was wandering around aimlessly. I had been told that Indians have a deep fear of any mental disorder. They believe that the unfortunate is possessed of a devil and can never be normal again. This attitude is shared by people of many cultures.

Given this information, try to imagine my dilemma when the chief, a lady, begged me to have CM committed to an institution at once. Apparently, he had requested welfare assistance over and above the amount allowed, and raised hell when refused. Hence the chief's plea.

I had never been faced with such a situation. My knowledge of psychiatric nursing was theoretical and I had had only very brief encounters with patients with postpartum psychosis. My reaction was, "Oh, Lord, what must I do?" Had a transfer been offered me that day, I would have grabbed it at once. But that was not likely to happen.

The next day I paid him a visit. Imagine my surprise when he opened the door. His appearance suggested that a breeze could knock him down. (The office staff were big, hefty persons and they were scared of this individual!)

I introduced myself, offering assistance—indicating, however, that I had no control of any welfare funds but could only recommend. It was fall; he had a thin blanket, no sheets, no pillows, a hard uncomfortable mattress, and nothing else. Those were his immediate needs. I spoke to the social services officer of Indian affairs and extra money was granted to buy the essentials.

During my third visit to CM I suggested a medical check-up and possibly a chest X ray as he was coughing frequently. Immediately he became hostile. "You want me to see a doctor because I have had TB and then you'll get me into that hellhole." (This was the mental institute.) I thought, Oh, dear, I have blown it. "No, CM. You are coughing; don't you think you need some medicine?"

He replied, "What kind of a nurse are you; don't you have cough syrup in your bag?" I said, "Sure I have, but cough syrups do not cure. They might relieve the irritation in your throat but that is all." With a little more courage, I continued, "I don't want you in the hospital. I don't believe you need to be admitted." CM said, "I know what your plan is. But you can make the appointment and let me know. I don't think I'll keep it anyway. I have no car, and I can't walk 20 miles to a doctor."

I concluded this visit somehow, leaving him a bottle of cough syrup, promising to notify him when the appointment would be, and also arrange transportation.

The last time CM had discharged himself from the hospital 2 years ago, we had received recommendations that he continue on Artane and one other drug. I called a doctor I knew fairly well and one who I knew would take time to listen to CM. I explained the situation and promised to send him a copy of the hospital's recommendations if he would see CM. Of course, CM never kept that appointment, nor two subsequent ones. He lied to me that he had seen the doctor but had lost the X ray request form. I knew better but gave no indication.

Then apparently CM entered a home on the reservation and took a guitar, and this was reported to the police. When they came to investigate, CM docilely handed them the guitar. That same day, now knowing about this incident, I met CM walking along the road. He told me he was going to see the doctor, then hitchhike to the city. I offered to take him to town. I stopped at the reservation office and was met by the chief, who was obviously disgruntled with my lack of action, and demanded that I have CM committed. I told her that it seemed he was leaving the community and that I was taking him to town.

Twelve miles from the reservation, a police car signaled me to stop. The officer asked if he could speak to me privately. He explained that he knew I had CM and asked where I was taking him. I told him, and also how I felt, that CM really meant no harm if only people would leave him to try to find himself. The officer assured me that they had no wish to prosecute him and if I had his confidence, they would leave me to cope as I saw fit. Naturally, CM wanted to know what the police wanted: I lied and told him it was about some other matter. He had no appointment with the doctor, but I knew the doctor would see CM, so we went.

Dr. H prescribed an antibiotic, Artane, and other medicines, as well as the chest X ray. Whatever the consultation consisted of I never inquired. However, it was too late for a chest X ray that day. He was given the antibiotic, the pharmacist promised that he would order the other medications (which unfortunately were not in stock), and CM was to fetch them the next day.

CM had his X ray, which was negative. He probably took the antibiotic, but never went for the other drugs. He knew what they were for, and later told me that if he took those pills he would, in time, be back in the mental hospital, and in no way could I get him to take them. (When Dr. B found out that I had never visited that hospital, he described the place as being very antiquated and depressing and said that he personally would never have a patient committed there if possible.)

Two years have gone by. I have never dared to discuss medication or anything related to his mental health with CM. Together a social worker and Indian affairs personnel and I have tried to get him into retraining courses. He never completes a course, giving poor excuses for dropping out. He does beautiful charcoal sketching and has visions of becoming a commercial artist, but has only completed grade 7 at school.

Have you thought of helping him get in touch with one of the native art outlets?

I have tried encouraging him but I have never been able to reach out to his inner self. He looks upon me as the only friend he has. But why am I so ineffective?

Am I afraid to become too involved? He comes to my office at odd times, just to talk. At times I have such pity for him that I have been tempted to invite him to my house. I have a 17-year-old son and a 15-year-old daughter. CM drinks when he can get alcohol and he has sniffed solvents. Am I afraid my children might try these things? But then they meet all of this in their daily contacts. I really do not wish to take my work home.

Am I afraid that I will be trapped by freely experiencing positive feelings toward CM that he might misinterpret my intentions? How can I motivate him to recognize his innate worth and believe in himself? Maybe he does recognize his latent qualities but no one will give him the chance he wants. I do not know how. I am not demonstrative nor able to express my feelings verbally, not even to my closest relatives. I am embarrassed to talk about my inner feelings. I choose to listen but offer no advice because I do not know how to give or express myself.

CM is presently serving a jail sentence for theft. The lawyer in charge of his defense agrees with me that, basically, he is honest, yet his mental processes are disordered. He wants so much to be wanted, he allows other young boys to use him to participate in thievery. Somehow he is always caught but cannot see that these fellows are not really friends.

I like to think that my lack of knowledge of psychiatry excuses my inability to cope with such circumstances. In other words, I am a cop-out. I find that others, both in the medical and paramedical professions, have thrown in the towel, saying that this boy is a hopeless case, a schizophrenic. I do not see myself accepting this. I like to think positively, that mental illnesses, like physical illnesses, can be cured. Maybe they cannot and I am involving myself with something that cannot be solved. Have I really given up but have refused to admit this to myself? When CM returns to his society, which I hope will be this fall, I will be there, it seems, and so will everybody else in that community. Even if those of us involved were to be transferred, records are kept and records are damning. One life is doomed. If only I could leave a record of some positive solution found, it would not seem so useless.

Attached is a copy of a letter CM wrote to me. (The handwriting in the original note was in extraordinarily beautiful script.) I felt good when I read it. Maybe I can still accomplish something and maybe there can be some hope for this pathetic soul.

Dear friend,

I guess I'll drop you a few lines tonight before I go "beddy-bye." I'll have to inform you that I am in jail at the moment.

I would like to thank you for all that you have done for me. I really am glad there are people like you who still exist. I should be out sometime this coming fall. I was worried about you leaving your job as the public health nurse. I hope you never do. I am in the hospital "check" at the moment awaiting my appointment, which I don't think was ever arranged. Can you tell me the doctor's name again? I want to move from this boring place to where I can do some work to occupy myself a bit. I'm sleepy right now and I'll have to say good-bye for the time being.

Your friend,

CM

8

UNMARRIED MOTHERS

Of the 550 cases in the study, 2% focus on Unmarried Mothers. Of the 10 cases that focus on Unmarried Mothers, 4 are described as Helpful, 6 as Unhelpful. Percentages shown for comparison only (see Tables 2.3, 2.4; pp. 32–35).

COMPARISON WITH ALL OTHER SITUATIONS

Helpful Factors

Highest Rating

- Nonjudgmental.
- Wanted to understand how patient felt.
- Took time to explain.
- Used physical closeness.
- Came to terms with own feelings; was able to enter into patient's problem.

Unhelpful Factors

Highest Rating

- Was disapproving, judgmental.
- Prejudiced toward group of which patient was a member.
- Afraid would break down and cry in front of patient.

Helpful Factors	% of Cases in Which Cited
1. Wanted to understand how patient felt	100
2. Nonjudgmental	100
3. Took time to explain	75
4. Helped patient express feelings	75
5. Used physical closeness	75
6. Was a sounding board	50
7. Gave moral support	50
8. Came to terms with own feelings; was able to enter into patient's problem	50
9. Initiated referral to another profession/resource	25
10. Liked the patient	25
11. Looked beyond patient's outward response/behavior to underlying causes	25
12. Positively identified with patient due to similar life/professional experience	25
13. Not unduly influenced by negative opinions of other staff regarding the patient's personality	0
14. Helped family members deal with the situation	0
15. Made this case the basis for overall policy change/improvement	0
16. Was trying to prove self to senior staff members	0
17. Discussed religion with patient	0
18. Used innovative rehabilitative procedure	0
19. Had received training in recognizing social-emotional needs of patients	0
20. Was honest with patient/relatives	0

Unhelpful Factors	% of Cases in Which Cited
1. Prejudiced toward group of which patient was a member	83
2. Was disapproving, judgmental	83
3. Did not want to understand	50
4. Treated the condition, overlooking the patient	50
5. Felt guilty but could not communicate	33
6. Purposely disregarded significant cues in patient's statements/behavior	33
7. Felt pressured (within self) into doing things rather than coping with feeling elements (tension present)	33

8.	Failed to look beyond initial negative impression of patient's personality	33
9.	Felt inadequate to enter into patient's problem because had not personally resolved the issue	17
10.	Breakdown of interprofessional communication/cooperation	17
11.	Afraid would break down and cry in front of patient	17
12.	Avoided needs of family members	17
13.	Rationalized actions and thoughts	17
14.	Self-image was threatened	17
15.	Disliked patient	17
16.	Short-staffed; too little time to devote to the patient	0
17.	Negatively influenced by opinions of other staff members regarding personality of the patient	0
18.	Lacked training in recognizing social-emotional needs of patients	0
19.	Overidentified due to being similar age to patient	0
20.	Incapacitated by own fear of death	0
21.	Failed to seek authoritative advice regarding innovation	0
22.	Disregarded own judgment because wanted approval of senior staff members	0
23.	Lost professional role: patient became friend	0
24.	Felt guilty but still would not communicate	0

"Carol, will you come in next, please?" I said, as I called in the next patient. Carol and her friend Susan had come to our family planning clinic that evening. Prior to the doctor's examination I was responsible for taking the patient's blood pressure, weight, urinalysis, and a hemoglobin test.

"Please sit over on that stool, by the counter. I am going to take a drop of blood from your finger," I remarked. When she was seated my eyes scanned her quickly. Her general appearance was most untidy. Her bleached blonde hair looked much like a miniature haystack; her eyes were heavily made up with black makeup. She looked rather pathetic.

Inwardly I recoiled at the thought of taking blood from her dirty finger. Attempting to make some conversation, I claimed that it would only be a mere prick, and she would scarcely feel it! "But I'm very nervous about it," she said, pulling her hand away. Her hand did feel clammy. She was just a bit of a thing, only 17 years of age, with an illegitimate child only a couple of months old.

It took me longer than was normal to get enough blood for the test. This annoyed me to no end. "How in the world could anyone be so dirty and unkempt?" I thought. "What a character! So young and carrying on the way she has been with the fellow—probably on welfare . . . ''

It was time to show Carol into the examining room. Closing the door behind her, I requested that she undress and get up on the examining table. She stood there, in this small room, looking rather uncomfortable and helpless. "What is the doctor going to do? I've never had this done before," she said rather nervously. Whom does she think she is kidding? I thought. These young girls! They only think of themselves—irresponsible. Impatiently I arranged the sheet over her abdomen and legs. What dirty feet! The odor nearly knocked me over. I felt repugnance toward this girl—this young slip of a girl—younger than my own daughter! Thank goodness Judy was not that type of girl.

There was little conversation while Dr. P did the routine pelvic and Pap smear. Gingerly I prepared the slide; there was suspicion of disease. "Have you thought of marrying this boy, Carol?" questioned Dr. P. "We are too young," she replied, with a wan smile. "My mother is taking care of the baby." Too young—my foot! I thought, indignantly. Why didn't she think of that before she got herself into this mess?

"You may get dressed now, Carol. Use this stool as you step down so you don't fall," I said, pulling out the footstool from under the table. "The doctor will discuss your needs before you leave."

She looked around, unsure of just what to do next. "You know it really wasn't my fault," she said. "My girl friend took my pills!" I was shocked and horrified. Opening the door I took her into the room where the doctor waited. Returning to the examining room, I thought to myself, Now to clean up this mess and air the room before the next patient! Am I ever glad that her type are few and far between in this place!

Normally I try very hard and manage to make each patient feel relaxed by talking with them or holding their hand in reassurance and support. Why was I so cool and indifferent to Carol? She had a need far greater than many others to whom I had given support. She needed understanding and patience on my part and above all warmth and love. I rejected her completely. She must have sensed it. My criticism of her actions were unjust. I was cold and indifferent toward her. I disliked her because she was so dirty, and because of what she had done. I had talked to her briefly, but I am sure she must have sensed my repugnance, my holier-than-thou attitude.

Here was a young girl whom I could have helped, except for the barrier that I placed between us. I could have done a great deal for Carol—but I failed her in every way. Whenever I recall the events of that occasion I am filled with remorse, and only wish I had the chance to relive that hour with Carol.

Not only are *prejudiced toward group of which patient was a member* and *was disapproving, judgmental* the most predominant responses in relation to the Unmarried Mother (5 out of 6 cases), these same responses also apply to the question of giving up the baby.

The Social Services Department had referred this case to the County Health Department, with the request that I make the visit, as I had known the family for over 20 years. The school principal had advised that Lucille, aged 14, was pregnant. He had hoped that Lucille and her family could be persuaded to place the child up for adoption. However, the social worker was not successful and hoped that I might meet with some success.

The family was the classic example of the multiproblem family: three generations of illegitimacy, alcoholism, unemployment, welfare; they were unkempt and unclean. However, with all this there was a certain amount of family solidarity and loyalty.

Willingly, full of confidence, I visited the family the following day. I had known the grandmother and been present at the birth of her last child. I had delivered a number of the grandchildren, visited when someone was ill, was on friendly terms with all three generations—in fact we were genuinely fond of one another! After a lengthy discussion in which I pointed out Lucille's youth, the advantages to the baby if it were brought up by two loving parents (the usual argument in this situation), I met with strong resistance and finally adamant refusal.

There are also advantages to one's own parent's love.

The family would accept all responsibility for the baby. Lucille told me that Mummy was pregnant when she married Daddy, Aunt Jane was pregnant when she married Uncle Jim. It was simply something that happened and was nothing to worry about or to feel ashamed of. I also learned that the father of the child was living in the home and marriage was not considered at the present time. Lucille planned to go back to school after the birth of the baby.

In subsequent visits I was not able to change their minds; my only small success was Lucille's willingness to come to prenatal class and her mother's agreement that Lucille would take "the Pill" if the family physician was agreeable.

Why did I fail? I went in with no thought of failure. I was full of confidence, which perhaps showed very plainly, and I think this immediately put the family on the defensive. Through the years my word and advice had been accepted, although perhaps in a limited fashion according to their capabilities. I had insisted for years on higher standards of cleanliness, health care, and nutrition and met with some success. However, when it came to the responsibility of a member of the family I was wrong, for in this lower-class family an illegitimate child was not the tragedy it is to me, a member of the middle class.

Also involved could be resentment of the establishment for taking away "one of us."

I think I was trying to impose my standards of life and morality on a class that does not think as I do. If I had visited with an open mind and not implied that this was a tragedy I might have been successful.

Or you might have discussed if the family had doubts of their own that may have been sublimated in their defense of themselves.

I wonder if I may even see the fifth generation of this family. Perhaps this child will not be suitable for adoption and in this case I would feel that the family was right and my middle-class ideas were all wrong.

Whether the child turns out to be suitable or not should not be the criterion for "right" or "wrong" ideas. I suspect you knew that this family actually had more warmth than many middle-class families—which may cause one to reassess one's own values as well.

*   *   *   *

I worked in a nursery in a large city hospital for quite a while; consequently I came in contact with a number of unmarried mothers.

At first I got myself in quite a state every time a mother was upset at giving up her baby, but finally I got myself adjusted to the idea as I witnessed how many of them didn't seem to really care.

One day a girl about 18 years old was admitted during the night and had a normal baby weighing 5 pounds 13 ounces. The baby had tiny perfect features, and the mother was quite delighted with her. This was strange as the baby was being given up, and most mothers in such cases never really wanted to see the baby. This mother was unmarried, and was a call girl. At first I thought this maternal interest was an act for the patient next to her, and was surprised to hear her say she wanted to breast-feed her baby.

My first reaction was to tell her if she did this it might be a little more upsetting when the time came to give the baby up. She was quite a cooperative patient, and she might have listened to me, but I told myself the baby needed it as she had to be fed every 3 hours.

Every day I watched the mother getting more involved and I never said anything to her. We both admired the baby and we were happy when she gained weight. I dreaded to think that it would soon be time for her to leave the baby.

Her social worker came and they both identified the baby, yet I'm sure she didn't realize she would soon be parting. When at last she was discharged and saw the baby before leaving, she became quite hysterical; the baby was taken away, while she was given a sedative.

Assessment

I feel I didn't help in the situation because I allowed the patient to become too attached to the baby. She was probably feeling guilty, and thought the best she could do was to try to make it up to her baby by giving and doing all she could for her. Maybe if I had just said a few words to her, or even her social worker, she might have been content to feed the baby a few times with the bottle, and not become so involved.

I thought of the baby, and not of the mother, finding excuses every time I felt guilty. If I had thought of my patient, I would have realized parting would be more painful, doing it her way.

As happens quite often, the decision to give up the baby was not thoroughly thought through and should have been given a good deal more time and care much earlier so that the plan regarding feeding the baby, etc., was understood by everyone before the birth of the child. You are quite right—close liaison with the social worker was absolutely essential.

All of the Helpful cases involve being *nonjudgmental* and *wanted to understand how patient felt.* Half of those who describe these responses indicate that it was because they *overcame own feelings to enter into patient's problem* that they were able to respond positively; in other words, they had consciously struggled with the issue of unmarried motherhood. In the following cases, the nurse is able to look beyond the doctor's superficial opinion that the patient "took it very well," and to take the initiative in helping the patient to surface her fears.

Miss H was a single girl, 18 years old, from a small northern town and presently working in the city. She had been admitted with complaints of hyperemesis. A routine pregnancy test proved to be positive. Miss H's doctor advised her of her pregnancy at the beginning of my shift, and, according to him, she took it all very well. Somehow, her reaction to this news seemed inappropriate to me. I immediately considered how upset I would have been. Thinking that a normal reaction to such news would have been denial, hostility, or guilt, I decided to look deeper into Miss H's placid behavior.

Twice I approached Miss H before supper that evening, once with medication and once to take her temperature. Neither time did I broach the subject, feeling that perhaps she needed time to gather thoughts and also wondering just what business of mine it was anyway. These latter feelings subsided as I gradually realized that I was capable of helping this girl during her crisis, and perhaps lessening the burden for her to carry.

Finally, after supper, she called me to readjust her intravenous drip. Having done this, I sat down beside her on the bed. I noticed she had been crying and used this as my cue. Touching her hand to convey my empathy, I said something to the effect of, "You've been crying. Has it something to do with what the doctor told you earlier?'' Looking back, I think that I didn't use the word pregnant because I neither wanted to be forceful, nor did I want to have my helpful advances rejected. Instead I tried to impart my knowledge of her condition by my manner.

Miss H seemed happy to vent her feelings. She sobbed out all her feelings of anguish, while I tried to comfort her and let her know that I understood. I have always felt that it is wrong to be morally judgmental of others. Unwanted pregnancy can happen to any girl, should the circumstances be similar.

I tried to help her sort out her present and future condition, encouraging her to think realistically and positively. When she brought up the possibility of abortion, I tried to help her examine it, and advised her to discuss it with her doctor. I have my own opinions about abortion, which I did not want to influence her, so I felt that the doctor might be better able to handle it.

Having one's own opinion should not necessarily mean that one cannot help another to begin to sort out a problem. (No doubt the doctor has his opinions too!)

I feel that this situation proved to be a success for both Miss H and myself. Miss H began to look at the future realistically with a certain amount of acceptance of her pregnancy. I hope I managed to give her some support during this crisis, and allowed her to vent her emotions. I gained in satisfaction, self-esteem, and pride by helping Miss H. I must admit that I felt very successful as a nurse who could diagnose and treat not only physical ills, but also emotional ones.

9
CONVALESCENCE

Of the 550 cases in the study, 21% focus on Convalescence. This is the highest percentage of occurrence, followed closely by Interpretation of Condition with 20%. Of the 116 cases that focus on Convalescence, 54% are described as Helpful, 46% as Unhelpful.

COMPARISON WITH ALL OTHER SITUATIONS

Helpful Factors

Highest Rating

• Initiated referral to another profession/resource.

Unhelpful Factors

Highest Rating

• Treated the condition, overlooking the patient.
• Failed to look beyond initial negative impression of patient's personality.

Helpful Factors	% of Cases in Which Cited
1. Gave moral support	62
2. Helped patient express feelings	56
3. Wanted to understand how patient felt	54

4. Looked beyond patient's outward response/behavior
    to underlying causes   49
5. Took time to explain   43
6. Initiated referral to another profession/resource   41
7. Nonjudgmental   29
8. Was a sounding board   29
9. Came to terms with own feelings; was able to enter
    into patient's problem   29
10. Helped family members deal with the situation   25
11. Not unduly influenced by negative opinions of other
    staff regarding the patient's personality   21
12. Liked the patient   11
13. Used innovative rehabilitative procedure   11
14. Positively identified with patient due to similar life/
    professional experience   11
15. Had received training in recognizing social-emotional
    needs of patients   5
16. Made this case the basis for overall policy change/
    improvement   3
17. Discussed religion with patient   3
18. Used physical closeness   3
19. Was honest with patient/relatives   3
20. Was trying to prove self to senior staff members   2

Unhelpful Factors	% of Cases in Which Cited
1. Treated the condition, overlooking the patient	68
2. Failed to look beyond initial negative impression of patient's personality	58
3. Was disapproving, judgmental	47
4. Self-image was threatened	42
5. Did not want to understand	40
6. Purposely disregarded significant cues in patient's statements/behavior	38
7. Felt inadequate to enter into patient's problem because had not personally resolved the issue	28
8. Disliked patient	25
9. Negatively influenced by opinions of other staff members regarding personality of the patient	19
10. Avoided needs of family members	15
11. Short-staffed; too little time to devote to the patient	13

12. Felt pressured (within self) into doing things rather than coping with feeling elements (tension present)   13
13. Lacked training in recognizing social-emotional needs of patients   13
14. Prejudiced toward group of which patient was a member   12
15. Felt guilty but still would not communicate   13
16. Rationalized actions and thoughts   11
17. Felt guilty but could not communicate   11
18. Breakdown of interprofessional communication/ cooperation   9
19. Failed to seek authoritative advice regarding innovation   8
20. Afraid would break down and cry in front of patient   4
21. Lost professional role: patient became friend   4
22. Overidentified due to being similar age to patient   2
23. Incapacitated by own fear of death   2
24. Disregarded own judgment because wanted approval of senior staff members   2

Gave moral support is cited as the most common Helpful Response to convalescing patients (62% of cases). It is very evident, however, that this is a far more complex activity than many of us have imagined. This is clearly illustrated in the following two cases in which the nurse makes special efforts to bend hospital routines hoping to offer and demonstrate her moral support. The results—for the two patients—are diametrically opposed.

The patient, Mr. T, age 37 was diagnosed as a severe cardiomegaly with heart failure; he was awaiting a heart transplant. For the first few days, Mr. T was swamped by the specialists and the labs for work-ups. This intense concern for him seemed to give him new hope. He was the focus of important debates and concerns. However, as the weeks passed and there was no available donor, Mr. T became weaker and very demanding. He was often eliminated on doctors' rounds because there was nothing more to be planned for him. Some of the nurses were impatient with his many little requests, and resented it when they were assigned to the section he was in.

Mr. T was angry and hostile at times and would complain that he wanted his night sedation at 11:00 P.M., or that his food was cold, or that it was not what he wanted, and so on. I felt his appetite was poor, but also, this was a chance for him to express some of his anger. I would listen to him and then offer to order him something else on his salt-free diet. The same was true with the routine of the day; if I could accommodate him, I would, as I felt that he must feel as if the most important aspects of his life were slipping out of his control. Besides, for me, it was a way of saying that he was important and that I was glad to put myself out a little for him.

As time went on he gradually came to accept his situation. The absence of a heart donor was no longer translated by him as evidence of no one caring. I think that my being willing to bend hospital routine a little helped him to know we cared and to make this adjustment.

The patient, Theresa, age 18, was diagnosed as having terminal kidney disease. She had been in the hospital intermittently since the age of 11. She suffered from chronic kidney disease, which eventually led to her having both kidneys removed and a kidney transplant done. She later rejected the transplant, and after approximately 6 months, she had the transplanted kidney removed and was placed on hemodialysis twice a week. Theresa had very little to hope for in the future. She was not a candidate for another transplant, and had a life expectancy of 2 to 5 years.

If Theresa complained I usually tried to remove or lessen what was annoying her. She used to cry easily and rather than have an emotional upset I used to let her do what she wanted within necessary limits. She liked to go to bed late and sleep until 10:00 or 11:00 A.M. each morning, and I would let her do this. I thought I was affording her an opportunity to be an individual.

However, she showed little interest or cooperation in her treatment. Later I learned that it was because she felt no one cared if she progressed or not—even temporarily. In not being required to follow the rigidities of hospital routine, she felt she had been written off.

Much has been written about the good patient role. In the following cases the nurses' expectations of their patients and their particular approach to giving moral support actually constituted a barrier in the relationship.

Mrs. S appeared depressed. She had been in Hamilton three weeks with her son while he had major (very successful) renal surgery. Her husband telephoned from home to say that he would be in Hamilton on business.

I was excited for Mrs. S and helped her plan an enjoyable visit, thinking this would be a happy occasion for her. Upon her husband's return home, Mrs. S still appeared depressed and I felt this was understandable.

It would have been so easy to have left it right there. We are not often given a second chance to correct our errors.

1. I assumed Mrs. S to be depressed by her unaccustomed inactivity and enforced separation.
2. It was I who was excited about Mr. S's imminent visit.
3. It was I who had played the major role in planning the visit, compensating for, without noticing, Mrs. S's lack of enthusiasm.
4. I assumed she was depressed by her husband's return home.

I feel my main error was in imposing my own values and not being objective. I saw what I wanted and expected to see, and acted on what I would have felt.

I realized correctly Mr. S was the predisposing factor, but failed to recognize that after his arrival Mrs. S was not elated. I was so busy feeling happy for her I didn't notice she wasn't happy at all.

It appears Mrs. S neither looked forward to nor enjoyed the visit with any degree of excitement. Indeed my thoughtless excitement merely helped further convince her that she obviously didn't love her husband, that she had no normal feeling for him at all. Later I learned that separation papers had been signed.

No wonder the poor lady was feeling depressed on his return. I wonder, if I had been able to listen, instead of imposing my own picture of the perfect marriage, whether indeed I could have helped them in some way.

Mrs. F, who is 35 years old, has been suffering from cancer for the past 5 years. It started as breast cancer and has advanced to a stage of multiple bone metastasis. She has a family of 9 boys ranging in age from 14 years to 6 months. Up until the last 2 months she has been able to do nearly everything for herself. However, since the cancer has metasticized to her neck, pelvis and femur, she is dependent on other people for her care, and at present is in Delta Convalescent Hospital.

On inquiring what she had been thinking about, she stated she was getting extremely restless and she wished she could get her strength back and stop feeling so helpless. All her life she had been a very independent and industrious woman. She had cared for her nine children with little help from anyone and now circumstances were such that she had become dependent on other people for even her personal needs. This was a complete change of role for her. When I nodded understanding, she started to explain some of the inadequacies she was feeling.

As Mrs. F was explaining her feelings, I noticed that she was beginning to lose control and cry. Therefore I interjected to change the pattern of discussion.

You really asked her to open up and then when she did, you may have prematurely "put the lid on."

If I had encouraged her to cry she would have been embarrassed as our conversation was taking place in a sitting room far from the seclusion of her own room. Moreover, crying for her in front of me would be a threat to the independence she was attempting to rebuild.

Perhaps Mrs. F really needed to tell you all her fears about her inadequacies in order for her to name and face them in the open—even cry about them (perhaps better in private, but she could have been helped by a feeling from you that crying is absolutely natural and isn't a helpless or weak thing to do). As you point out, Mrs. F was going to be struggling to adapt to a more dependent life—new roles and new perceptions of herself. In order for her to do this she shouldn't have felt she had to keep up a front—reinforced by you—of being her same independent self by not crying; i.e., she needed to know that her loss of control in crying made her no less worthy as an individual in your eyes than her loss of control in other physical tasks.

Treated the condition, overlooking the patient is cited as the most common Unhelpful Response (68% of cases) in cases of Convalescence and has the highest rating of this Response among all Conditions.

Mrs. R was a pale-looking 23-year-old young woman. She had been in a car accident. Her father was killed and her 5-year-old son was left with minimal brain damage; the patient herself received bilateral hip dislocation. This was supposedly corrected with a spica cast, but she was left with a piece of soft bone, which was supposed to decay on its own, floating around the right hip joint. The patient couldn't bend over and was to have a physiotherapist come to her home three times a week.

Mr. R worked in a casket factory and was away all day until 7:00 P.M. There were two children, 5 years and 3 years of age. The family had recently relocated into a hall they had purchased. Their previous dwelling had been condemned after they moved out. The hall remained just that—complete with stage and oiled wooden floors—and minus indoor toilet facilities.

Four months earlier, Mrs. R's mother had been on her way to visit them and had died en route. Previous to the accident Mrs. R's father had been living with them, and they all missed him terribly. Their life had been one trauma after another, and their dwelling had to be seen to be believed.

After the initial shock of the insurmountable problems and sorrows of this family, I was very keen to help them in whatever capacity I could. The family physician was very understanding and sympathetic to this family and encouraged me to do all in my power to ensure the utmost in health care. He was concerned with basic health rules such as cleanliness, and wanted me to show the patient the proper care of teeth, for herself and her children.

Mrs. R related quite openly to me, telling me her past misfortunes. The two children were quite obnoxious on the first visit, and all Mrs. R would say, without moving, was, "Do you want Mommy to get the belt?" She was obviously a nervous woman, and as I looked around at the chaotic mess of the hall I couldn't help but wonder, "Where am I to start?"

For subsequent visits I concerned myself with the physical needs of the patient and family in general. They didn't have enough bedding, so I obtained some for them from the Salvation Army. Mrs. R had been working before her accident and had made three application claims for unemployment insurance, all to no avail. So on her behalf, I wrote to the representative from our area, and he saw that she did receive unemployment benefits.

Next, I set about to clean the children up. Because they had no bathtub I announced proudly that I would bathe the boys in the sink. What a fight that was! They screamed, yelled, kicked, and finally the 3-year-old bit me! I can honestly say I didn't know how to react. My first impulse was to give the child a good slap, but I quickly regained my composure and said, "That wasn't a nice thing to do, David. Now let's get you bathed." Mrs. R sat wide-eyed and said what a naughty boy David was, but that was all the response there was from her.

As time progressed I found my visits were of shorter duration, as I hurried in, asked a few questions, and left. Eventually, through physiotherapy, Mrs. R was rehabilitated, and was discharged from home care.

But alas! Three weeks later she had had an epileptic seizure, had been hospitalized, and was once again readmitted to Home Care. When I heard the news I said, "Oh, no—not again." So I resumed my rushed visits, observed the children being very disobedient (but cleaner), and rushed away. I even suggested to the home care office that my visits be cut to once every 2 weeks, as I felt I had no more to offer Mrs. R or her family.

I must confess I did feel guilty at the time, realizing that I was short-changing this patient. Not being realistic, I think I had visions of rapid improvement in their physical set-up, and didn't accept them as they were. I thought I was going to change them, I suppose. Mrs. R was obviously undergoing a tremendous physical strain, plus the fact that she was mourning for the father she'd lost.

Did you talk about this with her?

She seemed to ignore the antics of her children, and they pretty much did what they wanted. I could have been of assistance by helping her to learn consistent care of her children and more adequate methods of coping with discipline.

Rather than listen, and discuss and teach basic health rules, I went ahead full-steam, bathing the children, ending up being bitten. Rather than being patient and consistent in my visits, I became frustrated and decreased the frequency of my visits, when help was so obviously needed. Generally, I felt uncomfortable, and therefore wasn't useful in the manner I should have been.

I found it easier to work with their physical needs, and in so doing was avoiding the very real emotional needs of this distraught mother with her young children. No doubt the mother sensed my attitude, communicated by my abrupt visits.

As time went on, I was aware of what I was doing, but rationalized and said, "I can't do anything more for them anyway." I decreased my visits and in so doing alleviated my immediate anxieties and frustrations—thus depriving this family of the total care they deserved.

*   *   *   *

It is hard to realize and admit that one's self does not function positively in all situations. It makes one feel frustrated and angry with oneself, but the blame is inevitably projected onto the patient.

Mr. White was a 69-year-old man living with his only relative, a sister who was 80. They lived in a three-bedroom, semidetached, two-storey home in deplorable condition, situated in an upper-middle-class area.

Initially I was sent on a home care referral in relation to the sister. She needed iron injections and someone to teach her brother to apply dressings to ulcers on her ankles. I parked in front of the house at about 2 o'clock in the afternoon and remember wondering, in disapproval, why people would keep their drapes closed during the day. My attitude was negative before entering the home, probably because the grounds were unkempt. More is expected of people in the middle class.

Mr. White took ages to answer the door. When he did my first reaction to him was disgust, not only because he hesitated to let me in, but because of his appearance. He was a thin, short, dirty man, with about 2 weeks growth of beard, and long gray hair to his shoulders with a braided band around his forehead. He apologized for the condition of their home before I was allowed to enter, and when I did I was speechless.

The stench, the garbage, the flies, the darkness—just everything sent me into a state of shock. It must have been at least 30 seconds before I noticed the little old lady in the corner. My feelings changed, but only long enough to gather my thoughts and ask how they were managing.

Mr. White quickly answered that he did not know how the doctor expected him to learn how to do these treatments, because he also had very sore legs. I asked if I could examine them. His slippers were stuck to his feet and when he raised his pant legs, I began to panic. His legs and feet were weeping, swollen, and appeared gangrenous.

I then became very angry and impatient. I wondered why an investigation had not been arranged by the hospital coordinator before Miss White was discharged. I guess I had to blame someone for putting me in this situation. From this point on I used myself even more negatively. I became a dictator. I blurted out, "You just have to get to a hospital, Mr. White. I will make arrangements for your sister, and get a doctor to see you in emergency." I realize now that I could have prevented their extreme anxieties that followed. I should have taken more time to sit and talk, and explain their situation to them. Within the next hour Miss White was on her way to a nursing home, and Mr. White to the hospital. While making these arrangements little communication occurred. My anger grew because of the condition in the home. I had made up my mind (dictator again) to call in the sanitation department. As Mr. White left for the hospital I told him that I would arrange help to get the food garbage out of his home. I did nothing to alleviate their fears. In fact, I created cause for further fear. By the end of my visit I was totally exhausted and glad to leave.

Five days later Mr. White returned home and required teaching of treatment to his legs. I can remember being angry once more, this time at the office, for sending me instead of the regular nurse for that area. Mr. White requested that I return because I knew his situation. Teaching was accomplished in a few days and the sanitation department had initiated their actions. I was still appalled by his surroundings and his hesitation to improve them. I referred the case to the Public Health Department, leaving Mr. White to grope for answers from another source.

I should have realized that Mr. White was asking for my help when he requested that I return. He must have been ashamed because he only hesitated to let me enter: he did not ask me to leave. I gave no concern for his or his sister's general well-being, nor to their feelings. Mr. White in particular was made to feel that he was bad and neglectful. I cut off all channels of communication and gave neither of them an opportunity to express their problems as they saw them, or to participate in solutions.

Among all Situations, the Response of *disliked the patient* receives the second-to-highest rating where Convalescence is concerned. In these cases the nurses point to this factor as the reason for *failed to look beyond initial negative impression of patient's personality* (58% of the Unhelpful cases). This is the highest rating of this Response among all Conditions.

This case concerns a patient in the Bayview Convalescent Hospital. This incident proved to be a lesson to me never to say things on impulse. Mrs. H was termed a problem patient due to her past psychiatric history and her present erratic behavior. She was in our hospital for physio following a knee operation. Among her problems was one of obesity, and Mrs. H had put herself on a strict 100-calorie diet. The result was a very weak Mrs. H!

Did anyone support her in her effort to improve (i.e., diet)? It seems she was trying, however ineptly, to do something.

She was often childish and demanded a great deal of attention. This often annoyed the staff, who were usually hard-pressed for time.

This particular incident occurred late at night (about 10 P.M.) after a rather strenuous and busy evening. I was in Mrs. H's room settling her down with the nightly back rub and reminding her to use the bathroom before taking her sedation. This suggestion was punctuated with a statement to the effect that "The night nurse is busy enough without bringing bedpans to you at midnight." (This comment was prompted by a complaint from the nurse the previous night.) The result of this was a hysterical sobbing and loud screaming that we were unfair and out to get her. Mrs. H did not settle down for hours, and kept half the floor awake as well. At one point I threatened to put her into the sunroom.

My attitude was very poor in dealing with this patient. The odd thing is that my regret was in her reaction to my words, not that I said what I did to her. Why did this woman often get on my nerves? Why did she repulse me at times? Perhaps I felt that she was childish and that any adult should know better. Every now and then a nurse finds she can take just so much abuse from patients who take her for granted and often treat her like a common maid. This is degrading at times and difficult to ignore. Mrs. H had problems, many of them. Normally I was able to humor and help her. However, if any pressure mounted on the floor, as in this case, I indirectly took it out on her.

I recognize my failings and I know that as a nurse I should not give in to such destructive criticism, especially of a patient. One must remember that patients are people, and often not themselves when sick.

* * * *

The following is a case in my professional life, which leaves much room for improvement.

Jim was 20 years old, a typical hippie in appearance. Having seen him around the small town where I lived, I already had pre-formed opinions of him before he was admitted from the operating room to the surgical floor where I worked, following a motor vehicle accident in which he had sustained a fractured right femur. Whenever I had seen Jim in the past, he had always been with a rowdy gang of noisy young men.

His pain threshold seemed very low, and although previously sedated, he screamed loudly when assisted by the orderlies into bed. We positioned Jim as comfortably as we could and left.

As Jim's long stay with us progressed, his behavior went from bad to worse. He refused to be bathed in the morning because he wanted to sleep, and profane language could be heard coming from his room when a staff member brought his breakfast tray in.

In the beginning I tried to be friendly by asking Jim about his work and his friends, and his plans for the future. Sometimes he would answer with a grunt or a shake of the head, but more often he would ignore me. He had one demand: "Leave me alone." He didn't want us to touch him or to talk to him and he didn't want contact with other patients. Jim was so hostile that his roommates quickly asked for a transfer.

Eventually Jim was watching TV most of the day. I well remember one of the many attempts I made to talk with him. "Jim," I said, "I'd like to explain the medication you're on." With a scornful look he reached over and dumped my entire medication tray.

Another day, when a nursing assistant and I were making his bed, Jim punched her with all his might as she gently positioned his leg. She refused to enter his room again.

It was not long before all the staff, including myself, avoided Jim as much as possible. The hostility he displayed was matched by the staff's hostility toward him, going in a vicious circle. I remember telling him in no uncertain terms just what I thought of 20-year-old tyrants. Was I aware of my negative feelings toward hippies in general, and Jim in particular, with his long hair and his rebellion against the values of society? As I reflect now I am sure some of my feelings must have been evident.

I realize now that in my mind, I was comparing Jim to Barry, a 17-year-old, extremely likable young man recently on our ward, who had been diagnosed as having leukemia, with 2 months to live. Barry was the pride of his parents, an intelligent boy who had planned to make a career in the field of biology. And here was Jim with what was to me a minor injury in the sense that it would in the future not disable him in any way. Did he not realize how lucky he was?

No, of course not. What I should have remembered is that each patient's response toward his illness is unique. The same illness can hold different meanings for different individuals. The severity of the illness can vary when seen through different eyes. Jim, normally a healthy person, had been active in car racing before his accident. Perhaps he feared he'd never be able to participate in this activity again. His physician had an abrupt, rushed manner, and Jim may have been harboring fears of permanent disability about which he was afraid to question his doctor. If I had spent more time with Jim, and showed more patience, perhaps some of these anxieties could have been dispelled.

Jim had quit school after grade 10 and left his hometown, apparently to get away from a very demanding mother. It is highly possible that the dependency of the hospital situation made him feel very threatened because of his previous experience with an overbearing mother.

The dislike that the staff felt for Jim may have posed a threat to an already threatened self-image. He had had to fight all his life to obtain independency, and now in the hospital his equilibrium was upset.

When looked at from these angles, Jim's behavior becomes explainable, if not acceptable. If I could have seen this picture earlier, my approaches to him would have been modified, not expecting instant rapport, and perhaps I would have worked harder and more intelligently at obtaining it.

As professional persons, we should be aware that in all of us there are certain prejudices that are at work. Certainly we need to realize what our particular ones are if we wish to form a helping relationship with our patients.

In this case, the nurse was able to recognize and admit her own anger, assess how much of it was justified—and begin to turn the relationship around.

I would like to tell you about a situation in my experience as a visiting nurse in which I was most unhelpful in meeting the needs of a patient of ours. Miss G is a 60-year-old lady who is blind and terribly crippled with arthritis; she has had both conditions for many years. She is able to live by herself, in a low rental one-bedroom apartment, with help from friends and the visiting nurse.

Miss G does not consider her blindness a handicap, as she states she once had vision and is able to "see" things through other people, recalling images she has stored from her sightful days. She is able to get around, but walks with a shuffling gait; it takes her a good 10 minutes to get her from the bedroom to the living room. She depends on her friends to do her shopping and laundry, and transport her if she needs to get out. The visiting nurse is required to assist her with a sponge bath (her hands are also badly crippled), dressing, special foot care (she has numerous corns and callouses), and a dressing to a stasis ulcer on one ankle. It was decided with the patient that 3 days a week would be sufficient for her to maintain good hygiene. It didn't take too many visits to realize that there were going to be many problems in working out an acceptable routine, both for Miss G and the nurse.

The first problem was that of time. Because of her slowness in getting about, I couldn't give her care in the length of time I thought I should allot for her visit. Miss G thought I should use the time that it took her to get ready by doing a few chores for her. Some of these chores were watering her plants, cleaning out her toaster, winding her clock, squeezing her some orange juice, mopping the floor, etc. I found myself getting more and more irritable as the list got longer, and to compound the problem, she would ask as many as three times if I had done everything exactly as she had asked. Giving her care was a problem in itself. If she was persnickety about her apartment, it was nothing in comparison to herself. One towel had to be used for her back, another for her legs, and somehow she knew from the feel of the towel if you weren't using the right one. She has nylons with seams in them, and getting the seam at precisely the right spot was a project all in itself. She had me cutting up bits and pieces of tissue to wind around her toes so that her shoes wouldn't rub.

I had this terrible feeling that I was being manipulated by her, and rather than confront the situation, I found myself doing things purposely to annoy her. She liked her care at a certain time and I found myself purposely coming later. I would try to get things done as fast as possible, so I could get out of her apartment, but she always decided that she just had to have a few more things done that day, so I ended up staying longer. The conversation was very sparse, as I was usually seething mad after I had been there only a short time. I found myself arranging to be off on days that she needed care, so someone else could do her, which upset her further as they didn't know her routine.

I took the problem up in team conference a few times, but handled that badly as well. I don't think I was really looking for a solution so much as pity for myself, having to look after this terrible patient. By doing this I was making things worse for her because anyone filling in for me started off not wanting to go there from all my moaning about what a terrible call it was.

All the while this was going on (9 months) I kept feeling like a creep. I tried to get myself to look at the good side of her—how much better she was able to function with such handicaps than I ever could—but 5 minutes inside her apartment the hair was up on my back and I was ready to come to blows with anything she said. It sure wasn't a very pleasant way to be, and if I thought I was badly off, imagine how she must have felt, as the care was a necessary part of her routine in order to be able to live as independently as possible. I kept wondering what had happened to my so-called empathy, and then I began to realize that empathy came easier when I dealt with an easy patient—someone who was pleasant and easy to get along with—but when I was put to the test with a more difficult patient I failed badly.

I dealt with this lady in the same manner for 9 horrible months. Then, this New Year, I made a resolution that somehow I was going to turn the situation into something positive and it's one resolution that I hope to see through. I haven't accomplished this yet, but I hope I am on the way.

I sat down and tried to put together some of the positive things about her life-style that I could work with. I knew there was no way that I could ever get her to be a relaxed, easygoing person, as her disabilities are a part of her life-style, and if anything, would get worse as time went by. She couldn't see things to check them out for herself, so that was part of why she triple-checked everything I did, and she certainly wasn't going to walk faster, so I knew I was going to have to work within these limitations. I also knew I was going to have to work doubly hard at establishing a relationship due to the terrible mess I had made of it up to this time. But this is what I've done.

Since I usually started off on the wrong foot, having to wait until she got to where I could give the care, and this was the time she used to have me do her chores, I suggested to her that when possible I would come around a certain time. This would enable her to get set up before I came, and we could get right to her care when I came. I told her I didn't begrudge her the time, but I did have to see a number of patients during the day, and perhaps the quality of the time I spent with her was more important than the quantity. I also explained to her that I would do some of the chores she wished done, depending on how my day was. I also suggested to her that perhaps we could find someone in the community who could do some things for her, for a little money, and that she could spend more time in chatting and visiting with her friends rather than assigning duties. I could tell she was mulling things over in her mind and I decided to give her a bit of time to see how much she could initiate on her own.

Well, within a few weeks, she had contacted the Girl Scouts, and had found two 12-year-olds who would do some odds and ends for her for a small charge (she was living on a pension and had to count her pennies). After going a few times at our agreed-upon time, and finding her not yet ready, I would leave and do another patient and come back when she was ready. This only happened a few times before I found she was all set at the agreed-upon time. I still found I had to constantly battle with myself to keep my cool, and not damage what was beginning to happen.

I began to see that part of the reason why Miss G tried to keep me as long as possible was a growing awareness on her part that she was becoming less able to care for herself—that if someone didn't do these things for her she would be forced to consider chronic care. I also began to see that there was a lot more to this lady than I had ever let myself find out. She had a very alert mind, was more up-to-date than a lot of people in areas of current affairs, had quite strong opinions on political and economic situations, from listening to the radio and chatting with other people, and was extremely well informed. I also found out that she just loved talking about recipes, and ones that appealed to her I copied for her. She had one of her friends make them up for her, passing on her friends' recipes to me. She also took delight in hearing about my outside interests—she seemed to be able to live a part of these, knowing about them. I still find it hard to know how much of myself to reveal, so that when a situation occurs that calls for professional handling, I have not become too much of a friend to be able to function in the capacity of nurse.

The last few months have become an interesting and enjoyable experience, not only for me, but because of the changes in Miss G. I don't wish to give the impression of living happily ever after, as there are still many times when her persnickety ways try my patience, as I'm sure some of my ways irritate her. But we are building.

Purposely disregarded significant cues in patient's statements/behavior (38% of the Unhelpful cases) is described as a reaction to feeling inadequate to cope with the patient's problem and thus retreating behind a very constricted nurse role.

I was assigned five patients, four of whom were extremely sick and could do nothing for themselves. The other was Mrs. Bench, a private patient, who was operated on for a hysterectomy 7 days earlier and was due for discharge the following day. She was known to be spoiled, difficult, and demanding.

She was 35 years old, an attractive, well-groomed woman. She was married and her husband seemed devoted to her. They had two children, aged 5 and 7 years.

I was in a hurry when I went to see her and when I greeted her she barely replied; she seemed haughty and aloof. Hurriedly I gathered her toilet articles together and requested her to get up and wash in the bathroom and left her. My approach was unsympathetic and bigoted. I failed to establish rapport.

I returned after 20 minutes and she refused to get out of bed or bathe herself, saying that she was tired. I pointed out the importance of ambulation following surgery, but to no avail. Angrily, I hurriedly got the basin of water and bathed her in silence, making no attempt to disguise my displeasure. She was uncooperative. She was well; she was going home tomorrow. She was taking up my time when others needed me more. I did not recognize that she might have been depressed and although she was physically able she was probably not mentally able to carry out these functions.

While silently bathing her she suddenly offered, "I had this operation because I did not want any more children." I thought this was a very callous and distasteful thing to say. I did not reply and left the room. I failed to recognize that this was her attempt to tell me that she needed help.

During the day she rang the bell several times, making petty demands such as pulling the curtains, raising the head of the bed, and so forth. After each encounter the hostility increased. Finally she said that the hospital, the nursing care, and services were deplorable. I was angry and irritated at this woman who I thought was pampered, spoiled, and privileged—who seemed to have everything, including a happy home life. Again I was unaware that her attention-seeking behavior was in fact a plea for help.

I was upset about the day's events and when I went home I reflected on the

situation. My attitude was prejudiced. I did not show her any kindness or understanding. I had been blind to her emotional needs. I wondered why she was
hostile. Perhaps she had wanted to talk to someone, but everyone, including
myself, was too busy or uninterested. Perhaps only now did she realize the
enormity of the operation and she might not have been accepting it. Reviewing this, I tried to talk with her the following morning, but it was too late; she
stared at me in silence.

She did have problems. Not long afterward she divorced her husband, gave
up custody of her children, and became an alcoholic. I have always regretted
that I was not kind to her and purposely disregarded her cry for help.

*   *   *   *

While changing the dressing on a patient after the removal of a breast, she remarked, "I can't stand to look at it." She turned her head to the side and
spoke about having to have the dressing changed with disgust. She also commented that she had this "dirty, smelly dressing on all night."

In retrospect I can see the mistakes I made in this situation. While changing the dressing I tried to explain to her that the incision was clean, and a very
neat job done by the surgeon. This didn't answer her need. She was completely disgusted with the surgery. She didn't want reassurance about the neat job
done by the surgeon. This woman cried out because her body had been muti-
lated. She undoubtedly was concerned with her husband's reaction to the incision—whether he would still look at her with love in his eyes, or disgust.

If I had really listened when she commented about the "dirty, smelly dressing," I would have had a cue. But I missed both the verbal and nonverbal
behavioral messages. I was busy changing the dressing and thinking of what I
had to do next. Even if I had listened I don't think I could have dealt with this
situation adequately. I would have tried to reassure her and give her understanding and sympathy. I don't think I had the knowledge or ability necessary
to get the patient to bring her problems out into the open. I didn't really think
it was my place to get so involved with her personal feelings.

I assumed she wanted to be reassured that the incision was neat. I assumed
she wanted my professional opinion on the appearance of the incision. I made
no attempt to find out what really was bothering her. I didn't know then that I
wasn't listening to her. I didn't realize that I had missed behavioral clues. I
wasn't really aware of them as such. I looked on her actions as reactions to the
surgery—feelings that she would overcome in time. I didn't see my reception
of these actions and feelings as part of the nursing process—assessing total
needs, recognizing the signs of crisis, and intervening in a crisis. I didn't see
her actions as part of a traumatic experience following mutilating surgery. I
didn't see them because I didn't want to.

This head nurse understands the cues but retreats behind an authoritarian function.

Mrs. Brent, an elderly lady, was admitted to our small hospital having suffered a stroke with considerable paralysis involving her throat and speech. She was conscious. Mrs. Brent was on a high-calorie fluid diet, fed small amounts every 2 hours.

The Brents had no living children and were retired farmers. Mr. Brent visited every evening and fed her large amounts of orange juice; after he left she vomited with a great deal of choking. The doctor witnessed a vomiting spell and ordered the orange juice to be discontinued for fear of aspiration.

I was the charge nurse on the 4–12 shift when I met Mr. Brent at 4:05 P.M.

Nurse: Good afternoon, Mr. Brent.
Mr. Brent: Good afternoon, nurse—where is Mrs. Brent now?

He appeared upset. His tone of voice made me aware that something was bothering him and set me on the defensive.

Nurse: In her usual room, I expect.

I immediately began going through the files—they indicated no change.

Mr. Brent: No, she's not; they moved her.

I was irritated at the 8–4 shift for not keeping the files up-to-date and annoyed they had not informed me of the move at report. He would think I did not know my job. I wanted to confirm what he had said.

Nurse: I'm sorry, I'll walk down the hall with you.
Mr. Brent: Never mind, they're always moving her. That's why she's worse than when she came in.

This was not true—what was he leading up to? I realized this could be misplaced criticism. My feelings were hurt as we had worked very conscientiously with Mrs. Brent.

Nurse: What do you mean?

Mr. Brent did not respond. He was not communicating at all. I had to establish rapport as the orange juice problem still had to be discussed. He was irritating me.

Nurse: I expect she was moved to this room to comply with your insurance coverage. Did you ask the secretary for a private room?
Mr. Brent: Yes, I talked to the secretary. She shouldn't have been moved.

I wondered if he didn't understand what the secretary had said, or if she had communicated with him.

Mr. Brent: I lost my son, and she's all I've got.

He wasn't really upset about the room, but about his wife's condition. I felt very sorry for this old man, all alone. I understood how he felt—he was frightened.

As head nurse it was my duty to discuss the orange juice situation with Mr. Brent, as the doctor ordered, but I was reluctant to speak to Mr. Brent when he was obviously so upset about the move. I was afraid and anxious with regard to both the doctor and Mr. Brent, and would have rather stayed securely behind my desk. As my defense I became very remote and businesslike.

Nurse: Mr. Brent, I really must speak to you about giving Mrs. Brent the orange juice. She chokes so. Could you leave it with us, and we'll feed her?

There was no answer.

Rapport was never established due to conflicting feelings of both parties. We were not able to solve any of our problems.

You had the answer but perhaps felt that if you really opened up and showed him how you understood, it would make it less possible for you to be businesslike. As I'm sure you realize now, it might have actually freed him to feel far more a part of your helping team.

In spite of the fact that the child was actually the identified patient, the following case illustrates the nurse's insight in picking up the parents' cues and including them as the basic units of help.

Four-year-old Sandy P was a regular visitor to our pediatric unit. Despite frequent periods away from home, she appeared happy and well adjusted. Her acute attacks of allergic asthma were becoming more frequent and severe.

While evaluating Sandy's condition, I became concerned with the expressions of Mr. and Mrs. P. They were always terribly upset on Sandy's admission, but this time I noticed an expression of frank hostility in Mr. P and an expression bordering on fear in Mrs. P. Sandy was indeed in severe respiratory distress but she had been worse and certainly responded rapidly to therapy.

As soon as it was clinically possible to leave Sandy, I talked with the Ps in private. Mr. P readily unleashed a torrent of dammed-up emotion. It seemed

Mrs. P was struggling with the dust-free room technique prescribed by the allergist, which was by no means easily accomplished as the Ps have three children under five years of age. Sandy was scarcely home before she commenced wheezing. Mrs. P appeared to feel very inadequate concerning her care of Sandy and felt that her husband somehow held her responsible. She appeared to have been running around in circles trying to appease him and give adequate care to her daughter.

Sandy's affliction had been described to the Ps as being allergic in origin and different areas had been explored to ascertain specific problem areas. Mr. P, however, seemed unable to accept this. He appeared to need something concrete as a reason for Sandy's persistent sickness and Mrs. P's supposed inadequate care was the target.

This was the first time Mr. P had actually expressed this feeling in words and it sounded dreadful, so much so that he finished almost apologetically. Mrs. P seemed to shrink away. I hastily explained that although it sounded dreadful, once admitted as a basic problem something could be done about it. Smouldering tensions merely exhaust everyone.

Mrs. P related how she gave Sandy her medicine and never left a wisp of dust anywhere. Mr. P explored areas he felt she could have missed. His own mother never sat still; she was always flitting around gracefully with a duster. It all sounded so petty but it was good to get it out in the open and over with, so that something constructive might be achieved.

From the type of reaction Sandy was having she had to be allergic to something at home. I chanced to ask the Ps if they smoked. They both answered in the affirmative. I explained that it was not uncommon for a child, or even an adult, to react this way to cigarette smoke. The Ps took to this prospect readily. Any answer, right or wrong, was better than no answer, or the impossible impasse of blame and guilt that they were living with.

Even if the cause was not the smoke I felt I had helped the Ps by: (1) observing problematic symptoms of tension; (2) taking time to explore the cause; (3) encouraging them to vent their feelings; (4) encouraging them to seek their own ideas of cause; (5) offering them a theory to work on; (6) promoting self-help. I feel my major contribution to this family was in facilitating and promoting communication. The Ps worked together and successfully stopped smoking. Sandy has been admitted only once this year.

In the following accounts, the nurse points to her labeling of the patient as the basis for *was disapproving, judgmental* (47% of cases) and *did not want to understand* (40% of cases). Here, the nurse identified the patient with a relative of hers, and expected the patient to be the same.

One summer, while doing relief duty at our local hospital, one of my assigned patients was a 70-year-old blind man. He had been admitted a few weeks earlier for tests after being diagnosed as a suspected heart attack. Since admission, according to the report, he had been withdrawn, having to have everything done for him, from washing him to feeding him and taking him to the bathroom. He had been blind for some years, and, according to a daughter with whom he lived, had been able to manage quite adequately while she was at work all day.

After report, I went around and introduced myself to the patients I was to take care of, and when breakfast arrived, I made sure I delivered his tray and helped arrange the meal so he knew where everything was. I then told him I was going to help deliver the other trays and would drop in every 5 minutes to see if he needed help. When I returned the first time he was still exploring his breakfast; the second time he had his head back against the pillows in a resigned way, and he had hardly touched anything. I encouraged him to continue, asking about his likes and dislikes. He continued but quite slowly. Each time I returned I made sure he knew of my presence.

When breakfast was taken away, I asked if he wanted to wash right away or later. "Right away," he said. I readied him for his bath, then told him the exact position of each article: towel, soap, etc. I told him I would return to wash his back. When I returned he had not started his bath, stating all the other nurses had bathed him. I questioned the need for this, since the doctors stated he was able to do his own routine care. He was quite indignant, saying I was lazy and inconsiderate: how was anyone to know how helpless he was—here he was stuck away in the hospital with these blankety-blank nurses to look after him. I became quite angry when he started using choice words. I told him that even if he didn't respect himself, he should respect me enough not to talk to me like that. Even though I hadn't been blind, I told him that I had lived with my grandfather for 10 years or more and he had been blind all that time, but that he was the type of person who was independent. I also suggested some other nurse could look after him and went to consult the head nurse. She suggested I stay with him, since this was the only spark he had shown since admission.

Good, since he could have felt this was another rejection of him.

Apparently, he thought his daughter had put him in the hospital because he was too much trouble and he became very depressed. The other nurses hadn't questioned this and tended to all his needs, making him feel more useless.

This is a good example of human nature. When he felt valued and loved (as he had been at home) he had the will and strength to be independent. But when he felt his daughter was rejecting him, it destroyed his spirit and his feeling of being worthwhile. So he tried for attention through dependence.

He gradually came to see that hospitals are places to help people get better, not a place where they go to die.

I had been angry, because when I knew I was to have a blind patient to look after (my first) it brought back fond memories of my grandfather. I guess I tried to see my grandfather in this patient and he did not meet my expectations. It was such a shock for me to find someone just the opposite of my grandfather, I became indignant and tried to push him too fast, for the wrong reasons, into doing things for himself.

In this case, the prejudice existed on both sides.

Mr. Pace was 56 years old, a habitual drinker with arteriosclerosis and right hemiplegia. He was able to do a great deal for himself, but chose to be uncooperative and difficult. He had a sour, miserable personality, and his behavior was so belligerent and aggressive that the staff avoided him most of the time. When I began working on his ward he was labeled as the most unapproachable patient there, and had been passed from nurse to nurse without any progress; he was handed over to me to see if I could motivate him.

He was a real trial. He never had a civil word to say to me, and for one month I took all his abusive words and uncooperative behavior while boiling inside most of the time, checking my reaction, remembering that I was the nurse, showing instead outward calm, trying to maintain my position as a nurse on the floor, and coping with an aggressive patient.

This patient finally succeeded in breaking me down. One sunny morning in the fall I walked into the bed area where Mr. Pace was lying, as usual smoking, disregarding the rules, and intentionally doing so. I offered him the usual morning medication, greeting him with my pleasant, tolerant smile; he jumped out of bed shaking his left fist and in between his shouts and obscenities, he made me know in no uncertain words that he was not taking the blankety-blank medication from any nigger nurse. I saw red, not because of the obscene language, since I was used to that by now, but the word *nigger* triggered me off. I said to myself, "You have had it with me, buster; who do you think you are, lying around in bed, making and breaking rules to suit yourself, coming in late, intoxicated nearly every night?" I was steaming inside. I felt like sending him to Mars, but very calmly, and icily, I said to him, "Well, Mr. Pace, I am not wasting any more time with you. I am sorry you feel that way about nigger nurses—that I cannot help you with—but you can take your medication or leave it. If your conscience decides that you should take the medication from me, I will be in the medication room." With that statement, I crisply turned and walked out of the room.

I avoided Mr. Pace like the plague most of the time, just doing the bare essentials for him. After a couple of days, I noticed that he was actually trying to be pleasant in a disgruntled way. He was out of bed after breakfast with his bed made, which was surprising. I would hear him saying to the patients, "Here comes my nurse, she is the best one around here." I never commented or let on that I heard. I continued to give him the cold shoulder.

About one week after that incident, I was preparing the morning medication when Mr. Pace came into the room, asking if he could talk to me. He wanted me to help him make up his mind as to whether he should try to go to the workshop or go out. Instead of listening to him, I quickly brushed him off with the excuse that I was busy. I knew that this was my chance: the situation had reversed; the patient was trying to reach out to me for help—and this would be the ideal time to make a breakthrough with him. Instead, I was so prejudiced against him that I blocked out my reasoning.

That was the last time I saw Mr. Pace. His body was found the next day in Lake Ontario. The post mortem showed that the patient had ingested a considerable amount of alcohol. Now, whether he fell or jumped into the lake, we will never know. His death came as a shock to all of us. There was no history of suicidal attempts, and we all knew that he was able to hold his liquor. It bothered me: did he really commit suicide, or did he have an accident? I felt very guilty.

Allowing oneself or not allowing oneself to be *influenced by the negative opinions of other staff members* regarding the personality of the patient is obviously critical in Convalescence. These factors rate second-highest among all Conditions for both Helpful and Unhelpful cases.

Marie, a middle-aged lady, was admitted to the hospital with extensive bed sores on her back. Apparently she was cared for by her husband at home without the help of a visiting nurse. However, things got out of hand and she had to come to the hospital. Marie was a typical Londoner, with a strong cockney accent, outspoken, cheerful, and now bedridden. Unfortunately, the head nurse was her opposite: well spoken, cold, authoritative, and snobbish. What she said was law. She was feared by the nursing staff and relationships were quite unnatural. Although it never came out openly, there was a feeling among us that Marie's behavior, if not the woman herself, was frowned upon by the head nurse. Somehow Marie did not fit in such a clean, well-run, and silent ward. All this made for a strained atmosphere where patients and nurses spoke only when spoken to in front of the head nurse. But behind the screens much whispering and winking of the eyes went on.

Marie's care had to be done frequently; therefore, she was placed in a bed at the far end of the corridor and we were told that we would find this more convenient because it was nearer to the equipment room. On such occasions much chatting took place on Marie's part and it was always about her favorite subject—horse races. She eagerly waited for her husband to visit so that she could hear the latest about the races. Unfortunately, her excitement did not communicate itself to the nurses. To make things worse, whenever her care took longer than necessary the head nurse peeped through the screens with further orders for us to carry out. Marie reacted to this by talking rather crudely about her relationship with her husband whenever that nurse was nearby. We ended up by caring for her in silence. Gradually Marie stopped bothering with the nurses and became quite friendly with the maid, who spent a lot of her time just dusting her locker, but all the while talking happily about the races.

Then one day Marie discharged herself from the hospital; this came as a shock to the nursing staff and a well-deserved shock it was. We had put our fear of displeasing the head nurse before our responsibility to the patient. I myself, as a very inexperienced nurse, had felt quite insecure as to what to do in such a situation and weakly followed the example of my senior nurses. We were all affected by an authoritarian system that militated against a therapeutic climate vital to the patient's well-being. Our fears of incurring that nurse's sanctions prevented us from examining objectively the disastrous effects that our behavior and practices were having on the patient—we ended up by doing our work mechanically and lost sight of the patient as a human being. We rationalized the fact that hospital routine left very little time for socializing with patients, thus ignoring their fundamental needs. Occupying the patient with meaningless activity became just busy work. We rationalized our guilty feelings by saying that the maid had lots of time to talk to Marie, while we could not do so because of a shortage of staff and because of the head nurse's strict supervision.

Needless to say we all learned a lot from Marie; most of all we learned to accept the patient as he or she is, to adjust our schedules to meet his or her special needs, and to provide an atmosphere of receptivity to the patient's needs.

In this account, the nurse faces the meaning of her prejudicial judgment, and her anger toward her patient.

Last year, I worked as a staff nurse on a male surgical floor. One day we admitted a young man, in traction, who had been injured in a car accident. This person happened to be acting leader of the local Devil's Angels motorcycle gang, and certainly looked the part—scarred, overweight, club sign tattooed on one arm.

The general reaction of the staff to this person was repulsion and fear of what he represented. Everyone avoided him as much as possible, as he often raised embarrassing scenes in order to get what he wanted. I, too, avoided him, feeling disdainful of his rude mannerisms and fearful of being embarrassed by him.

One day he was especially upset because his water—which he had been pouring down his leg cast to relieve the itch—was taken away from him. He told me that he was going to use his urinal and pour that down! Suddenly I felt very angry and told him how I felt about his manners and said, "Go ahead if you really want to—it's your leg!" To my surprise his response was not the usual insulting remark. He said nothing.

That was what started me thinking. I felt that had I indignantly flounced off, he would have continued to act out about the situation. Then I tried to put myself in his position. He must have been feeling very isolated and rejected in this strange place. Maybe his loud rudeness was his way of saying, "Notice me. I'm sick. I need attention, too."

Yes, or, "I will live up to the only reputation I have."

That afternoon, I went and just started to talk to him about general things, the accident, and eventually about himself. He became quite receptive, and told me fascinating things about his life as a gang member. I found that underneath that tough exterior, he had great feelings of insecurity—especially about his future.

I wondered whether he had accepted my earlier angry outburst because it was the first show of any expression of feeling toward him as a person that he had received from any of us. Anyway, I know that after I had aired my feelings, I was able to see and accept him as an individual, in spite of his mannerisms. My honest expression of feeling had been of value to me. After that I was able to approach this person without fear or repulsion—as a friend.

Sometimes it isn't appropriate to air one's feelings to the patient quite so directly! In this case, at least, it cut through the indifference and silent treatment he had been given up until then. Sometimes one has to air one's feelings only to oneself (or trusted colleagues) and thereby go through the same process of facing and coping with one's anger. As you point out, the object is to open oneself to being able to consider the situation from the patient's point of view as well.

Basic to many Unhelpful Responses, nurses explain that their *self-image was threatened* (in 42% of the cases). Here a nurse vividly describes a most difficult situation and the agonies involved in failing to meet her expectations of herself.

Just recently I decided that it would be a challenging experience to nurse patients in a setting other than the hospital. I chose public health, thinking that I would take my nursing experience to the home of the patient. A patient would be more relaxed in his own home. After all, the hospital atmosphere was so formal. I was sure a patient would be more receptive in his own environment. Little did I realize that I was not prepared. There would be times when my nursing care would be totally inadequate.

My first week at work had gone very well, I thought. It was my last visit of the week. I looked at the visiting card to review the case and drove into an area of the city with which I was not familiar. It was a shabby area of unkempt rooming houses. I remember thinking, All these poor people, I'm going to make a special effort to provide all the help I can. The brief history on the chart described Mr. D, a 28-year-old bachelor, "depressed, not working, on disability pension because of an apparent back problem and recurrent skin infection. The patient needs emotional support and encouragement to resume work."

I entered the house and walked down the hallway until I found his room. I knocked on the door and a voice from within shouted, "Come on in, the door is open." I opened the door and quickly glanced around. The plaster was coming loose and the paint was peeling. There was only one dresser, and a bed on which the patient was lying. His clothes were soiled, the bed linen was grey and dirty and piled in a heap at the end of the bed. I was shocked. I had never seen anything so hopeless. I recall the feeling that I did not want to enter the room. I stepped only a few feet inside the room and did not close the door.

"Hello, I'm Mrs. S, the new nurse. I will be taking Mrs. B's place." "Oh," he remarked, "I wondered what you would look like. Not bad, not bad at all. Come on in, sit down; sorry they didn't give me a chair." I said to myself, "This guy is kind of fresh, I don't like his manner."

I felt uncomfortable being in his room. I replied to Mr. D that it was quite alright, "I would rather stand; I've been sitting in the car all day." Mr. D replied, "Boy, you must have a neat job if that's all you do is sit in the car all day." I was really being obvious, I thought; he knows that I'm reluctant to come into the room. He could sense that I felt uneasy. I walked a little closer to the bed and tried to appear more relaxed.

I asked about his back. He remarked that it was still painful. "I know you people don't believe me. You think I just want to loaf around." This thought had been expressed by the other nurses, but I didn't want to get into that conversation. He was so open and abrupt. I thought of my own inadequate feelings at the moment. I could not cope with this problem now. I changed the topic of conversation to his skin infection.

Mr. D mentioned that he had just been to the drug store. The doctor had given him a prescription for ointment. "You're a nurse," Mr. D said. "How about putting this stuff on my face?" His face was covered with boils; many of them were open and draining. I felt nauseated; how could I touch his face? I didn't even have sterile gloves. My aversion must have been obvious in the expression on my face. "Hey, what kind of a nurse are you, you've seen worse than this!" I knew that I had insulted him. How could I be so unfeeling? I said, "It doesn't bother me. It's just that I don't want to cause more infection by touching your face with my hands. I really should use a sterile technique." Mr. D said, "I don't have any sterile forceps either. What did you expect me to use?" I asked him to show me where I could wash my hands and then I would apply the ointment.

He directed me to a washroom down the hall. When I opened the door I was sorry that I had offered to help. The sink was filthy. I couldn't back out now. I washed my hands as best I could and returned to the room. I did have a package of sterile gauze in my bag. I demonstrated how the ointment should be applied, put the remainder of the gauze on the dresser and said that I would return at the end of the week to see how he was managing. He remarked as I was leaving, "I don't think you will be back." I affirmed that I would and rushed to the washroom to soap my hands again.

As I walked out of the building I said to myself, "He is right; how could I ever go back there again?" I was repulsed by his manner, the sight of the room, and the appearance of his face. My disgust was apparent.

How naive could I be to think that everyone lived in a middle-class environment? I would not have been so repulsed if I had been caring for Mr. D in the nice, clean surroundings of a familiar hospital ward. And yet I was quite aware that people do live in the same environment as Mr. D. I had failed. I had not acted in any way like the compassionate, empathetic nurse I had been trained to be. I was supposed to be helping this man and all I did was show my aversion. He sensed this from the minute I walked into the room. I failed to establish any rapport. The mere fact that I was hesitant to enter the room showed the patient that I felt insecure in the surroundings. My negative facial expressions were also quite apparent to the patient when he asked me to apply the ointment. How could I expect him to trust me as a nurse? We are told that it is important in establishing a rapport to convey to the person that he is important and that someone cares; the health professional must try to develop or maintain the client's feelings of self-esteem. I failed to do this. I let my middle-class values interfere with my purpose for visiting Mr. D.

We are told that it is important to accept people as they are regardless of social class: allow people the freedom to be themselves. In this way the nurse can maintain her own personal standards without being shocked by others. I did not remember this when I entered Mr. D's room. I let my personal feelings enter the situation. I could not overcome my shock and disgust sufficiently to deal with Mr. D as a person and a patient who needed professional help.

The report said Mr. D was depressed. He needed emotional support and encouragement to resume work. I had consciously avoided the topic of work. Mr. D said that the nurses felt he was just loafing around. He was angry. I felt incompetent. I did not want to deal with this problem. His anger had caused me to become slightly apprehensive so I changed the topic of conversation. I put my feelings ahead of his feelings. No wonder he was angry. I wouldn't have wanted to return to work if my face looked anything like Mr. D's face. No wonder he was depressed. Why couldn't I see his depression and his not wanting to return to work were related. He needed emotional support and I did not provide it.

I increased the patient's anxiety when I very obviously gave the impression that I was anxious to terminate my visit. I conveyed a lack of concern and a lack of time to give adequate care. I left Mr. D with the feeling that I would not return for a second visit.

As I drove back to the office I wondered how depressed Mr. D was feeling now. My visit had been totally wrong. I would have to show Mr. D that I would return and that I really did want to help him.

As previously noted, across all Situations, *initiated referral to another profession/resource* rates highest in Convalescence. Often making a referral is perceived to be a somewhat mechanical task, if not a covert way of dumping onto another professional. Because the patient has been ill prepared for the referral, it may not "take," though the initiating source may or may not ever follow through enough to know the results. The following case is an excellent example of the crucial work that must precede many referrals.

My initial encounter with Mrs. C was when I visited her home at the request of the school principal to investigate the reasons for increased absenteeism, offensive body odors, and discipline problems amongst her children.

Mrs. C, a widow, lived with her six children, ranging in age from 14 to 3 years, in a three-bedroom flat above a store. The older children were undisciplined, rude, and obviously lacking parental control, while the younger were whiny, sickly, and withdrawn. All six were suffering from eneuresis. Mrs. C was an extremely thin, pale, poorly dressed woman who chain-smoked constantly. The apartment, which reeked of stale wine, was in a chaotic state of untidiness, with filthy floors, and garbage and dirty dishes piled high. Mr. C was suspected to have committed suicide 12 months previously. The general picture presented was that of a multiproblem family with little potential for improvement.

When I arrived Mrs. C appeared nervous and fidgety as she apologized for the mess of the house. She said she had no problems and felt it unnecessary that the nurse should be visiting. Even though this distraught woman was verbally denying the need for help, her nonverbal communication came through to me as a woman crying out for someone, anyone who would care enough to take time to listen. So, drawing on every resource of my limited professional background, I sincerely attempted to appear nonjudgmental and empathetic as I encouraged Mrs. C to first discuss the most evident and superficial problems such as the children's clothing, diet, enuresis, and so on. I discovered the scar that some agencies, such as Social Services Department, had left on this family through previous dealings, and so I tried to pose as little threat as possible in my endeavors.

Having myself come from a broken home where my mother raised six children alone, I was conscious of her manifold problems and was able to appreciate her conflicts and the need to express them to a neutral outside person. I obviously did indicate a desire to understand, because Mrs. C slowly began to relax and become more expressive with each visit. Her favorable response to my initial efforts gave me encouragement or personal reward so that I was willing to strive even harder for her sake because she met my own basic drive to feel needed.

My long-standing philosophical belief in the dignity, worth, uniqueness, and irreplaceability of every human being was reinforced by this family's progress and prompted me to feel that Mrs. C and her children were important enough to warrant the time and resources they demanded of me at that time. Even though I was extremely busy in my district, I tried not to appear hurried so that Mrs. C would feel free to confide her fears and talk out her frustrations. I returned every week on the same day; maintained my noncoercive attitude of acceptance and carried out all of my promises to her so that she would not lose faith that I was trustworthy and dependable.

Through successive visits, gradual improvement was noted in the cleanliness of the apartment and Mrs. C's appearance, and it appeared to me that Mrs. C was striving to meet my approval. The teachers at school reported that the younger children were arriving more frequently, more suitably dressed, and with diminishing odor. I gave continued support and praised Mrs. C's smallest efforts, encouraging her to keep up the good work.

More and more Mrs. C began to express her deeper feelings until finally, one day, she discussed her husband and his death. She confided that he had been a terrible, dogmatic man, who beat her and the children in his rage. Mr. C apparently had threatened for months to kill himself the day before Christmas, and this was exactly the day on which he died. She described every detail of the happening and how she and the children had stood by and watched without sending for help.

I was pleased with this revelation and felt pride in my success of bringing Mrs. C to the state emotionally where she could trust my confidence enough to reveal this to me, a person outside her family. The family physician's diagnosis of the cause of death was that of a heart attack, but both Mrs. C and the children were experiencing overwhelming guilt feelings concerning this traumatic experience. Mrs. C referred to the incident as the family murder.

Recognizing this as a major step forward, I attempted to establish, with Mrs. C, some concrete goals for the family. I was convinced that my sincere love for these poor people, which involved responsibility, respect, and knowledge, motivated my concern. So, acknowledging the limitations of my ability and assessing the stability of our relationship, I suggested the inclusion of another agency. Mrs. C agreed and the entire family was referred to a mental health clinic where they were counseled on a weekly basis by a psychiatrist, social worker, and child psychologist.

I was aware of personal growth and an increasing adequacy to work perceptively as I sought to feel and experience with the patient, but I also facilitated a growth relationship within the C family. Even though giving warmth and interest, I was able to maintain my own separate identity and emotional objectivity while still achieving predefined goals.

The outcome of this family was truly a success story, because they all responded well to therapy. Mrs. C still phoned to have me visit, but as she became more independent I decreased the frequency of my visits, and she moved back into the family circle to exercise parental discipline over the older children and give much-needed affection to the younger. I realized, though, that before she was able to give of herself in the manner expected of a mother, she must first receive from me. The children regained respect for their mother and began to function as a family unit again to overcome their problems and face life anew.

A very sensitive use of your own personal background, insights, and desire and ability to give—thus a highly integrated piece of service.

Across all Situations, *short-staffed; too little time to devote to the patient* is cited second-most often in the Situation of Convalescence. Here it is the patient who picks up the nurse's cue.

I was working on a very busy surgical floor where the staff shortage was acute. I had a large number of seriously ill patients who required most of my time and attention. I also had a few convalescent patients, including an old lady who had had a lumbar sympathectomy the week before in an unsuccessful attempt to relieve her arthritic pain.

Throughout the hectically busy evening this lady frequently rang for me and finally, about 15 minutes before I was to be relieved by the night staff, she rang again. She said she would like her pillow arranged more comfortably, but she really wanted to talk. She told me of her son, who was living elsewhere, what a wonderful son he was, how he tried so hard to visit her but was so busy with his business and family. I was filled with sympathy for her; I realized her loneliness and how long and dreary the night must have stretched out before her. As she talked on, I suddenly realized the passing of time; my charts were to be signed off, medications to be recorded, the report to be given to the night staff; then, without even thinking, I surreptitiously glanced at my watch. In that moment she saw me and the animation faded from her face. Her happiness in speaking of her son was forgotten, and she was back in that hospital room again. We said goodnight and I left with a deep sense of guilt to privately curse the paper work that awaited me and my own stupidity.

Almost every history of nursing text at some point refers to the ministering angel image of the nurse. Some accounts would place this role not more recently than the First World War, relegating it to the unsophisticated pre-era of nursing as a science. Others believe it is only as this image is reinstated that nursing will maintain itself as an art. The following is an almost classic illustration of the nurse in this role.

When I was working at the Southside Hospital, on surgery, there was a car accident patient whom I specialed. The patient, Robert, was a young married man about 28 years of age. When Robert arrived on the ward he was unconscious and there was absolutely no response from him. I specialed Robert for 2 weeks, and he was a patient I'll never forget. It was the first time that I really felt that a miracle had been performed.

Every day when I nursed him, I hoped that I would get some kind of response from him. He was the only patient that I had for 2 weeks so I was able to give him very thorough nursing care. From the time that I first walked into the room, I talked to this young man, telling him who I was, explaining procedures to him, asking him to respond for me and generally commenting on the weather and his devoted wife. Whenever I left the room, I always made sure that I told him that I was going and always announced myself when I came back. I really believed that Robert would one day respond in some way. I felt very discouraged at times, wondering if it was all worth it, but I continued on anyway. I knew that he couldn't talk because of the tracheotomy tube that was inserted, but I felt if I kept asking him to respond by some movement that someday he would. I felt sorry for him, seeing him lying there. It only made me more ambitious to try harder.

Whenever I was about to do a procedure, such as give him a bed bath, I was very careful to explain what I was about to do. I felt that even though Robert didn't respond, he was still able to feel and to fear the unknown. I made sure that I exercised all his limbs, so that when he did regain consciousness his muscles would be in fairly good condition. When I was doing exercises for him, I put myself in his place, asking him if it was hurting him if I thought it might be. Again, I watched closely for some reaction, but there was none.

When the morning routine of care was done, I sat with Robert and told him things I thought would be of interest to him. I wanted him desperately to be in touch with reality. I felt guilty at times because he wasn't responding to my care. I wondered whether or not it was all worth it. When I looked at him, so helpless and young, I continued on. I thought that even though he couldn't respond, he could hear. I told him of the weather outside, the news, and his wife's visit in the afternoon.

His wife was very devoted to him and never lost faith. She came in every afternoon to talk to him. She would tell him family news and carry on as if he were responding. At times, it made me angry because I wondered, Why did this have to happen to them? His wife really believed, as I did, that Robert would respond soon.

I was careful not to talk of Robert's condition in the room. Outside, I encouraged his wife, saying that she was a great asset to him and that her presence meant a great deal to him. Actually, we both supported each other.

The days went by and still no sign of communication from Robert. One day, as I was exercising his leg, he blinked. I just couldn't believe it! I asked him to do it again, and he did. I knew then that he was on his way to recovery. Now I couldn't help but talk because I knew for sure that he had heard me. I told him how happy his wife would be. When I told his wife, we both had tears in our eyes. She said, "Thank you."

Robert's progress was rapid from that time on. In a month, he walked out of the hospital with his wife. For me this was a miracle. I knew that my methods of communication had worked and were very important. I supported and encouraged Robert and his wife and they supported me. We all believed that one day Robert would walk out of the hospital.

10
ALCOHOLISM

Of the 550 cases in the study, 2% focus on Alcoholism. Of the 9 cases that focus on Alcoholism, 4 are described as Helpful, 5 as Unhelpful. Percentages shown for comparison only (see Tables 2.3, 2.4; pp. 32–35).

COMPARISON WITH ALL OTHER SITUATIONS

Helpful Factors

Highest Rating

- Was honest with patient/relatives.
- Discussed religion with patient (same rating as Cultural Adaptation).

Unhelpful Factors

Highest Rating

- Avoided needs of family members (same rating as Death/Dying, Cultural Adaptation).

Helpful Factors	% of Cases in Which Cited
1. Gave moral support	75
2. Helped patient express feelings	75
3. Looked beyond patient's outward response/behavior to underlying causes	75

4. Nonjudgmental	50
5. Came to terms with own feelings; was able to enter into patient's problem	25
6. Helped family members deal with the situation	25
7. Wanted to understand how patient felt	25
8. Discussed religion with patient	25
9. Used innovative rehabilitative procedure	25
10. Positively identified with patient due to similar life/professional experience	25
11. Was honest with patient/relatives	25
12. Took time to explain	0
13. Was a sounding board	0
14. Initiated referral to another profession/resource	0
15. Liked the patient	0
16. Not unduly influenced by negative opinions of other staff regarding the patient's personality	0
17. Made this case the basis for overall policy change/improvement	0
18. Was trying to prove self to senior staff members	0
19. Used physical closeness	0
20. Had received training in recognizing social-emotional needs of patients	0

Unhelpful Factors	% of Cases in Which Cited
1. Was disapproving, judgmental	80
2. Treated the condition, overlooking the patient	60
3. Prejudiced toward group of which patient was a member	60
4. Did not want to understand	40
5. Failed to look beyond initial negative impression of patient's personality	40
6. Avoided needs of family members	40
7. Self-image was threatened	40
8. Felt inadequate to enter into patient's problem because had not personally resolved the issue	20
9. Breakdown of interprofessional communication/cooperation	20
10. Purposely disregarded significant cues in patient's statements/behavior	20
11. Rationalized actions and thoughts	20

12.	Disliked patient	20
13.	Felt guilty but still would not communicate	20
14.	Felt guilty but could not communicate	0
15.	Short-staffed; too little time to devote to the patient	0
16.	Felt pressured (within self) into doing things rather than coping with feeling elements (tension present)	0
17.	Negatively influenced by opinions of other staff members regarding personality of the patient	0
18.	Lacked training in recognizing social-emotional needs of patients	0
19.	Afraid would break down and cry in front of patient	0
20.	Overidentified due to being similar age to patient	0
21.	Incapacitated by own fear of death	0
22.	Failed to seek authoritative advice regarding innovation	0
23.	Disregarded own judgment because wanted approval of senior staff members	0
24.	Lost professional role: patient became friend	0

It is obvious that *was disapproving, judgmental,* or *nonjudgmental* are key Response factors. These Responses are cited in 4 out of 5 Unhelpful cases and 2 out of 4 Helpful cases. *Prejudice toward group of which patient was a member* (alcoholics) is named in 3 out of 5 cases. Only prejudice toward Unmarried Mothers exceeds this ratio.

This experience does not relate to a special situation or any one individual, but to a group of individuals, and my attitude toward them. The group that I refer to is alcoholic patients.

Although I do not overtly profess this feeling, secretly I have always had an intense dislike for anyone who was an alcoholic, whether it was someone on the street or a patient in the hospital. On several occasions throughout my nursing experience I have had to nurse a large number of these patients who were brought into the hospital in varying levels of inebriation or delirium tremens.

My first encounter with the alcoholic patient was during my student days. He was a man of 40, and I was asked to admit him to the ward. It was a very difficult and traumatic experience, and one I have always remembered. The man was obnoxious, verbally abusive, his language loud and profane, and he was physically brutal, throwing at me whatever was within his reach. He shouted constantly at me to leave him alone and this I would have gladly done, had someone else been available to care for him. I was to find out later and throughout my career that this was the general behavior of most alcoholic patients, both men and women.

Aside from alcoholics' hospital behavior patterns, I saw and nursed the battered child, the beaten up woman; I saw fear in the eyes of relatives; I knew of the destruction of family life: all were the result of someone's drunkenness.

I had no sympathy whatever for alcoholics and found very little that was likable about them. Although my nursing duties were adequately administered and my manner pleasant whenever they were recovered enough to be civil, I found that I did not make it a part of my duty to sit down and talk to them and be as friendly as I was to the other patients. I failed to realize that they were ill patients, many of them with pressing problems severe enough to make them want to drown their sorrows in alcohol, to the point where they were no longer able to control their actions. I realize now that I could have put away my prejudices and seen, instead, their needs. I can remember now that most of them wanted to be friendly, and with some petty excuses I had denied them those occasions. I realize that I could have been more understanding.

In *The Transparent Self,* Sidney M. Jourard [1971] refers to the patient who is in a certain range that the nurse dislikes. Jourard goes on to say, "Patients outside the restricted range are a puzzle or a threat to her and she does not want to get to know them. She takes care of their bodies but not their whole selves . . . there are nurses who cannot take care of people whose behavior is at first bizarre and incomprehensible" [pp. 202–203].

I do not know that my attitudes toward the alcoholic patient will suddenly change, but I realize now that I will have to work hard at it. I am sure I will always remember that quote.

*   *   *   *

Miss X, a 65-year-old, was admitted to the center because of alcoholism and epilepsy. Her therapist was on vacation and I was covering for her. It was Monday morning and doing your own work plus some other person's is not fun and games. Mondays are not my best days of the week.

I was sitting in a conference and could hear Miss X shouting and she sounded drunk. I thought this conference should go on all day so I would not have to face Miss X. The door of the room flew open and who should come storming in but Miss X, shouting, "Hey, you, are you looking after Miss S's patients? If so I want you right now, or you will be sorry." Well, I saw red and decided not to respond, because my name was not "Hey, you." Miss X shouted, "If you do not come I will have a fit and then you'll be sorry." The way we were sitting in the conference I was boxed in, so luckily for me the male staff member nearest to her responded, and the two of them left the room.

I thought, I should go—then, No, I am not going to be blackmailed. I waited until the shouting had died down and reluctantly went into the room where she was with the male staff member, explaining that she hated female therapists because they were stuck up. He glanced up and saw me as I was turning away and called after me. In the meantime, Miss X decided to have a seizure as threatened. I got her a foam cushion to have it on. She started shouting how cruel it was of me making fun of her having a seizure. She was so angry she forgot to have the seizure and left the center.

This lady usually came in twice a week, but now every morning she would be there with a problem. If I tried to talk to her she would shout or threaten to have a seizure. I got to the stage where I would set up my home visits in the morning so that I would be away from the center and could avoid her.

She would complain that no one liked her. As she walked into a room the other patients would leave. I wanted to tell her that if she stopped drinking, people would be nice to her, and the staff would try to help her, but it was me she was after. Sometimes she would call to see if I was there and if I was she would start shouting at me on the phone. She knew I was avoiding her and she would not have that. With other patients I would usually make an effort to understand the reason why we could not communicate, but with this lady I just wanted to give her back to Miss S with no questions asked. I really did not care for her and I did not try. I reassured myself that I cannot like everyone, especially people like Miss X.

I have chosen this case because it was one of the times I really failed as a nurse: I started off by seeing the work load and not the people with problems. I had an attitude of "I could not care less," and did not bring myself to meet her half way. I was very distant because I detested alcoholics and their attitudes. I could not accept her calling me "Hey, you," and manipulating me by having fake seizures, even though it was her way of reaching out. My aloofness created an explosion whenever we met. Rather than working it through, I ran away from her. I never really knew this lady or showed her empathy. I was insecure with her.

This big mistake was the turning point for me. Over the years I have learned to analyze my own feelings and behavior toward others. In handling people like Miss X I sometimes tell them that they are making me anxious or that I feel uncomfortable with their behavior. I know I cannot like everyone or be helpful to all, but I can try.

*   *   *   *

I worked in a distant rural area. A week before I went to Santa Fe I was called by a teacher-husband requesting me to go see his wife, who was very depressed and needed help immediately. He had not thought it urgent enough to stay with her until he had checked with me to see if I would be available to make a house call. I was the only nurse in the office at the time and had some important meetings lined up for the afternoon. It was almost 1:00 P.M. and I had not had time for lunch, so I was not too interested in seeing Ms. M at her home, which would take more time than if she came to my office. She was unable to do so, I was assured. I rationalized I was too busy, but the real fact may have been that I had difficulty communicating with Ms. M. Frequently she was drunk and for one reason or another I found her behavior unacceptable. However, I had guilt feelings about not seeing her, so I quickly left instructions with my secretary and made my house call, very much aware of my feelings toward her and the pressures of the day.

I found Ms. M at home in her living room with a friend who had just arrived and felt the situation might prove a bit awkward. After a few minutes of social talk I asked Ms. M if she wanted to see me in private. She immediately began crying and led me into her bedroom, where she began confiding in me. I could see how badly she wanted and needed to talk. She was very open about her home problems and spoke of her own feelings of inferiority toward her husband and almost all her friends. She trusted me as she spoke of confidential matters and I felt very guilty about my previous opinions of her. I really had not known this woman before. I had often felt sorry for her husband for having to cope with a wife who frequently embarrassed him when drunk. That day, as I listened to her, I perceived the situation in a different light. She was a quiet Indian woman; he an aggressive, educated Caucasian. He was always busy with extracurricular activities and other people. She felt very bitter and resentful and I knew she needed help. She felt she had a good relationship with her two school-age children.

In a few days I would be leaving the area so I planned to meet with both her and her husband at different times that evening. Together we worked out a plan for them in hopes of bringing about better understanding between them and to help Ms. M to learn to gain more confidence in herself.

Although this may seem like a simple problem, to me it was much more than that. I know I did the correct thing by going to help and by going to her home to do so. I am not saying that my initial feelings were not justified. Frequently we are under pressure and our true feelings seem to emerge as our defenses break down. However, the force that took over and made this into a therapeutic relationship was the understanding on my part, brought about by past memories. I am prejudiced against drunkenness, in spite of the fact that I know that it is an illness. (I am not assuming that Ms. M is an alcoholic.) I just know that when she let down her defenses I was struck with reality. Not long ago I was unable to shake off the inferiority complex that dominated my frame of mind. Someone helped me to see my own sense of worth and as I sensed that Ms. M really needed help I wanted her to find her sense of worth as well. She needed to examine the ontological dimensions in her life and find meaning for her existence. Although my sessions with her were limited, she felt much better having talked to someone she trusted and thought could help. I encouraged her and her husband to seek out the help of the new nurse when necessary.

Often we get so wrapped up in our technical and administrative duties that we forget about the real reason that we are in a particular job. Feeling guilty and threatened (not accomplishing much in a limited time period) at the same time, my initial attitude was selfish. Once realizing the problem, I wanted to show my patient that someone did care about her.

Along with the Conditions of Death/Dying and Cultural Adaptation, Alcoholism occasions the highest ratio of *avoided needs of family members*.

Mr. Paul C is a 40-year-old man of Polish origin. He was born in Michigan, where he grew up, married, and fathered four children. He separated from his wife 5 years ago, and came to work in Detroit as a mechanic. For 4 years he has been living with Anita, who has a 19-year-old daughter. He was referred to a clinic by his employer for treatment of alcoholism on a mandatory basis, his job being on the line.

At first Paul was withdrawn and did not initiate conversation, but he was always pleasant when approached. He stated that he did not understand what was going on in group therapy; therefore, he was not participating. He was presently deep in debt and his relationships with his common-law wife and stepdaughter were strained; both problems were related. Paul, who was working generally between 55 to 70 hours a week, had entrusted his wife with the budgeting and financial administration of the household. She proved to be inefficient: bills were left unpaid and Paul wondered where the money went, so he took the administration in hand. This whole situation bred a lot of hostility, resentment, and distrust.

Paul depicted Anita as a calculating, domineering person, out to get every penny she could from him. He intimated that she would rather see him drunk and unaware than sober and assuming responsibilities in the household administration. The fact that Anita stopped visiting him at the clinic and refused to be involved in his treatment (we always tried to involve spouses in treatment) appeared to confirm Paul's assertion. However, he was not ready to make any move regarding his marriage, so my immediate goal at that point was to keep him sober, thus preserving his job, and assume a wait and see attitude about his marital situation. He was put on a deterrent drug, disulfiram (Antabuse), and returned to work. His employer was very satisfied. Good . . . but far from being good enough.

While it is all right to trust people, I should have been more alert to the possibility that perhaps there were two sides to this story and put more effort into getting his wife's side. There was no home telephone and it was not customary to do home visits; if I had done a home visit, it might have reinforced her defensiveness. Anita, I learned later, felt that Paul had given her a very bad reputation among staff and patients and that already everyone was against her.

What then? The involvement of the public health nurse could have been the answer. She might have introduced herself into that home in a "I'm the district nurse; I was just passing by" kind of visit. Having been clued in to the situation she would have known what to look for. Well, I failed to use that resource. I allowed Paul to continue to play the alcoholic game, as described by Dr. Eric Berne [Berne, 1978]: Paul was the alcoholic, Anita the persecutor, myself the rescuer and the dummy alternatively. I assumed the role of the dummy when, for instance, I was understanding how painful it was for him to endure the silent treatment from his wife and still maintain sobriety.

In reality he was drinking every day and was not taking Antabuse. The reason his wife would not talk to him when he came home was that she knew instantly when he was drunk just by the way he slammed the door, and she knew that whatever she would say would trigger a fight during which he would become verbally and physically abusive to her. (I learned her side of the story several weeks later, when she called for a joint interview out of frustration, for to her dismay his attitude toward her was worse than ever.) In this particular case I would agree with Dr. Berne's [1978] theory that the ideal treatment would be for all the people who are important to the alcoholic (wife, employer, friends, therapist, etc.), to break away from the game itself instead of merely shifting roles, thus getting the alcoholic to stop playing the game altogether.

It is significant that it is primarily in the Situations of Alcoholism and Cultural Adaptation that *discussed religion with patient* is an important factor. As Alcoholics Anonymous is known to have a religious component, so do cultures, and this may free nurses to feel more comfortable in discussing this aspect of life than is otherwise the case. In the Situation of Death/Dying, for example, discussion of religion between nurse and patient is never cited.

The situation that I wish to discuss and in which I felt personally involved in a helping situation involved an adult male alcoholic. When I first met him on the medical ward he was in a state of delirium tremors, physically restrained, and having visual hallucinations.

However, daily he improved and quickly developed a ravenous appetite. He seemed grateful for the extra-large servings of food obtained for him and this became somewhat of a mutual joke between us. From then on he seemed more open and I sensed a certain change in his attitudes. Although he had quite a good sense of humor, he seemed depressed. When the opportunity presented itself, I asked him if he wanted to talk about it, and he seemed willing. He began by stating he had been involved in a car accident prior to admission and was to be jailed for it. It had apparently happened during a 10-day memory lapse. His whole conversation was very negative and included attitudes toward church, family, local poverty, and his job. The facts, as he presented them, indicated he had had a history of tuberculosis and that his drinking habit developed during his stays in a sanitorium. I welcomed his negativism at that time, hoping he would feel more free to talk.

During the next few weeks, we talked several times and each time he seemed more at ease and slightly less negative. On one of these occasions, I asked him, when he was discussing his problems, if he would agree that most of his problems related to his drinking habits, and he agreed. Prior to this he had referred to his habit but had not elaborated on it. It was then he told me about rare visits to Alcoholics Anonymous in another city, but he said that he could not make their theories work for him and that he just could not control his desires for this habit.

Later we talked about AA's 10 steps for the alcoholic and its reference to a higher power. He came back to the higher power idea several times. On one occasion I suggested that even though one can be turned off church, one may still have confidence in God, and reach out to him for help. He did not seem impressed or antagonistic.

It was good to pick this up, as he was obviously searching this question.

He was discharged shortly after. This man later became a friend of our family and settled in our small city. He did find the help he needed in his dependent state. He works diligently for AA, has a managerial position, and attends the same church denomination he criticized. He invited me to his third-year AA anniversary, and related the account just written with no negative overtones. He expressed gratitude that someone had been sufficiently interested to help him and that he intended to do the same for others.

11
ELDERLY

Of the 550 cases in the study, 6% focus on the Elderly. Of the 31 cases that focus on the Elderly, 52% are described as Helpful, 48% as Unhelpful.

COMPARISON WITH ALL OTHER SITUATIONS

Helpful Factors

Highest Rating

- Liked the patient.

Unhelpful Factors

Highest Rating

- Disliked patient.
- Negatively influenced by opinions of other staff members regarding personality of the patient.

Helpful Factors	% of Cases in Which Cited
1. Helped patient express feelings	69
2. Wanted to understand how patient felt	69
3. Gave moral support	56
4. Took time to explain	50

5.	Was a sounding board	38
6.	Looked beyond patient's outward response/behavior to underlying causes	38
7.	Liked the patient	31
8.	Initiated referral to another profession/resource	25
9.	Helped family members	25
10.	Used innovative rehabilitative procedure	25
11.	Positively identified with patient due to similar life/professional experience	25
12.	Came to terms with own feelings; was able to enter into patient's problem	19
13.	Was honest with patient/relatives	19
14.	Nonjudgmental	13
15.	Used physical closeness	13
16.	Not unduly influenced by negative opinions of other staff regarding the patient's personality	6
17.	Had received training in recognizing social-emotional needs of patients	6
18.	Made this case the basis for overall policy change/improvement	0
19.	Was trying to prove self to senior staff members	0
20.	Discussed religion with patient	0

Unhelpful Factors		% of Cases in Which Cited
1.	Was disapproving, judgmental	67
2.	Failed to look beyond initial negative impression of patient's personality	53
3.	Did not want to understand	53
4.	Self-image was threatened	47
5.	Purposely disregarded significant cues in patient's statements/behavior	40
6.	Disliked patient	40
7.	Treated the condition, overlooking the patient	33
8.	Rationalized actions and thoughts	33
9.	Breakdown of interprofessional communication/cooperation	27
10.	Felt inadequate to enter into patient's problem because had not personally resolved the issue	20
11.	Felt guilty, but still would not communicate	27
12.	Negatively influenced by opinions of other staff members regarding personality of the patient	20

13. Felt pressured (within self) into doing things rather
     than coping with feeling elements (tension present)   13
14. Avoided needs of family members   13
15. Prejudiced toward group of which patient was a
     member   13
16. Short-staffed; too little time to devote to the patient   7
17. Lacked training in recognizing social-emotional
     needs of patients   7
18. Failed to seek authoritative advice regarding innova-
     tion   7
19. Lost professional role: patient became friend   7
20. Felt guilty but still would not communicate   7
21. Afraid would break down and cry in front of patient   0
22. Overidentified due to being similar age to patient   0
23. Incapacitated by own fear of death   0
24. Disregarded own judgment because wanted approval
     of senior staff members   0

A nurse describes her experience as a nursing consultant to the senior citizens' branch of a national foundation.

For over 3 years we collected data; visited approximately 200 homes; talked to residents, administrators, and nursing personnel; assessed facilities and residents regarding load of care, organization of nursing unit, staffing needs, activation programs, etc. Then we evaluated the data and set up guidelines to assist in developing, maintaining, and/or upgrading the programs in nursing units (e.g., the need for staff in-service education to provide greater job satisfaction and a safe, optimal level of care for residents). We presented workshops to assist the staff in homes for the aged to better understand the elderly, i.e., their physical and mental disabilities, individual needs, etc. Although a number of nurses expressed interest in developing programs in their facilities, the majority of homes for the aged and staff we had hoped to reach felt that they were already too busy to start something else, too short-staffed, or their residents didn't like change. Many nurses commented on my attitudes and approach as being genuinely sincere, but said that "It would never work in our home" or "Sounds great but not attainable." Many, it seemed, had given up on trying.

A nursing supervisor describes her convictions about the importance of helping young nurse interns to face the issue of liking/disliking to work with the elderly.

When our geriatric ward was first opened (a unit in a large general hospital) it was all unhappy: the patients, the nursing staff, and the medical staff; morale was at an all-time low! The climate of this area permeated by word of mouth throughout the hospital and one could hear the ward referred to as the senility ward or, even worse, the vegetable patch. Gradually, this dreadful attitude changed through the support and understanding and encouragement given to the staff, positive attitudes began to rub off, and a mature philosophy of life evolved. Today it is a popular area of the hospital and the consensus seems to be that it is a great place to work, even though it is considered to be one of the busiest areas. It is a ward that is shown with pride to medical and hospital visitors.

In supervisory work, much can be done on a day-to-day basis in general conversations with medical and nursing staff, by attitudes, and by example. This is an ever-ongoing process. In working specifically with the nurse intern group (third-year university nursing students assuming administrative duties and responsibilities) I feel that I have helped them to feel the deep personal satisfaction that they can derive from caring for these patients even though responses of appreciation and gratitude are not often found. The young nurse can become sensitive to the patient's loneliness in this stage of life and come to feel that her care and interest are indeed comforting.

To the 21-year-old life is full of excitement, expectations, and opportunities; life to the 81-year-old is looking back instead of ahead. Even though they look at life from varying points of view, each can benefit from sharing ideas. In our society the emphasis is on youth, which widens the gap between young and old. Studies show that a great number of student nurses aspire to do pediatric nursing. They say the infants are lovable, even though they can be messy. What is so different about caring for the aged?

Working with the aged gives the nurse intern an opportunity to develop and verbalize her philosophy of life, which is helpful in the process of maturation. I feel very strongly that the nurse interns need this kind of help, and without support and understanding negative attitudes develop.

Yes, defenses to protect their own fears.

As a young nurse, I had feelings of depression at the thought of old age, futility when good recovery was not apparent, and helplessness and hopelessness at the time of death.

Much has been written documenting our society's unwillingness to really commit itself to caring about the elderly. That *liked the patient* and *wanted to understand how patient felt,* or conversely, *disliked patient* and *did not want to understand* are crucial factors in this area is confirmed by the fact that these Response factors rate highest and second-highest in relation to Elderly as compared with all other Conditions.

Almost inevitably, the question of the patient's dependence/independence becomes a focal point in the nurse-patient relationship. The following cases illustrate the conflicts and complexity of emotions that are involved as both patients and nurses struggle with these questions.

Mr. W was an elderly single man who was admitted to the hospital with a diagnosis of osteoarthritis. He walked with a cane, slowly and very unsteadily, and seemed always about to fall at the next step. However, he was living alone, cooking his meals, and going out when necessary to shop, etc. He was very independent and refused assistance at walking, his bath, etc. Eventually, he began to allow me to help him, to tell me about where he was living, about his illness and the difficulties he had had. He seemed to be a nice old man who was lonely and glad to have someone interested in him. However, when something happened to upset him, e.g., an orderly in a hurry who was abrupt with him, he became almost a different person. He became angry, using loud and rude language, and very independent, saying that he had a right to good treatment, he could have the orderly lose his job, etc.

A clue to his underlying fears: a loss of self-worth at the end of his life—he was determined to be as capable as the next fellow, perhaps all this man had was himself so he had to protect his image of himself, appearing well in command of himself and others.

My first reaction was to be annoyed at him for getting so upset about what seemed to be a minor incident. I tried calmly to explain that the orderly was not being rude to him in particular but unfortunately had an abrupt manner, although he was really very kind. (This was true.) Mr. W became less angry and seemed apologetic. We continued in this manner throughout Mr. W's stay in hospital, with him varying from being a kind and lonely old man, to a very difficult patient.

However, it became apparent to the medical staff that Mr. W was not able to live alone and look after himself. It was partly my job to discuss this with him and try to convince him that it would be a good idea for him to live somewhere he could have his meals and housekeeping services, but where he would be independent otherwise. Mr. W was completely against this. He began to talk about signing himself out of the hospital, for various reasons. When one reason was removed we discovered that he had another one.

In the meantime I spent what seemed like hours trying to convince Mr. W that he could not go back to his room. Sometimes he would seem to be listening and I would feel that I was making progress, then in the end he would refuse.

Sometimes he would do all the talking about why he felt the way he did and I could not get a word in at all. His mood would continue to change violently and unpredictably. When he was calm and quiet I would feel that he was just lonely and that I should be very patient and understanding. But I felt that I was spending more time than I could afford listening to the same story repeated, and getting nowhere. When Mr. W got angry I would get annoyed with him and feel that he was a stubborn and impossible patient who was causing more trouble than he had a right to. This feeling was strengthened by the fact that the other patients would get upset and angry when he was loud and rude. Also the opinion that he wanted to be independent in order to continue drinking made me less sympathetic to his feelings.

Mr. W finally signed himself out of the hospital, refusing an appointment to come back to the clinic. I still feel that he was a lonely old man, very proud and independent, who wanted help but was unwilling to accept it. Perhaps greater patience and understanding on my part would have altered the situation. Perhaps it would be necessary to work with him over a longer period of time than an active treatment hospital allows in order to gain his confidence and have him accept help. Although I may have helped him to feel that someone was concerned about his welfare, I was completely unsuccessful in helping Mr. W to accept the kind of care he needed.

*   *   *   *

One morning a phone call from a distant city requested a visiting nurse to call upon an old lady living by herself. It was her son who phoned. He told us he had not seen his mother for some time. There was a communication break between his mother and his family. That afternoon I made my first visit. I was shocked! The house was in a dreadful condition. The odor was indescribable. Old, moldy food was spread on every table in the house. Newspapers, several layers thick, covered all the floors. Flies were buzzing around. A little old lady, seemingly ill, was resting on a sofa. Her clothes were very dirty and obviously had not been changed for some time. She was weak, pale, and very thin.

I explained who I was and my presence there. I told her who had sent us. She said, "Oh, he never had time for me. I don't want him now, thank you; I am managing fine." She had a certain dignity about her. I agreed with her about managing fine, but said I would be back. She could not tell me the name of her doctor. "Haven't needed one lately," she said.

When I returned to the office, I contacted her son and told him about the conditions in his mother's house. He did not know her doctor's name and said he was sorry, but could do nothing for her. He would be responsible for our fee.

From then on I felt responsible for Mrs. P. After some phoning I located her doctor, who had not seen her in the last 10 years. He agreed to see her that evening. We met at Mrs. P's house, and he suggested moving her to a hospital. Mrs. P was not going to go anywhere. Her physician diagnosed her illness to be gastroenteritis. She would need special diets and lots of fluids, but Mrs. P could not be persuaded to leave her house. She would not let me give her a bed bath or change her clothing. She slept on the sofa. She was my first patient the next morning.

I visited twice the next few days, giving her fluids and some solids, trying to clean the worst of the dirt out of the house. She recovered rapidly and was very pleased with my visiting her so often. I decided she needed a housekeeper, but she was not going to have one! In the meantime the office had contacted her son again and suggested his mother be moved to a nursing home. He told us that an application to one had been made some time ago, but his mother had refused.

The next day, when chatting with Mrs. P, I mentiond nursing homes to her. She ignored this, but let me give her a sponge bath and change her clothing. She obviously was a little senile, but I became very fond of her. She had an old-fashioned vase on a shelf and I admired it. She said, ''Take it. I have not used it in years!'' ''Let's get some flowers and put it on the table,'' I said. She seemed very pleased and had recovered remarkably.

Every day I tried to talk her into leaving the house, pointing out the advantages of a nursing home. She refused. After some weeks I only went in every few days. At that time we began to be very busy and I looked after another area, but she was still my patient, as she was so used to me. I promised to drop by in 3 days. Five days went by until I went back.

Mrs. P was lying on the sofa. She had a winter coat on in spite of the heat. A small suitcase was standing beside her and the vase she always wanted me to have. Mrs. P had died! I could not believe it. The doctor said she must have died 2 days earlier. She had packed her case to go to a nursing home, after I had talked about it for so long. I had promised to be back in 3 days and had not come. She had the vase ready for me to take. I felt terribly sorry that she had died so alone while waiting for me. I had a strong feeling of guilt. She probably would have died in a nursing home very soon, but the fact that she was dressed and waiting for me made it terrible.

Yes, how very sad. And no amount of rationalizing about how busy you were can really help you. Yet you reached out to this woman in a warm, caring way, which, in turn, made it possible for her to realize that security could be found in avenues other than total independence from everyone. And that was a great gift.

In the following cases, the nurses point out that involved in the issue of liking and wanting to understand the aging patient is often an accompanying dislike of their relatives and therefore a breakdown in the patient's care.

I had as one of my weekly patients an elderly widow who lived alone with only her cat for company. Her only child, a daughter, lived with her husband and two children only a few blocks away, but they seldom visited her. Her daughter did, however, own the five-room bungalow in which this woman lived and assumed responsibility for the taxes, electricity, fuel, and phone. Mrs. W's only income was Social Security, out of which she bought her food, clothes, and medicine. The latter took up a good portion of her monthly check and was patent or prescription medicine of long standing. She was actually fairly comfortable as compared to many elderly people living only on a pension.

Since I was her only visitor, this lonely lady looked forward to my weekly visit, and over a period of time she came to depend on it so much that she resented any other nurse visiting in my place. Therein lay my first mistake. I should have maintained a more professional attitude with her so that it would be the nurse she awaited eagerly and not the person. I understand now that warmth and empathy could have been communicated within the nurse-patient relationship and not on such a personal level.

You were right, however, that this woman needed someone on a personal level.

As time went on Mrs. W confided in me her deep disappointment in her daughter. She believed that Elsie had always been her father's girl, and that when he died she couldn't be bothered with her mother. The occasional times that they were together Elsie would complain about how busy she was keeping house and looking after her two boys. I found this very hard to take, since I, as a recent widow, was bringing up three children alone, working, visiting my own parents regularly, and was the main emotional support of my widowed mother-in-law, who had lost her husband and son in the same year. I grew to almost hate this woman who had no time for her lonely mother and instead of trying to improve the relationship between them I sided completely with Mrs. W. I let my own personal feelings, because of my own situation, become involved. I also realize now it is not right to compare what one person does with what another can manage. Some people just simply have more energy or drive than others. There may have been some very good reasons why this daughter could not manage to spend some time with her mother.

Because of the seeming neglect of her family, I got into the habit of buying things for Mrs. W. What I should have been doing was teaching her to budget her money. Since she did have many of her needs looked after, such as housing, utilities, and fuel, the pension should have covered extras, like underwear and slippers, which she said she could not afford. The patent medicines were a complete waste of money and I should have been able to bring her to an understanding of this.

Mrs. W was constantly complaining about her lack of money, very upset about her daughter's indifference, and growing quite dependent on me. Had I not been so blinded by emotion because this woman's daughter seemed to have everything and yet withheld love and companionship from her mother, I might have worked more constructively. I could have tried to bridge the gap between them and I certainly should have encouraged Mrs. W to be more independent.

A very sensitive assessment of both yourself and your patient. It would be very difficult not to become overidentified with Mrs. W out of her need to place you in a substitute daughter role, and out of your own personal experience with loss and loneliness. It is very true that professionals often become so angry at the rest of the family (i.e., the daughter in this case) that we also shut them out. As you suggest, a reconciliation should have been explored here; failing that, someone who might have had the time (uncomplicated by a professional role) to be a daughter substitute might have been a solution (e.g., a lonely daughter who needed a mother substitute!)—sometimes such a person can be found even within the patient's wider family connections, or can be a volunteer visitor from a nearby church, etc.

*   *   *   *

This case concerns an 80-year-old woman, Mrs. D, and her 47-year-old unmarried daughter, Miss D, who worked at a part-time job.

The doctor at General Hospital diagnosed Mrs. D as senile dementia when she was there under observation. Our orders as visiting nurses were to visit 3 times a week in order to bathe her and to assist her in walking. Mrs. D, on observation, needed constant supervision because it was apparent by the bruises on her body that she had had numerous falls. Since Mrs. D was so senile, it was obvious that she was unable to do the simplest of tasks for herself. It was essential that her daughter help her, but unfortunately Miss D was not caring for her mother properly.

My immediate reaction to this case was that Mrs. D should be in a nursing home and this was confirmed by my supervisor and fellow workers. After discussing this with the daughter and getting negative results, I took a dislike to her and this, of course, set up a barrier between us. Apparently she did not want her mother in a nursing home because "they" would take her money and she felt that she deserved her mother's money.

Instead of trying to understand the daughter by discovering more about her, I talked to her in an authoritative, impersonal manner. Since my concern was for my patient, I should have at least tried to gain the daughter's confidence by offering to find out more about placing her mother in an inexpensive place or finding someone to be with her at home. Nothing seemed to go well and instead of getting closer to the daugher I was drawing further and further away, until eventually she thought of me as a threat.

Although I used some available resources, such as speaking to the public health nurse in the district and trying to find a family doctor, I didn't follow through and act as a liaison in order to establish rapport with Mrs. D and her daughter. After a few months I was able to get a doctor to visit Mrs. D and speak with her daughter about a nursing home. She finally consented, but Mrs. D died before going. It was discovered that she had an aortic aneurysm.

Being so preoccupied with the new experience of working with people in their own environment, I can see now that I was more concerned about how I was going to cope, rather than working with my patient, Mrs. D, and her daughter in reaching the best solution for them.

It is only relatively recently that there has been recognition of the elderly as people to whom sexual expression may remain very important and whose self-identity in this regard can become very undermined and threatened. That this area can pose a real problem to the nurse in terms of *liked the patient* and *wanted to understand how patient felt* is vividly described.

Mr. D is 80 years old, a healthy and energetic individual. Mr. D's wife, Edna, suffered a stroke 3 years ago, leaving her completely incapacitated. When Mrs. D was discharged from the hospital Mr. D refused to have her sent to a nursing home; he planned to manage her complete care himself. At the time of discharge Edna's sister was also in the home, but due to differences of opinion, left.

Visiting nurses found Mr. D a very opinionated man who at times was difficult to work with. He wanted his wife's care done in a special way, and he became quite hostile if he doubted any nurse's capabilities to carry out his wishes.

I began visiting Mrs. D, giving her nursing care three times a week. Mr. D started to trust me as time went by and a mutual friendship developed. He realized I honestly cared for his wife, and he was very grateful for this.

I started to understand Mr. D's feelings of antagonism toward nurses, myself included. Mr. D felt responsible for his wife's physical care, possibly because of guilt. He was very sorry for the amount of suffering Mrs. D had had, and wanted to make her as comfortable as possible. He was very kind and loving to his wife, always thinking of her well-being. He would often hug Mrs. D in trying to elicit some response, but often to no avail.

Mr. D became very cooperative and friendly, often helping me with Mrs. D's care. I quite enjoyed his company, as often the family will run away as soon as the nurse arrives to care for the patient. Mr. D would take my hand and thank me for my help, sometimes putting his arm around my shoulder. I felt at the time it was just a way of showing his approval. Later, however, he tried to kiss me on the cheek when I was leaving from a visit. After the second time, this did bother me, but I did not want to hurt Mr. D's feelings—or maybe even my own. (Like everyone else, I like to be liked, and maybe I was afraid of hurting that relationship.) I tried jokingly to tell Mr. D I had a very jealous husband who would not appreciate Mr. D's advances. Mr. D just shrugged and said, "Your husband won't care if you don't tell him."

The situation gradually went from bad to worse. Each visit was like a small nightmare to me as I hurried to get out of the apartment before Mr. D could get near me. As long as I was doing my nursely duties, he was a perfect gentleman.

I discussed the problem with my supervisor. Her only comment was that if I had not allowed Mr. D to call me by my first name when I started visiting I would not have had this problem. A lot of help that was! I needed to know what to do.

The climax came when one day, as I was getting on my coat, Mr. D grabbed me by the shoulders and kissed me on the mouth. I have never thought of myself as a prude but I can imagine the look of surprise on my face. All I can remember is mumbling good-bye and running out the door. How very professional!

For 2 days I dreaded the next visit. I made up my mind to take the direct approach. I could not be the sniveling child-nurse any longer.

On my day of calling, I coolly and calmly walked up to Mr. D, asking him to talk with me in private for a few minutes. I explained to him that I thought he was a very nice man, but that he had to realize I was the nurse and he was the patient's husband. (I wanted to convey to him that I thought he was an attractive man, and not at all repulsive—but I didn't want him to kiss me.) Mr. D looked rather startled at first, but said he would do whatever I wanted.

I had accomplished my purpose but I did not feel very proud of myself. I had not answered this man's need. He still needed someone to give and receive his affection as his wife was incapable of this.

Since my leaving the district, the nurse who has replaced me has also had problems with amorous advances by Mr. D. I guess he felt that with a new nurse "nothing ventured, nothing gained."

*   *   *   *

As a visiting nurse I do active nursing care on people in their homes. Mr. B was a 76-year-old bachelor, quite active, living alone in a rooming house. He appeared very lonely with few interests outside of watching television, playing chess with himself, and drinking beer at the hotel. (If he wasn't an alcoholic he was certainly a heavy drinker.) My role was to scrub his back and apply medicine to heal a large number of carbuncles.

The problem with this patient started when he began to touch me, I thought, unnecessarily. This made me feel very uncomfortable and defensive in his presence. I was firm with him, stating, "I don't like having you pat me, or kiss my hand, or try to kiss me. I am here to heal your back and that's all!" He would apologize afterwards and I would think maybe I was making too much of this. When I explained the problem I was having to our liaison nurse, she replied, "If he doesn't stop, we'll discharge him from home care." I felt sympathetic towards him—his family was all dead and he really had no one to care for his back—so I continued visiting. I felt that at my age, I should have been able to handle a 76-year-old man.

I found I started disliking him and felt repulsed by him, even though I felt sorry for him. I would avoid being close to him except when I was doing his back. If I became friendly at all, as I do with most patients, he would try to touch me again. I was very uncomfortable in his presence, and felt his touching was an invasion of my privacy.

Mr. B tried to please me during this time. He drank very little. (He was taking medicine at the time and it was better for him not to drink.) I should have followed this up in some way at this time to encourage him not to drink in the future, but I didn't. Because of my feelings, I spent as little time with him as possible.

He told me, "I become very depressed at times. I feel that there is nothing to live for." I replied, "What about your friends? They care for you." But I did not encourage Mr. B to talk about these feelings. I would leave quickly, because if I showed I cared he would reciprocate with some sort of body contact.

He often said, "I don't know what I'll ever do when you don't come any more." He would have tears in his eyes when he said this. I didn't want him to become dependent on me; I really didn't know how to handle it and so would reply, "Oh, you'll manage like you did before I came. You still have your friends at the hotel." There again I didn't encourage any personal feelings—his or mine.

At one point Mr. B said, "You probably think because I'm 76 years old I don't have any sexual feelings—but that's not true." At this point I became both repulsed and guarded and replied, "I hadn't thought that." There again I discouraged any further communication. I really let Mr. B down by not allowing him to express his sexual feelings—and this certainly would have helped for a better nurse-patient relationship. But because I felt repelled by this old man with no teeth and pimples all over his body, the last thing I wanted to get involved in was a conversation about sex. I see now I could not cope with such a discussion.

I encouraged him to go to a senior citizens' club. If I had investigated it further, and found someone to take him, probably he would have gone. But I let it go at just mentioning it. I also told him about the chess club a block from his home—but there again I didn't take any positive action. I was afraid of becoming too involved with this patient. How would I ever handle it if he became too dependent on me?

I feel now, if instead of being repulsed by his advances I had sat down and held his hand (sometimes touching someone is so important when one is alone) and listened to him, I would not have failed with this man. I would have shown him that I accepted him, and thus he could have accepted himself. This certainly would have helped his drinking problem. If I had been more concerned with his feelings and needs than my own, I would have been able to help him find a place in the social life of his peers, and he would have been lonely no longer.

A new director of nursing in a home for the aged makes a point of touching each resident.

As a matter of routine, I visited the residents in the dining room at breakfast and at lunchtime. As I passed the tables with four residents at each, I made a point to touch each resident on the shoulder or hand, and look at them as I made general comments and smiled. They responded, usually with a smile or hand gesture. I knew they enjoyed it. It was a good feeling! As the days passed the residents began visiting the nursing office and told me how glad they were that I had come to their home. It was all very reassuring, and I didn't really stop to think about what they were telling me. One lady told me that I was so warm and understanding, and she felt that someone really cared when I touched her each day—no one had done that for a long time. A single red rose was delivered to my office "to someone who cares from someone who says thanks"—it was from a 90-year-old gentleman who later said, "You will never know how pleasant it was to have someone touch me."

Compared to all other Situations, it is with regard to the elderly that the nurse most often allows herself to be *negatively influenced by opinions of other staff members regarding personality of the patient.*

I was working over the Christmas holidays. At the time there were approximately 22 patients on the floor and the situation I am going to describe occurred in the evening when the staff consisted of myself, an R.N., and a nursing assistant.

Mrs. G was an old lady of about 78, who was in the hospital due to diabetes, heart complications, and general problems related to old age. She was cantankerous, demanding, ungrateful, and stubborn, according to the nursing notes, so I immediately pictured the "pointed hat with the broom" image and poor Mrs. G didn't have a chance!

That night we were really busy with several very ill patients and were doing minimum amount of care on those who were not acutely in need of attention.

Mrs. G was immediately clumped in with the latter. When I was carrying IV bottles to the other end of the floor she'd be wailing for a bedpan. When I was giving injections to relieve pain, she'd have a dizzy spell coming on; when I was putting up blood she was sure she was going to die, couldn't I come and talk to her. Whine, ring, grumble, complain!

Finally, with nerves frayed (but not just by Mrs. G), I figured she was the only well person who could really take my anger, so I really let her have it. Who in the nursing profession hasn't uttered these lines before: "You're not the only one who's sick on this ward, you know. I have other people to look after too! After all, you've got a lot to be thankful for; there are a lot more people who are far sicker than you are, you know. Why can't you be more considerate of the other patients? Can't you see you're bothering them by always ringing for the nurse! If you don't stop ringing that bell for these little things, I'm going to take it away from you. It's only to be used in emergencies!''

With my speech completed, I left, feeling a small pang of guilt mind you, but I still left. Going up the hall 5 minutes later I noticed Mrs. G had pulled her curtains and her light was turned off. Being caught up again with routine activities I didn't think anything more about it. Toward the end of the shift I was making final rounds and left Mrs. G till the end, partly because I was sure she'd want something and partly because I was feeling uneasy, for she had not uttered a sound since I had given her my lecture.

Upon coming into her cubicle, I noticed her eyes were shut but she didn't appear to be sleeping. I asked very quietly if she was awake, with no answer. Feeling really uncomfortable by this time, for I had noticed two tears trickling down her cheeks, I made a pretense of fixing up her bedside table. Finally, a small voice said, "Nurse, I'm sorry I'm such a bother, sometimes I get really lonely." Her eyes were still shut.

At this point I really did feel miserable and not trusting my mouth (it had done enough harm) I held her hand for a few minutes. I felt so uncomfortable and ill-at-ease because of my own feelings of guilt that there was not one constructive thing I could think of to say to help this woman with her most obvious needs as she suffered feelings of fear, loneliness, and isolation. Quietly saying that I was sorry too, I left the room.

This could have been handled so much better professionally as well as humanely if I had not prejudged her, if after becoming annoyed with her many requests I had realized why she was making them and set some time out to talk to her about her feelings. Instead, I took my own frustrations out on her, causing her to have an even greater feeling of fear and isolation as well as guilt for being such a nuisance. Even at the end, because of my own guilt feelings I wasn't able to help her.

Any ideas as to what you might have said?

This, I feel, is one of the greatest flaws you run into in nursing—rationalizing that because you don't have the time you can cease to try and make the time for the little things, for they count just as much as the dramatic life-saving ones!

That being *negatively influenced by opinions of other staff members regarding the personality of the patient* sets in motion the circle of *failure to look beyond initial negative impression* (53% of cases); *did not want to understand* (53% of cases) and *rationalized actions and thoughts* (33% of cases) is very evident in the following account.

A common X ray procedure is the carotid arteriogram, which shows the blood circulation of the brain. It is a very uncomfortable procedure. Using local anesthesia a large needle is placed into the carotid artery located in the neck. A radiopaque solution is then injected into the artery accompanied by a hot sensation. The patient is placed on a table with his head sharply bent backward. Since the table is narrow—and also because the patient could grab the needle—his hands are tied and a strap placed over his legs. Intravenous sedation is given only (1) if the patient is fully conscious and apprehensive, or (2) if the patient is very restless and confused.

My patient arrived from the emergency department with a diagnosis of a possible brain hemorrhage. A radiologist walked by and commented, ''Hum, a classical case of dementia.'' The elderly man who was lying quietly on his stretcher did indeed appear confused. My first error was to assume that the patient was confused and I left with the rest of the room for a coffee break. No one spoke to the patient or explained that the procedure would be delayed a short while.

On our return, we attempted to move the patient over to the table. Although he understood our rather curt directions, he became upset and stated that before he would move he had to go to the YMCA and pay for his room. This was greeted with a few laughs from the people present. I did nothing to help the situation by stilling the laughter or by my own manner when I said, ''OK, as soon as this is over, then you can go.''

By this time many people were in the room so the patient was firmly assisted to the table. I did not explain the procedure to the patient as I still assumed that he was totally confused and would not understand me anyway. Therefore, the man suddenly found his neck extended and his hands tied against the table.

On calling the resident to carry out the procedure, I repeated the staff doctor's instant diagnosis and laughed and said that the patient wanted to pay his room rent at the YMCA. I also said, ''I suppose you'll want some sedation,'' in such a manner to imply that it was absolutely necessary in order to be able to carry out the examination. When the resident entered the room, he merely glanced at the patient. Almost always, even in cases of confusion, the doctors introduce themselves and give some explanation of the procedure. Undoubtedly, my recounting of the patient's behavior influenced the resident enough to convince him that the patient was "too far out" to bother.

At this point, we did the first thing right since the patient had appeared in X ray. Although without an explanation, we did give IV sedation so the patient slept throughout the examination.

At the end of the procedure I was noting the patient's insurance number, age, address, etc., for the records. Under address was written YMCA, 55 College Street.

I feel my reasons for my not being helpful in this situation are only too apparent. I should never have taken the staff doctor's statement regarding the patient's confusion as the absolute truth. Certainly the patient was confused but he could have received benefit from a simple explanation and some honestly expressed reassurance. I should not have been so definite in my opinions to the resident, as I influenced his assessment of the patient. My unprofessional behavior in the room (i.e., condoning the laughter, giving false reassurance) did not set a standard for the other staff members to follow.

I might add that the technicians and myself felt very badly about this situation with the result that more consideration resulted from our experience.

In this case, the nurse specifically asks herself to what degree she should be influenced by generally accepted nursing theory and practice as opposed to treating particular situations.

I will now take a look at a situation in which I do not feel as though I even got to first base, let alone tried to be helpful.

I visited an elderly gentleman by the name of Mr. M, aged 93, once a week to assist with a sponge bath. Mr. M was quite capable and would have been able to do his own bath if the bathtub was not on the second floor; he would have had to climb approximately 15 stairs. He took no medications whatsoever.

I usually tried to arrange my visit for 11:00 A.M. so that he might sleep late. He was always sound asleep when I entered his bedroom, but arose quickly when he heard me. When questioned about not sleeping well he stated that he slept soundly from 9:00 P.M. until 11:00 A.M. the next morning. After his bath he dressed himself and came to the kitchen to eat breakfast. His sister, with whom he lived, stated he slept until 1:00 P.M. the days I did not come, and even then she had to tell him to get up. After breakfast he sat in his rocking chair in the kitchen, staying there until supper, at which time he went to the dining room.

Shortly after dinner he retired to his bedroom. He did not read, go out for a walk, or even watch television, which at one time he had enjoyed.

I lightly brought the subject up one day of going out for a walk with me and he laughed and said he hadn't been out for 2 years. I asked why and he said, "There's nothing to go out for a walk for." I thought that possibly he felt unsure of his footing when walking by himself so I proceeded to order a walker. However, this arrived and sat in the corner collecting dust.

During several visits I emphasized the importance of fresh air and exercise and what would happen to his body if he continued to neglect it. I could have been talking to a brick wall and have gotten further.

During our training it was emphasized that there is great importance in getting a patient up and walking after surgery, and so it is with the elderly. We must get them socializing, playing card games, and the like. We do not listen to what the patient wants but we do what we know is best for the patient.

Have people Mr. M's age not had enough socializing in their time? Maybe they're quite content to just sit and watch the world go by. Mr. M could not see any reason in getting all this exercise and perhaps I should be asking myself the same question. Why should I be trying to make life miserable for him when he is quite content doing what he is doing—simply because I have been taught that we must keep everyone active? I am caught between my emotions. I see the relevance of theory in regards to exercise maintaining a healthy body, but I can also see my patient's point of view. What applies in theory does not always apply in practice. Another example would be not allowing a 95-year-old man apple pie because the crust is too high in fat content, which would increase his chance of a stroke. Why not give him what he wants; he may not have too much longer to enjoy it!

For us to be taught one thing but turn around and preach another is a very difficult thing to do. Even today I have not really come to grips as to what I should have done for Mr. M.

One is inclined to agree with your philosophy as long as you really understand what your patient is saying about himself and why, and that together you have examined all the alternatives and consequences.

12
COLLEAGUE RELATIONSHIP

Of the 550 cases in the study, 8% focus on the Colleague Relationship. Of the 43 cases that focus on the Colleague Relationship, 40% are described as Helpful, 60% as Unhelpful.

COMPARISON WITH ALL OTHER SITUATIONS

Unhelpful Factors

Highest Rating

- Failed to seek authoritative advice regarding innovation.
- Disregarded own judgment because wanted approval of senior staff members.

Helpful Factors	% of Cases in Which Cited
1. Gave moral support	61
2. Helped patient express feelings	61
3. Wanted to understand how patient felt	56
4. Took time to explain	50
5. Was a sounding board	39
6. Nonjudgmental	39
7. Looked beyond patient's outward response/behavior to underlying causes	28
8. Used innovative rehabilitative procedure	28

9. Positively identified with patient due to similar life/
    professional experience   28
10. Came to terms with own feelings; was able to enter in-
    to patient's problem   17
11. Initiated referral to another profession/resource   17
12. Not unduly influenced by negative opinions of other
    staff regarding the patient's personality   17
13. Helped family members   11
14. Made this case the basis for overall policy change/
    improvement   6
15. Was trying to prove self to senior staff members   6
16. Had received training in recognizing social-emotional
    needs of patients   6
17. Was honest with patient/relatives   6
18. Liked the patient   0
19. Discussed religion with patient   0
20. Used physical closeness   0

Unhelpful Factors	% of Cases in Which Cited
1. Failed to look beyond initial negative impression of patient's personality	44
2. Self-image was threatened	40
3. Felt guilty but could not communicate	32
4. Treated the condition, overlooking the patient	28
5. Did not want to understand	28
6. Was disapproving, judgmental	28
7. Felt inadequate to enter into patient's problem because had not personally resolved the issue	24
8. Breakdown of interprofessional communication/cooperation	24
9. Purposely disregarded significant cues in patient's statements/behavior	24
10. Rationalized actions and thoughts	16
11. Lacked training in recognizing social-emotional needs of patients	16
12. Failed to seek authoritative advice regarding innovation	16
13. Negatively influenced by opinions of other staff members regarding personality of the patient	12

14.	Disregarded own judgment because wanted approval of senior staff members	12
15.	Disliked patient	12
16.	Felt guilty but still would not communicate	12
17.	Felt pressured (within self) into doing things rather than coping with feeling elements (tension present)	8
18.	Prejudiced toward group of which patient was a member	8
19.	Short-staffed; too little time to devote to the patient	4
20.	Lost professional role: patient became friend	4
21.	Afraid would break down and cry in front of patient	0
22.	Avoided needs of family members	0
23.	Overidentified due to being similar age to patient	0
24.	Incapacitated by own fear of death	0

The influence of other staff opinions and the need for staff approval may prompt the nurse to *disregard her own judgment*. This response is highest across all Situations in the Colleague Relationship.

Until I joined the staff of the Corbin County Health Unit, I nursed part-time at our 63 bed, hometown hospital. In this type of setting most of the patients are repeaters and well known to the nursing staff. The nurses also know each other well and this leads to a type of familiarity about the patient and his needs that I don't think is healthy. Many times at report and in the time we were doing our charting for the day, the nurses would remark about how stupid a certain patient was or state he had nothing between the ears and similar derogatory remarks that had nothing to do with the patient's physical condition.

As the mother of a retarded child, these remarks really hurt me. As a nurse and as a mother I should have spoken up in the patients' defense. I was afraid to express my true feelings and I think I failed in my responsibility. I just hope that if my son were ever a patient there that the staff could see him as a suffering human being and not just a dum-dum.

I worried more about what the staff would think of me if I spoke up than I did of their two-faced nursing care.

Here the nurse explains the ways in which her (nurse) role and the image of the hospital as competent and caring were undermined by colleagues in the emergency department and again on the ward.

The two situations chosen for analysis of self in a helpful and unhelpful situation are recent occurrences, and for me particularly emotional occasions, as they highlighted a series of deplorable parent-nurse relationships that had besieged our floor, a pediatric isolation unit.

Peter, a formerly vigorous and alert 9-month-old baby, was admitted to our floor at mid-evening. He was unconscious and his respirations were becoming increasingly distressed. A diagnosis of encephalitis had been made. We had been expecting Peter and as the nurse in charge I had just managed to arrange competent nurse coverage, even though the patient assignments were extremely difficult for each nurse on duty that evening.

Peter was certainly no candidate for shared care. The nurse in emergency had not told me of his actual condition; she had said that he was irritable, but not critically ill. She had possibly confused names, as so often happens. We were aghast when we saw the condition of the baby and I was appalled when I saw his parents. They appeared dazed; they did not respond to anything in our official questions about Peter. They appeared frightened, anxious, and grief-stricken.

As Peter's nurse began to tend to him, my next concern became the parents. After a quick consultation with the resident, we agreed upon what realistic approaches we could define for the parents. I was to be allowed the use of cases in past occasions to make my point if necessary. Anything that would establish some hope was to be used. I urged them to come with me and we would leave the room for a short while. I told them that they could return to stay with the baby as long as they wished. They came quickly, saying very little in response to my quiet monologue about the nature of the isolation unit and the unusual techniques of gowning, masking, and restricting visitors, the latter to be waived in this situation.

At this time I was attempting diversion from the crisis and in my further explanations, I tried to make them feel that they would be helping us to help Peter. They appeared to be more relaxed as we settled into the lounge. Peter's father said to me as we sat down, "You didn't know he was that sick did you?" I had to reply no, and then I elaborated somewhat upon how frequently we do see children with this illness and how in time we become prepared for such emergencies. Peter's mother then told me that the baby had been well up to the morning of the day of admission, but she had been unable to arouse him from his early afternoon nap. They had then rushed Peter to the hospital and had waited about 4 hours for him to be admitted. In the interim there had been two brief visits from the doctor to give information about Peter's progress, but no visits from the nurses. The parents had been left alone with their imaginations, and their concern and fears became magnified.

I then told them that there would be several people in the unit who would be able to give them accurate current information about the baby's condition. I stressed that at first Peter's illness required the almost constant attention of the doctor and he might on occasion be less free to keep them informed. As they became more openly expressive of their fears, I was able to offer the realistic and yet optimistic points of view suggested by the resident. Encouraging and reinforcing their response with positive aspects appeared to relax them somewhat and I felt that we had successfully established a groundwork for communication in preparation for what was to come.

Several days later I did not support the family and in doing so allowed them to cast very well-placed doubt about the ability of the unit staff to care for the child.

Baby Peter's respirations at this time required the support of an artificial respirator. The nurse caring for the child had allowed blockage of the tracheal tube and Peter subsequently experienced a respiratory arrest. Fortunately a resident was immediate to the room and Peter's breathing soon returned to normal with technical assistance. In the room during this time were Peter's parents. They told me shortly after the incident that they had remarked to the nurse that the child was having respiratory difficulty and his color was rather pale as well. They suggested that she call a doctor. She refused, saying that Peter really seemed all right and that they were not to worry. Peter's parents were intelligent people, and were not passive. They had had experiences with brisk nurses and seemed to be winning the war of personalities. But they had on this occasion decided to remain calm and unobtrusive for there really might not be reason for overconcern.

As we discussed the incident in the corridor outside Peter's room, the clinical instructor walked by us and we heard her comment in passing with a young student, "Peter would never have arrested if there had been a student in there!" Peter's father asked me what she meant and I could reply only that I didn't know. They turned from me and without a word returned to the child's bedside. I had been honest in my reply, but the implications of the passing comment had left me completely unable to answer his question with tact and without demolishing the speaker who had placed me in this position.

It has been very difficult for me to analyze the use of self in each of the mentioned situations, so I have chosen the concept of role to make my awareness somewhat clearer. The public expect various set attitudes and responses from nurses in their roles and in my first meeting with Peter's parents I acted the role of the nurse as I, and I hope they, had felt it should be played. There were attempts to create calm, to seek a quiet atmosphere, and establish a receptive atmosphere for treatment. Such an atmosphere contributes toward opening up channels of communication through which parent and nurse can help each other to help the patient. If I had become visibly angry with the emergency department I would have cast doubts upon their competence and this would have negated any further efforts by the doctors and the nurses to help Peter and his parents.

There would have been a difference between your expressing anger at the emergency care and letting the parents know you could understand their feelings about what happened there.

I had chosen to stress the positive when I spoke of previous cases the unit had cared for.

As to the comments of the clinical instructor concerning the negligence of Peter's nurse, this threatened me and my staff and my interpretation of my role. How could I explain incompetence, rudeness, and disaster? The instructor was not someone I admired but she did hold a position of responsibility, of which the parents were aware. My role in relation to my profession, loyalty to the hospital, and my reactions personally were so contradictory that the result was paralysis. As yet I have not found a satisfactory alternative as a response within this situation.

Most nurses are motivated by care and concern for patients and staff. Perhaps when we realistically examine and expose what we really want for the public in relation to ourselves, we may resolve these conflicting roles and loyalties for mutual benefit.

The following two accounts raise the familiar issue of potential conflict between nursing service and nursing education colleagues. The first case is recounted as an example of *failed to look beyond initial negative impression* (the most common Unhelpful Response: 44% of cases).

I still cringe when I recollect the terrible result of my incompetence in handling this particular situation.

While I was still a fairly new supervisor, Mrs. Brown, one of my head nurses—quite perturbed—reported to me that an instructor, Mrs. Smith, from one of the affiliating schools of nursing, had, on more than one occasion, reprimanded her students in the patients' rooms. Her concern here was that many of her sick patients were upset by this behavior and had expressed sympathy for the students involved. Mrs. Brown also reported that this instructor had given orders to her students that were contrary to our hospital policy, without asking permission. She requested my intervention in this matter.

I should explain that similar complaints had been received by other supervisors regarding other instructors, and even though the nursing director was aware of this, no formal complaint had ever been lodged.

I failed in my duty because I immediately assumed without further investigation that the information that was communicated to me was true. I was judgmental and acted hastily by informing the assistant director and seeking her guidance in the matter. This, I realized too late, was the wrong approach. I should have handled the situation at my own level, in a quiet, objective, person-to-person discussion in my office. Thus, I would have developed rapport with Mrs. Smith and at the same time I would have enhanced Mrs. Brown's confidence in my own ability to handle situations of this nature.

I failed to accomplish either. The assistant director insisted on having a meeting that would include herself, our director of nursing, Mrs. Brown, the director of the school, Mrs. Smith, two other instructors, and myself. Instead of a simple, positive meeting for clarification and understanding, old grievances were aired and all other errors of other instructors were discussed in a manner that made Mrs. Smith bear the brunt of it all.

In my estimation the meeting ended disastrously because Mrs. Smith felt singled out for persecution and was in tears. I blamed myself because I had lacked the ability to cope with the situation on my own. I did not help because I not only injured the instructor but I embarrassed Mrs. Brown and myself, as the situation ballooned out of proportion. I failed to establish rapport with Mrs. Smith and my method of solving this problem only widened the gap between us so that subsequent encounters were a source of embarrassment to both of us for a long while after. This was not my intention, but that makes me no less guilty, in that I did not weigh the possible results of my action.

It is also unfortunate that the assistant director did not consider offering consultation to you—a new supervisor—rather than running ahead with it. She made a mistake similar to yours, really.

In this case, an outside nursing instructor speaks quite candidly about her subtle attempts to influence the quality of nursing service care.

Our nursing-assistant students make preclinical visits to one of the city's long-term care hospitals. Each instructor in turn accompanies a group of students and so several weeks might elapse between visits. This may make the instructor unfamiliar with the patients on any particular visit and can pose a problem, as she often finds it necessary to check some point of a patient's care with the untrained staff who work in the area, without accepting their method. An instructor is also aware that the staff subtly pressure the students to follow their example by making a reference that the instructor is out of touch with reality. The instructor, in turn, tries to influence the staff wherever possible as she realizes that the most important focus should be the best service that can be given to the patient.

On one visit my student was assigned a 44-year-old man with muscular dystrophy who had regressed to such a point that he was unable to move or feed himself. At report we were told that he had been admitted 4 days previously and had done nothing but complain and demand his pills for pain. As we planned his care, we agreed that there were many reasons for his complaining attitude and felt that we could accept this if it should appear. I also reminded the student that we had noted on previous visits that breakfasts appeared rushed, yet the food carrier remained with the dirty dishes long after the meal was over. In actual fact, nobody would be delayed if Mr. A took longer over breakfast than the generally accepted time.

The student appeared unhurried and the meal went smoothly, yet in fact Mr. A finished eating before the trays were collected from the wards. Mr. A then asked my student for a cigarette and remarked in front of the staff that he dearly loved to smoke, especially after breakfast, but as he could not manage this for himself he had had to go without. The student helped him with the cigarette after finding his supply, which had been locked away at the time of admission.

A little later I said to Mr. A, "You know, I've been thinking about your smoking problem. As you have realized, the staff here are much busier than we are, but I'm sure they could manage to help you enjoy your cigarettes if we could only think of something." Mr. A said, "Well, nobody need stand by the bedside and hold it like she did; I could wait between puffs." The floor nurse joined in at this point and said, "It would take about three cigarettes to get one good smoke at that rate." Mr. A said, "What's wrong with that?" I smiled at the nurse and said, "Let's see how it goes this morning, shall we?"

Before I had my little chat with Mr. A about the smoking, I had tried to interest the staff in Mr. A by pretending to talk confidentially to my student while making sure that they were within earshot. I had complimented my student on the fact that Mr. A had felt so comfortable with her that he could ask her help with the cigarette; I asked her how she felt that she had managed this. The student said she thought it was due to the relaxed mood of breakfast, to which I agreed and reminded her that it had taken no longer than any of the other patients' meals.

I had already found out that Mr. A was a veterinarian and had four children, so during the bed bath I started to ask questions based initially on this information. I made sure the questions and replies were heard by the staff in the room, as I hoped that if they knew more about this patient they might feel more sympathy for him. He seemed happy to talk to us, as his replies were full and expanded. We soon learned about his family, his profession, and the problems of a professional man who was unable to work at his profession. By discussing his present weight we were able to talk about how he looked before his illness, and also to get some idea of the bitterness he felt toward the doctors who had been unable to cure him or provide sufficient relief for his pain.

We knew he was in pain, although he did not mention it specifically, nor ask for any pills. Before we went to coffee I asked him if he would like a sedative as his doctor had ordered it for him and it was well overdue. He replied that he was uncomfortable all the time, but he would prefer to wait till later.

When we returned from coffee, we were happy to see the orderly assisting Mr. A with a cigarette, between making beds and chatting to him about the various breeds of dogs.

I felt that I had been helpful by surmising that the staff had stereotyped Mr. A and were not really seeing him as an individual person. I felt that Mr. A had perceived this for himself, resented it, and was reacting in the only way possible for him. I hoped to make him realize that the best help we could be to him was to act as a bridge to his regular nurses. I think he understood this and that was why he responded so eagerly to my questions, almost as if he were grateful for the opportunity to introduce himself.

I wanted the staff to realize that Mr. A had taken cognizance of the fact that they were busy and that was why he hadn't bothered them with asking for help with his smoking, but also that he could go without pills for pain q.h.4 provided that he got some support. I felt that the staff were ready to listen to our suggestions, albeit second-hand, because we had also appreciated their difficulties and not gone in like do-gooders, in a rather supercilious fashion. I felt I made the experience a meaningful one for my student because I had helped her to resist staff pressure in the first instance and she had not tried to speed up breakfast by the usual methods. Then she had been reinforced in the rightness of her care when Mr. A related to her in such a positive fashion.

During the following week the student came and told me that she had found out that Mr. A had died and that she was so glad that she had been able to be of some help to him.

Failed to look beyond initial negative impression was cited in 44% of Unhelpful Colleague Relationships cases. One of the catalysts behind this response appears to be related to factors of social class, stereotyping, and preconceived notions concerning groups in society to which the colleague may belong.

The following involves an interaction in our visiting nurses' office between a colleague, whom I will call Mary, and myself over the chart of a patient, whom I will call Sue. Mary and I had on occasion a few differences of opinion, which were effected by the 20 years difference in our ages and our different cultural backgrounds. I preferred to avoid contact with her (as did the other staff) on days when I was tired and tended to more easily get into an argument.

This interaction occurred on such a day. I had just returned from my lunch hour, during which I received some upsetting personal news. I had decided to work on some charts, as I knew I was upset and wanted to work on my own.

The situation occurred while I was in the nurse in charge's office, getting some charts. Mary came into the room in her usual flap and asked me for Sue's chart, as Sue had just moved from my district into hers. This patient had made a serious suicidal attempt a few months ago and I had since been working closely with her under the supervision of a psychiatrist. A few days before this situation Sue had contacted me for the first time on her own. It seemed as if after all these months she was beginning to trust and relate to me.

Mary: I need Sue's chart: she is in my district now.

Myself: Oh, I know she is in your district now that her husband is out of jail, but she still stays with friends in my district much of the time.

Mary: That doesn't matter—she lives in my district and I want her chart.

She showed some annoyance in her voice. I was starting to feel angry that she was so stubborn over such an issue. I wished she would leave as I did not want to talk with her this afternoon. I deliberately tried to talk calmly.

Myself: Mary, I would like to follow Sue as I am just starting to get somewhere with her.

Mary: You think you are the only one who can do mental health nursing; you don't think I can handle her!

I felt humiliated and was becoming very angry. I was so pleased with the progress of Sue and now Mary was going to take her. I was also concerned as to whether she really could handle her.

Myself: That's not the point. We need to think of the patient's needs and it seems she needs consistency. I think it would be difficult for her now to be readjusted to someone just when she is beginning to trust me.

Mary: You just think you are better. She is in my district and I want her chart.

Mary, too, was very angry. I felt frustrated and defeated, and wondered how she could be stupid as not to try to recognize the patient's needs.

Myself: OK. You take her chart—I don't care—that's it!

Mary got huffy.

Mary: Well, you don't need to get angry—that's a pretty negative attitude you have.

I was very angry at her and myself now. I tried to control myself and spoke very firmly.

Myself: Mary, take her chart and leave me; I'm busy.

I got my charts and went into my office. Within minutes, I was the only person left in the office. I felt embarrassed and ashamed of myself for acting in such an unprofessional manner at work.

I was preoccupied with my personal problems and allowed them to interfere with my functioning in a professional manner. I realize that one cannot always prevent this. Even though I was aware I was upset, I was unable to tell Mary that I was upset. I could have suggested that we discuss the issue the next day. In this way I could have compiled my thoughts and perhaps proposed a compromise. Instead, I projected some of my uptight feelings about my personal problems onto Mary, which in turn put her on the defensive. I think my voice tone and facial expressions revealed my feelings more than the actual words that were spoken.

I felt very angry toward Mary when she said I thought I was the only one who could handle mental health nursing. This statement threatened me and I was too angry to consider that perhaps I was giving that impression. Ever since we started working together, I have felt inadequate as a nurse around Mary. It seemed she was always letting me know that she had her public health diploma and that she knew more than I did. Mental health nursing is my specialty and the one area that I feel I can handle well. I think I reacted to her statement as a personal threat in that she was taking away a part of the area in nursing in which I felt confident. Also, I was more vulnerable to this interpretation because of my insecurity concerning my personal problems.

At the end of the situation I felt frustrated and defeated. I angrily gave up the patient, just to terminate the discussion. At this point, I was not considering Sue's needs at all. I believed she needed consistency and encouragement in building up a trusting relationship, but I was unable to follow through on this belief because of my anger.

It seems there was a definite generation gap and personality conflict between Mary and myself. I had been aware of it for a long time and had discussed the conflict with my nurse in charge, who also had conflicts with Mary. If we had sat down earlier and discussed our differences, perhaps this situation might have been avoided.

The following two cases describe the issue of prejudice to blacks in Unhelpful Colleague Relationships.

While on the 4–12 tour of duty in the nursing office of a major teaching hospital I received a call from the nurse in charge on one of the non-surgical floors. She said that she was sick and tired of the orderlies in that hospital. They never came when they were called and when they finally did come, they raised a big fuss about everything that they were asked to do. She also said, ''No one ever does anything about it; they just let them get away with murder.'' I told her that I thought she was exaggerating a little, but what was the problem tonight? She told me that she had asked the orderly to take Mr. Z in room 701 off the bedpan. She said that normally because of the difficulty in finding an orderly, she would have gone ahead and done it herself, but this patient was an extremely heavy man and was also very sensitive about females looking at him. As I knew this patient well, I knew that what she said was true. I asked her what the trouble was with the orderly and which one was it? She told me that it was Jack, and that he had been very rude to her for calling him something that she could have done herself when he was busy elsewhere. When she said that it was Jack who was causing the trouble, I recalled that there had been quite a few complaints lately about his work, lateness, and absenteeism. He was the black orderly on our staff and had a rather sullen manner. I told the nurse that I would look into the problem and went up to the floor to investigate.

When I arrived back at the nursing office, after speaking to the patient and the other nurse on duty, I called the switchboard operator and asked her to have Jack come down and see me. After about 20 minutes he arrived, and I could see that he had a very large chip on his shoulder. He was aware of why he had been called down and immediately started to justify his conduct on the basis that he was always being picked on and inferred that it had something to do with his color. He also said that he couldn't understand why the nurses couldn't take the patient off the bedpan when he had so many more important things to do.

I told him that the major concern of the hospital was the patient and the patient came first over all personal feelings. I also told him that Miss D was in charge of the floor and would not call him needlessly. I explained to him that this was a sensitive patient and also a heavy patient for a nurse to manage. In the back of my mind, I really felt as I talked to him that there was wrong on the sides of both the nurse in charge and the orderly. This particular nurse had a very unfortunate manner with personnel and antagonized people with her very brusque way. I felt she could have handled this situation with a little explanation and a little tact as well as a pleasant manner. However, I did feel that my loyalty lay toward her, rather than to the orderly.

Really to both, as well as to subsequent patients of theirs.

This particular orderly when he had first come to us had been an excellent orderly. He had a better education than most and showed signs of great capabilities. I felt that this laxness on his part lately had come about from disinterest in the job, which he felt was beneath him. There was a position coming vacant in the hospital in the near future that I knew he was interested in, and probably would have done well at, namely, the position of inhalation therapist. It only needed a word of recommendation to the proper authorities to have procured the job for him. However, although I have always felt that I am not prejudiced against blacks, I was slightly reluctant about recommending them for any responsible position. Thus, I did nothing constructive for Jack, just gave him a lecture and reported him to higher authorities. This made the third complaint that had been placed against him and because of it he was fired.

When I look back at the situation now I can see that I did nothing to help Jack for two reasons. One was that I guess I have more of a prejudice than I thought I had and the other was a purely selfish reason. I did not wish to get involved in recommending him for a position where there was a chance that he might not work out, as this would have reflected back on me.

But now, after listening to the lectures in medical sociology and the importance of not just hearing the words that people say, but rather what they are saying underneath, I realize that I failed in another way that did not even occur to me at the time. This was in the case of the nurse in charge. Reflecting back on the situation, I can see that she too had problems and when she complained about the orderlies and how difficult they were to get along with, she was really saying, "What is the matter with me, that I have so much trouble with personnel?" I should have realized this and tried to do something for her and I did nothing.

*   *   *   *

During the first week of my new assignment, a meeting was arranged for me to meet the entire staff in the nursing unit (day, evening, and night shifts). I expressed the desire of us working as a team, in attempting to meet the individual needs of the residents; welcomed any suggestions the staff wished to make concerning the program in the nursing unit; assured them of my support in providing safe optimal resident care; requested the staff to submit a list of the duties being performed, so that I could appreciate their load of care; encouraged anyone who was interested in upgrading or continuing their education to discuss it with me for necessary recommendations, etc. After the meeting, a nursing aide approached me and said that she was interested in upgrading herself. She had a family to support and wanted to achieve more professional status, to increase her income. She said that she had taken the practical nurse course, but it was not recognized in our locale, so presently she was attending an evening R.N. course and needed every Monday evening off. I discussed the time sheet with her, made tentative arrangements for her days off, and assured her that I would make an inquiry in regard to her course so that perhaps we could be more supportive to her. She thanked me and said that she would appreciate any help she could get.

The next day, I spoke to the coordinator of the R.N. school. She checked the records and told me that I had been led down the garden path! Records indicated that the aide had dropped out of the practical nurse course before the exams; had attempted screening for application to the R.N. course and failed twice; and on inquiry had not completed elementary grade school. I was utterly amazed to hear these reports, because I trusted the aide and was interested in helping her. This had been one of my previous responsibilities, to encourage upgrading of nursing personnel!

I was in the nursing office when the aide arrived on duty. She asked me how I made out. I asked her into a separate room and discussed my findings with her. She admitted the reports were true, that presently she was taking night school to upgrade her marks so she could try again—but then she said she knew I was prejudiced, and that she was being given a hard time because she was black. I tried to assure her that color did not matter. To this point, I had worked with a variety of cultures, and the important factor to me was that they carry out their responsibilities and attain job satisfaction.

I attempted to help this woman, but to no avail. I did not knowingly feel any prejudice toward her initially, but due to her continual insistence that I am prejudiced, I am now beginning to wonder. At this point, communication is strained and the prospects of helping her are diminishing.

In this situation I trusted the aide at face value, and offered to help her. When I told her my findings she was disappointed and demoralized and used the defense mechanism of accusing me of being prejudiced. I reacted inside to her inference about my being prejudiced and in turn used this as a defense mechanism against my feelings of failure to help her. I felt angry and frustrated. Presently I have failed because I have nothing objective to offer her regarding upgrading. She still occasionally refers to me as being prejudiced. I feel now that the negative reinforcement of being accused of being prejudiced is presenting an obstacle in our working relationship. This in turn is creating another obstacle, because termination of her employment may have to be considered to remove an unacceptable attitude of staff; this again creates a threat to me in not being successful in solving the problem.

Self-image threatened in one form or another is cited in 40% of the Unhelpful cases. The following describes the untenable position for both student and instructor of a student being encouraged to share a personal problem with an instructor—only to be routinely referred on through the nursing school hierarchy.

As a teacher of nursing students we have a responsibility to educate the students in technical skills and communication skills, among other things. To do this, the teacher and student must be able to communicate with one another. When such communication ceases, there can be little gain by the student from any experience arranged by the teacher. I would like to describe an experience I had in which communication between a student and myself went beyond the usual boundaries and resulted in not a closer relationship, but a complete breakdown of all communications between us.

Mr. X was a senior nursing student, considered by most of us to be a poised, sophisticated young man. In residence he was a leader of a similar group of students. At the time in question, Mr. X had just arrived on the surgical unit for a 6-week tour of duty. By the end of his first week, it was apparent he was having more difficulty adjusting to routine and responsibilities than was usual for a student of his experience and previously proven ability. Because of this I made an appointment to see Mr. X at 3:00 P.M., before he went off duty. He arrived promptly at the appointed time.

I asked him if there was some situation on the floor that was preventing him from coming up to my expectations of what was an acceptable performance of duties. I told him that I knew that at times there were personality clashes among nurses and if this was the case, perhaps talking about it might help us find a solution. To my surprise, Mr. X began to sob and then told me what his problem was. It did not involve his work situation at all, but was a home problem. His father had died a few months earlier and since that time Mr. X's mother, who had always been a fairly heavy drinker, had increased her intake of alcohol and had almost stopped eating completely. Mr. X's family belonged to the upper-middle class of society, so that his mother's drinking did not produce any financial problem. She was cared for by a housekeeper who had been with the family for many years, so her safety was not too great a worry to Mr. X.

The crux of the problem seemed to be that Mr. X felt that he should be able to assist his mother to overcome this problem. Due to his student role, he could not be home every evening, but because of his son role he felt he owed it to his mother to be with her constantly, a situation that his mother would not allow.

Also, Mr. X, as a nurse soon to graduate, wanted and needed to see himself as a professional with skills that would reach his mother. And so far he had failed.

I allowed Mr. X to talk about his problem but could not help him to any extent because resolution of his entire role conflict would have to come from himself with the help of the director of the school of nursing, who insisted upon carrying out all student counseling herself. I suggested making an appointment with the director, but Mr. X said he would decide after he had come back from his weekend at home. Our interview ended with Mr. X going off duty and with me feeling that I had been of little assistance except as a shoulder to cry on.

The following Monday morning, when I went on rounds, I met Mr. X, greeting him, I felt, as I usually greeted any student. He replied very briefly, politely but coolly, and excused himself quickly. That afternoon he asked to be excused from our usual staff conference. Since he was caring for some very ill patients and the staff were busy, I gave him permission to stay with his patients. Tuesday morning was a repetition of Monday, but at the conference, Mr. X rarely contributed and then only if asked a direct question. I began to feel that he was uncomfortable in my presence and instead of doing anything constructive and intelligent I began to avoid contact with Mr. X, except as was absolutely necessary.

To the relief of both of us, Mr. X was assigned to the night tour of duty for the remaining 3 weeks of his term on the floor. I saw him before he left for his progress report. During this final interview, neither of us referred to our previous interview.

To analyze the situation, it is necessary to look first at Mr. X's view of what had happened. He saw that he had told things to me, an authority and evaluating figure, things that he felt diminished his value and worth in my eyes. His self-concept, that of a poised, controlled person, had been shattered in his own eyes by his confidence of that Friday afternoon. As a result, he withdrew from me, refusing anything more than the most brief communications.

It may also have been that he had asked me to help and I had only suggested that he see the director and again tell what he probably considered his terrible secrets!

Looking at my own responses, I can see that I made things worse than they needed to be. As he became increasingly remote in his contacts with me, I withdrew from him. I did nothing concrete to let him know that his image had in no way diminished in my eyes. We were both unwilling to accept the fact that such intimate information could occur without changing a student-teacher relationship, which in this case was the truth.

Yes. You had asked him to tell you what the problem was, then couldn't follow through (a most unfortunate policy on counseling!), which created a real problem for you. Actually, in your own way, you were having role conflicts too. Perhaps this is one reason you weren't able to discuss the incident with Mr. X again.

Again, threatened self-image and perceived prejudice account for being judgmental and the response of *felt guilty but could not communicate* (32% of Unhelpful cases).

A situation in which I was not particularly helpful involved a conflict between myself and a co-worker, a nurse. Briefly, she was leading a discussion about unwed mothers in a manner that I felt could be more suitably applied to pornographic literature. As a nurse, I felt she was an agent of negative propaganda to the community. I objected strongly to her hostile attitude of social condemnation. As far as she was concerned, an unwed mother was a criminal. My own opinion was that an unwed mother was a person in desperate need of moral support and encouragement. As a woman, with personal experience with the problem of unwed motherhood, I could only say that I was sick and tired of listening to her expositions on the subject. I failed by my silence: because I was so wrapped up in righteous indignation and a fear of personal censorship, I could not bring myself to relate positively to this nurse. I wanted to help her to realize that an unwed mother was a real person in a situation that compounded her fears and problems. Under the influence of my own hostile reaction to her hostility, I could do no more than protest. I resent this failure on my part. I feel that had I calmed down and tried to help this nurse, I would have stopped one more voice of condemnation and started one mind and tongue on the road to a more positive view of unwed mothers.

Yes, your hostility to her was then compounded by your guilt at not handling this professionally yourself. Obviously, your co-worker wasn't handling it professionally either. For both of you this was a subject that carried with it very deep personal feelings and bias.

The following account illustrates the most frequent Helpful Responses: *gave moral support* (61% of cases); *helped patient express feelings* (61% of cases); *wanted to understand* (56% of cases); and *took time to explain* (50% of cases).

Miss A was admitted to the hospital with a diagnosis of advanced cancer of the left breast and a radical mastectomy of that breast was performed 3 days after admission. She was 53 years of age, a graduate nurse, but no longer employed full-time, working only part-time occasionally. She had a very pleasant personality and seemed to enjoy opportunities to speak to people and took a genuine interest in them. This could have been partly due to the fact that she lived alone. Since Miss A had no dependents, her illness did not cause any family problems. She did not appear to have any financial worries since she had not found it necessary to maintain a full-time job.

I was working the day shift during Miss A's stay in the hospital and nursed her pre- and postoperatively. Since she seemed to enjoy company it was extremely easy to make conversation with her and she was also a very interesting person to talk with. It did not take long to notice, however, that she was a very nervous person, since she had an intention tremor of head and arms.

It is difficult to pinpoint the exact reason why I took a special interest in this patient, as there are many possible reasons: the fact that she lived alone and she could be lonely; she was undergoing major surgery; a mastectomy had a lot of psychological impact; she was a nervous person and therefore needed someone to talk to; since she was a nurse I may have felt common professional ties; statistics show that 1 out of every 25 women will develop breast cancer, so I may have thought perhaps one day I'd be in her place. Probably a combination of the preceding reasons is why I felt an extra desire to try and be helpful to Miss A.

Shortly after having made acquaintance with the patient I recalled the fact that, although a mastectomy is major physical surgery, the psychological surgery she would be undergoing was as major, if not more so. Being a nurse herself, she knew what type of surgery she was about to have, but she needed someone to discuss the matter with. Even though she didn't have to worry about how a husband would react to this mutilation, the breasts are an identification with femininity and she had to be reassured that she would be as much of a woman as before. Extra reassurance had to be given because it is believed that single women feel more deprived than married women with children, whose breasts have served their essential function.

Preoperatively I concentrated on building a good rapport with the patient, so that she could have someone to confide in when she felt the need to. Postoperatively, while giving physical care, I made an effort to give as much psychological help as possible. The first few days she needed rest and then gradually rehabilitation exercises were commenced. As a nurse she understood the importance of exercise in order to regain the use of her arm but I found praise helped her to be faithful to the prescribed exercises.

Even though she had seen many scars I exposed her to her own gradually, so she would have less tendency to shun it once she got home. Looking at a scar on someone else and looking at one on yourself are two different things. We also discussed the type of prosthesis she could wear, once the scar had healed and she could be fitted. In the meantime we devised a way of padding her bra without interfering with the healing process. I tried also to give her opportunities to discuss anything else she might be worried about.

Miss A recovered from the operation with no major complication, only slight edema of the left arm. She was discharged after 17 days of hospitalization. As this patient was very nervous I felt that it helped her a great deal when I took time to talk with her and let her express her anxieties outwardly. I believe I was helpful, mainly because I always kept in mind the great psychological trauma she must have had and tried to find ways to lessen this trauma. Also, I did not take for granted that, because she was a nurse, she did not need reassurance.

Yes, very important, and you were not dissuaded by the fact that she was many years your senior and therefore should know it all.

For those in administrative authority, the balance involved in helping colleagues to achieve their own potential on the therapeutic team
and at the same time assessing one's own use of authority is obviously
an area of very real difficulty, as evidenced by the higher percentage of
Unhelpful accounts regarding Colleague Relationship. The following
illustrations span the major response factors cited.

I was puzzled by my lack of success in the use of self with my assistant head
nurse. She was cooperative, but uncommunicative, and often moody. I could
not reach her to discover what the trouble was. I wondered if it were jealousy
of me. From the time I assumed leadership of the floor, I used the permissive
approach with all my staff, hoping for a truly satisfying participation in patient care. Yet no one could work happily with this nurse. She could only be
satisfied by achieving her goals independently. She worked so hard that I was
concerned not only about her rejection of help by others, but also for her
health, because she exhausted herself. I tried reassigning the workload to relieve her, but that only seemed to make her feel that I questioned her competence, and she insisted on carrying what she considered her full share.

Returning from days off, when she had been left in charge, I would sometimes find that there had been serious incidents between her and the orderlies,
or occasionally another nurse. The atmosphere was so bad that I lost one of
my best orderlies because he could not tolerate her demands, which he simply
could not meet. I knew she drove herself to achieve perfection, and I was
grateful for the quality of physical care she gave our patients, yet I could never
make her understand that she could not drive others to the same extent.

I could never foster good interpersonal relationships between her and a
member of staff or a patient who did not meet her conception of what he or she
ought to be. I did not know how to break down her rigid moral values. Nor
could I take sides in their quarrels, and not knowing what to do, in order to
hurt no one, I often fell back on the excuse that perhaps one of them was tired,
and things would be better soon. After pointing out the good qualities of who-
ever was under attack, I did nothing except try to soothe feelings and let the
situation subside. I wondered sometimes if I should take a more authoritarian
attitude toward her, but because she was much older than I, and had been
there long before I arrived, I still feel it would have been a mistake. I had no
wish to alienate her from me, or from her job, which seemed the most important part of her life.

I thought perhaps the atmosphere of a busy floor where we seldom had
much time to really communicate was interfering with my efforts to reach out
in a personal way to this woman. Consequently, I invited her to my apartment
for dinner several times.

Do you think she thought she was being asked for herself or for the problem she was?

Invariably the conversation would come around to our work, but still I could not seem to form the ideas of interpersonal relationships so that they had any real meaning for her. She verbalized about the concepts as well as I did, but could not seem to put them into practice.

I did succeed in getting her to talk about herself, however. When I learned that she had spent her childhood in various foster homes, and had sometimes been used as a farm helper in the process, it increased my sympathy for her, but did not enable me to help.

She talked about her history, but had you realized what this meant to her, do you think you could have helped her to talk about herself—her fears as a child, etc., to help her open up and be accepted as a person, rather than a performer of tasks, which apparently was her only criterion for acceptance as she grew up and which she had now internalized for herself and others.

I did not realize at that time what this experience could do to her ability to form a satisfactory relationship, and, although I tried my best to hide it, I continued to be frustrated by her inability to fit into the floor smoothly.

Even with the little extra knowledge of psychology I am now gaining, I doubt my ability to really accept her inadequacies when they mean disruption for the rest of the staff and patients. I am fairly certain that I could do so if I alone were concerned, but a head nurse must try to meet the needs of many people, and perhaps there is just no way in which certain personalities can be accommodated suitably.

The only way I could see of solving the problem would be to have her transferred, but I could not bring myself to stigmatize her. Consequently, I continued to let her work alone as much as possible, but kept her away from anything but superficial contact with our problem patients, and brought her many good qualities to the attention of others whenever possible in an attempt to engender a better atmosphere. This nurse had already been discussed with me by my supervisor before I came to know her, and it was obvious that no one else understood her problem either, so I made no efforts at gaining help from that source, and felt that I was meeting her needs as far as I could. But was I?

She may have been so severely hurt emotionally that her actual ability to change very much would be limited. However, I am not sure that a transfer if handled with her would necessarily have been more stigmatizing than it was on the floor where she remained. She would be fully aware of your ploys (necessary certainly from your point of view, but still very hurtful to her whether she showed it or not). Was there any area (intensive care?) where her tireless

and efficient physical care would have been an advantage that could be ap-
plauded, yet where there was a minimal need for the characteristics she lacked?

The following account is the second part of the successful Situation
related on pages 134–135. There the nurse describes her move as the
first female nurse to an all-male psychiatric area, where she initiated a
program of arts and crafts for senile, retarded patients who had heretofore been offered no recreational program whatsoever.

In many ways in this same innovative situation I failed miserably. I never
managed to get the attendant staff interested in approving of or helping with
this program. Of all the team members, I was most closely involved with them
and I never made a dent in changing their way of thinking.

This was a period of great change in the hospital. Change and reform brought
trauma and insecurity. Until this time the attendant staff had been in complete
charge of the male side. Now new nursing supervisors and area nursing supervisors were being appointed and the attendants felt their position and chances of
advancement were threatened. Most of these people had limited training and
their work consisted entirely of custodial care. A quiet patient was a good patient.

In my account of the new program I greatly oversimplified the process of
change. It involved weeks of preparation, doing baseline studies on patients,
and many meetings with the staff team. The attendants didn't like this at all.
It was threatening to their whole idea of custodial care. It meant more work
and also meant changing their whole attitude toward the patients. They offered great resistance, both passive and active. Their defense mechanisms
worked overtime.

We had many more meetings with them; we appealed to their better na-
tures. We quoted incidences of mental disease in terms of family and self
("Would you yourself like to be isolated from the community and sit and do
nothing the rest of your life, or would you like your parents to?"). We told
them that the success of the program depended on them; that it must become
internalized and they were the most important factors. We gave them responsibility but they wouldn't take it. Nothing helped.

I was so frustrated I could have screamed. I thought they should all be
replaced with people who would see it my way. I guess I pushed them too hard
and expected them to adopt ideas of patient care completely foreign to them
without intensive retraining. I knew I would be leaving and was too anxious to
get the program firmly established before I left. I didn't stop to think that they
were not ready for all these changes at once. I probably did too much myself

and didn't expect enough of them. In short, I failed miserably with them in this area.

In defense of the attendants, I must say this was the only area in which they didn't cooperate with me. In all other situations they would almost bend over backward to help me or please me.

You were trying to appeal to their rational side when they were too caught up with a threat to their emotional equilibrium and status—very difficult.

*   *   *   *

I had recently arrived in Canada and was working for the federal government, in charge of a nursing station in a semi-isolated small town. The population was predominantly Indian. There were enough citizens in the surrounding area to justify also the existence of a small provincial health unit, manned by one nurse. She was a sporty, outdoor type, in her late 20s, a second-generation Canadian, pleasant and down-to-earth, and I liked her. We met during office hours and discussed various mutual concerns in the area where our work overlapped or where liaison was necessary, and we had made plans for joint educational projects.

Until that time, we had not really got to know each other as people, as I was out of town a lot, since my area consisted of around eight Indian reserves, scattered within a radius of 60–70 miles—some of them reached only by rowboat, overhead cable ferry, or on horseback. It was a busy, challenging life, since I was a widow with three small children. She had said that she spent most of her spare time hunting and fishing, and she had a large German shepherd dog, whom she really loved. After we had both had a chance to settle in and get to know our areas, I asked her over for dinner and we started to socialize a little, whenever possible. She started to have problems with accommodation, because of the dog, and wanted to move in with us, but it was not permitted.

After that things seemed to go wrong with our relationship and we found it difficult to communicate. A series of incidents over the dog being left at my place without notice, and a general taunting and needling over government policy, child-rearing, you name it, prevented any close personal relationship. I would always rise to the bait, springing to the defense of my own or government policy and we would end up in a wordy battle, leaving me emotionally drained, but seeming to give her a measure of satisfaction. Needless to say, our relationship deteriorated rapidly, so much so that it affected our liaison at work, to the detriment of the community, and from then on we each worked in our separate spheres.

In a small town with a mixed population of native Indians and whites, it is difficult to achieve a happy balance of people living in harmony. To have two different health promotion outlets was bad enough; that they were funded and manned by two different governmental agencies was worse; but to have two community health nurses being uncooperative was indefensible. Try as I might to make things better, workwise, at least, and she made overtures to me too, it always seemed to come right down to crazy issues, like my not being able to accept her dog as a person, or how our service spoon-fed the Indians! Looking back, I realize we were both needing help with our several problems.

In trying to adjust to a new country, new status, and life-style, I was blocked in with self-pity, hurt and on the defensive, like a mother bear, ready to spring to the defense of her cubs. The "noise" that was impeding our communication as nurses was our several deep needs as women, which were not being met. She had need for a family, or perhaps even for sexual identification, and for the release from jealousy and the oppressive feeling of deprivation she had inherited from her family's experiences. For my part, I had not fully accepted the loss of my husband and with the adjustments to change, the decision making, and the financial burdens of raising a family alone, and helping them adjust, it was not easy for me to respond without hostility.

We both considered ourselves to be good nurses, dedicated, hard-working, and conscientious. But were we? Were we both perhaps in that isolated area because we were trying to escape from facing reality, by becoming immersed in the all-absorbing pattern of giving to a difficult community, as to a patient? But were we too blocked in to be able to give of ourselves in a meaningful way? Had I been able to see through the fog of my unresolved problems or to listen with my "third ear," I would have heard what she was trying to say and we could have helped each other as women. Having recognized our several needs and the resultant hostilities, we could have taken steps to change things and we would have had more to give as nurses to the community.

13
CULTURAL ADAPTATION

Of the 550 cases in the study, 3% focus on Cultural Adaptation. Of the 14 cases that focus on Cultural Adaptation, 4 are described as Helpful, 10 as Unhelpful. Percentages shown for comparison only (see Tables 2.3, 2.4; pp. 32–35).

COMPARISON WITH ALL OTHER SITUATIONS

Helpful Factors

Highest Rating

- Was trying to prove self to senior staff members.
- Used innovative rehabilitative procedure.
- Discussed religion with patient (same rating as Alcoholism).
- Came to terms with own feelings; was able to enter into patient's problem (same rating as Unmarried Mothers and Adolescence).

Unhelpful Factors

Highest Rating

- Self-image was threatened.
- Avoided needs of family members (same rating as Death/Dying and Alcoholism).

Helpful Factors	% of Cases in Which Cited
1. Used innovative rehabilitative procedure	75
2. Was a sounding board	50

3.	Gave moral support	50
4.	Came to terms with own feelings; was able to enter into patient's problem	50
5.	Nonjudgmental	50
6.	Wanted to understand how patient felt	50
7.	Helped patient express feelings	25
8.	Liked the patient	25
9.	Helped family members deal with the situation	25
10.	Looked beyond patient's outward response/behavior to underlying causes	25
11.	Was trying to prove self to senior staff members	25
12.	Discussed religion with patient	25
13.	Used physical closeness	25
14.	Took time to explain	0
15.	Initiated referral to another profession/resource	0
16.	Not unduly influenced by negative opinions of other staff regarding the patient's personality	0
17.	Made this case the basis for overall policy change/improvement	0
18.	Positively identified with patient due to similar life/professional experience	0
19.	Had received training in recognizing social-emotional needs of patients	0
20.	Was honest with patient/relatives	0

Unhelpful Factors	% of Cases in Which Cited
1. Was disapproving, judgmental	70
2. Self-image was threatened	70
3. Did not want to understand	50
4. Failed to look beyond initial negative impression of patient's personality	50
5. Avoided needs of family members	40
6. Felt inadequate to enter into patient's problem because had not personally resolved the issue	30
7. Treated the condition, overlooking the patient	30
8. Lacked training in recognizing social-emotional needs of patients	30
9. Felt guilty but could not communicate	20
10. Purposely disregarded significant cues in patient's statements/behavior	20

11. Prejudiced toward group of which patient was a
    member   20
12. Rationalized actions and thoughts   20
13. Breakdown of interprofessional communication/
    cooperation   10
14. Felt pressured (within self) into doing things rather
    than coping with feeling elements (tension present)   10
15. Failed to seek authoritative advice regarding innova-
    tion   10
16. Disliked patient   10
17. Short-staffed; too little time to devote to the patient   0
18. Negatively influenced by opinions of other staff
    members regarding personality of the patient   0
19. Afraid would break down and cry in front of patient   0
20. Overidentified due to being similar age to patient   0
21. Incapacitated by own fear of death   0
22. Disregarded own judgment because wanted approval
    of senior staff members   0
23. Lost professional role: patient became friend   0
24. Felt guilty but still would not communicate   0

Of the cases describing Cultural Adaptation 10 out of 14 are described as Unhelpful. This is the highest ratio of Unhelpful to Helpful
cases of any Situation.

The following account describes the distance that can stretch so re-
lentlessly between nurse and patient.

The house was a modern one-floor bungalow, which, at a glance, appeared
the same as all the other houses on the block. Once up into the driveway, however, I noticed there were no curtains at the windows. The front step was
unswept and the lawn was ragged with last autumn's uncut grass.

Nurse: Hello. My name is Pat Hern. I'm a nurse from the Health Department, and I've come to talk with you about your new baby.

Mrs. M was a woman in her late 20s. She held a young child in her arms and
three others stood around her. She eyed me with suspicion.

Nurse: May I come in?
Mrs. M: Yes.

The living room was carpeted with what was once a red broadloom. It was now stained and filthy. There was a sofa placed at a careless angle in the middle of the room. The walls were unpainted, the plaster chipped and soiled. A foul smell permeated the air. She spoke to the children with a harsh voice, using the language they understood, for they quickly took up positions in front of the TV.

Nurse: Well . . . you have a large family.

Mrs. M: Yes; when we came from Lebanon 2 years ago we have three kids—now five!

Nurse: It's a lot of work to care for five children.

Mrs. M: Yeh—and too many girls. My husband want five sons and we got four girls and one son.

She was sober and thoughtful.

Nurse: Well, they're very pretty girls and they'll be able to help you one day with all of the work in the house.

We sat in silence for some minutes.

Nurse: Do you like living here, Mrs. M?

Mrs. M: No, don't like it here. Lotsa money but no good. Too cold out . . . everything.

She shrugged, an annoyed expression on her face.

Nurse: Where does your husband work?

Mrs. M: Electrician. Why are you here?

Nurse: Well, I'm a community health nurse. It is my job to visit people like yourself to show them the newest and best ways of looking after babies and children. I would like to help you with any problems you might have in caring for your family.

Her dark eyes flashed at me. She was almost hostile in manner.

Mrs. M: I'm from old country. I have my ways—not same as yours. Everything here OK. My husband's mother here now—she help me.

Nurse: Well, could I see the baby?

Mrs. M: OK.

She called upstairs and her mother-in-law, wearing a white muslin headdress, came into the room carrying the baby girl. The baby was wrapped in wide strips of soiled cloth and was screaming at the top of her lungs.

Mrs. M: Cry, cry all the time. Should be a boy, not girl. I feed her all the time but she cry, cry.

Nurse: You breast-feed her? I mean—you give your own milk to the baby?

Mrs. M: I know what you say—I know English OK! In Lebanon everybody feed baby themselves—no bottles.

She was indignant now.

Nurse: But maybe you don't have enough breast milk to satisfy her. You work so hard caring for the other children that your body may not be producing enough milk.

Mrs. M: Ach . . .

She glanced at me disdainfully.

Nurse: Do you have a family doctor?

Mrs. M: Yeah.

Nurse: Did he tell you how to feed the baby?

Mrs. M: I know how to feed the baby.

Nurse: Sometimes a baby needs to have milk from a can too.

She got up from the sofa quickly and brought me back a can of formula and a box of cereal (samples given to her at the hospital). I offered to show her how to prepare the food and we went to the kitchen. It was in worse condition than the living room. There were few utensils with which to demonstrate the preparation and I felt very frustrated. One surprising item in the kitchen was a padlock securing the refrigerator door. She saw me glance at it.

Mrs. M: I lock all the time—or kids drink all the milk.

When we went back into the living room I attempted to speak to the older woman but was interrupted.

Mrs. M: She speak no English.

Nurse: Please tell her I wish her a pleasant visit in this country. It must be hard to look after a visitor as well as a new baby and the other children.

Mrs. M: No. Not hard.

We sat in silence, then I spoke briefly to the children, commenting on the TV programs. They smiled but averted their eyes.

> *Nurse:* I'll be on my way now. If the baby keeps crying I hope you'll offer her the extra milk and the cereal. Then perhaps she'll sleep longer.

Mrs. M gave me a skeptical smile.

> *Nurse:* I'll be in this area on Friday. May I come to visit you then? I'm interested to see how the baby accepts the new foods.

There was a long pause.

> *Mrs. M:* I'm OK with baby. No trouble her. She will help me. Don't come.
>
> *Nurse:* Well, here is a card with my name and phone number. If the baby cries too much, call me. I'd like to come over to help you.

I walked to my car defeated and downhearted, knowing Mrs. M would never call me.

Analysis

I went to Mrs. M's house with a sincere desire to help her. My purpose was to learn about her and her family, gather necessary data and then to give her instructions as needed.

I intended to achieve these tasks through tactful questioning and active listening. But we were never able to establish rapport. Our cultural backgrounds were vastly different. When I saw the condition of her home, I made every effort to conceal my distaste. She knew, however, that her life-style and mine were far apart. She watched TV so she knew of our customs, as they appear on the surface, at least. They must have seemed as strange to her as a woman wearing a veil, a swaddled baby, or a padlock on the refrigerator seemed to me.

There was a language barrier and I underestimated her ability to comprehend English. I therefore oversimplified my message, which she found insulting. My assumption that she was deficient in knowledge created anxiety and resentment in Mrs. M. She felt I could never understand her or her customs, so she tuned me out, predicting that anything I might say would never have any meaning for her. She was skeptical of my methods and on the defensive about her old-country traditions.

She was, in fact, in need of knowledge. She needed to learn modern methods of child care and money management so that she and her children might integrate into the community. Most important, she needed to learn how to obtain and use our medical services, so easily available.

I believe I perceived her problems to be so monumental that I didn't know where or how to begin working with her. I was aware of my need to learn further interviewing skills and felt inadequate.

Another factor of which I am now aware is that Mrs. M was culturally biased against my country and projected that bias on to me. She was experiencing culture shock in a land of cold climate and strange ways. The fact that she had better housing and increased income meant little to her when she didn't know how to use the money and hadn't family or friends with whom to share what we call the good life. It frustrated me that she had so many of life's good things at her disposal and yet she refused help in learning how to make use of them. I believe this factor created a personal bias in me against Mrs. M.

The population of any city or town is made up of people with varied cultural backgrounds. It is essential then, for me to examine any cultural bias I possess and hopefully resolve the problem through further study and understanding. Only then will I be considered effective as a health professional.

If you had heard the cue this woman put out to you at the very beginning of the interview—"too many girls. My husband want five sons and we got four girls and one son" and later, "should be boy, not girl"—you might have found that bridge you were searching for.

Of all Conditions in the study, it is in Cultural Adaptation that *self-image was threatened* most frequently occurs. It and *was disapproving, judgmental* are cited in 7 out of 10 of the Unhelpful cases.

The following case refers to my public health work in a northern community that was half made up of Métis Indians. I had found in one school that 95% of the children had head lice. I excluded all of those children from the school and sent them home with printed directions for clearing up their heads before their return.

In this situation I showed a great lack of understanding of the community, of mothers, and of the problems in a mixed community. I realize now that I had a real fear of the situation, and wanted to be involved as little as possible. I made no attempt to understand the emotional factors involved. I acted in such an authoritarian way that I was bound to alienate everyone in the community. I rationalized my actions by saying that I was saving time by handling the situation that way. In fact, due to my own upbringing in a middle-class home, I felt that the whole situation was terrible, and in spite of my own knowledge could not help but associate lice only with lack of care and filth. In many cases—especially where the severest problems were—the mothers couldn't even read the forms. I disregarded this problem as I knew I would feel uncomfortable if I tried to handle it personally. I felt inadequate in my ability to speak to large groups so I ignored this means of educating the community entirely. I knew that I wouldn't be available directly if there were repercussions as my office was several miles away. I felt very safe. By grouping all of the children together I didn't try to understand either the Métis, with their special problems and lack of facilities, or the more affluent white members of the community.

If I had taken time with the mothers who had made an attempt to care for their children, I could have shown them that I could understand how a child could go to school spotless in the morning and return with lice at noon. I would have saved them from all the feeling of stigma attached to the exclusion. If I had also gone in and worked with the mothers who had such poor facilities and helped with this problem, I would have made far more progress. Instead I managed to antagonize the whole community through my lack of understanding and 3 months later 95% of the children in the school still had head lice.

$$* \quad * \quad * \quad *$$

The type of situation in which I find myself repeatedly not helpful is in dealing with children of Italian or other Mediterranean nationalities, who are brought up with a great dependence on their parents. I realize that many of our middle-class standards, including the stress on early independence, are peculiarly North American and must not be imposed on other peoples. Yet, I find myself treating such children with unnecessary impatience when they do not do for themselves what I think they should be able to do, even while recognizing that the children have had no say in the way they have been brought up. These children—who, because of their greater dependence, need extra attention, time, and evidence of affection while in a strange hospital setting—I find are the very ones I scold more often, leave alone for longer periods, and display more impatience with, certainly not providing for a positive psychological hospital experience.

As well as wanting to impose my standards of independence, there is mixed in a feeling of defeat. Many children refuse to take food or medications from staff members, in which case parents are heavily relied on, but when a child is able to effectively refuse his parents as well, there seems no other direction in which to turn. When such parents arrive to visit, my attitude of impatience is directed at them, or an attempt is made to avoid them as much as possible during their stay—yet these people have probably more concerns and questions than the majority of other parents and might benefit from additional health teaching.

Perhaps the whole idea of independence is even more important to me than I realize, for this is the area in which I have the most difficulty overcoming my own negative feelings toward people in order to provide the assistance or mere listening that they may be searching for. In realizing that this attitude I have is a culturally acquired one I have tried reading and thinking about Italian culture and practices, but seemingly to no avail.

Yes, I think it may be a combination of cultural and psychological factors, as most of our reactions are.

Confronted with the above type of situation I forget everything I've tried to understand and want to shake both parents and children. I want to convince them that the child must be taught within the protection of his home to stand on his own feet or his initiation into the world outside will be a cruel one.

It may be that watching this inhibition of independence in others is a threat to my own security or my own independence, which I have worked hard to achieve and which is very important to me. Nevertheless, I find it very difficult to react in a positive way to a practice I personally feel is wrong, resulting in clinging, insecure, and unadventurous children.

This is an honest and realistic self-analysis. You are willing to look beyond more acceptable excuses for your behavior and to search for less comfortable answers.

*   *   *   *

In September 1965, a classmate and I were sent to Vellore, South India, by the Board of World Mission, United Church. We were the first nurses to be sent who did not have postbasic training in nursing. Our objective was to work alongside the Indian nurses, to illustrate to them what all around nursing care involved. We were to work as staff nurses. I consider that my first experience on a private ward at Vellore was a failure in that I failed to meet the objective.

My first reaction was one of shock. The nurses did not seem to be interested in the welfare of the patients at all. Good nursing care, if known, was not carried out. Their negative attitude toward their fellow Indians from different states, and toward those suffering from Hansen's disease (leprosy) was very annoying. After all, I was quite willing to give nursing care to all.

It was the custom for relatives and servants to accompany the patient to the hospital, and to give some care to the patient while in the hospital. This was most frustrating to me. I was always tripping over them in doorways, or returning to the room to find that they had contradicted my orders to the patient.

The patients assigned to this particular ward were never very ill. Therefore, my nursing duties were very simple, and were often boring. A day's work consisted of making beds and of taking temperatures. Any attempt that I made at introducing an easier method or procedure was blocked. If I helped the pune carry water, the nurses just dismissed it as my poor Western upbringing.

Soon, I became very discouraged. What was the point of my worrying about the patients? I had come up against a stone wall. They had been doing things their way for thousands of years, and I was not going to change anything in my 2-year stay. I became bored and disinterested, and somewhat depressed. I had not achieved my objective.

In analyzing my reactions of shock, I realize that, although I had been well informed of the culture, I could not begin to understand it without living in the land for many years. My frustration was also initiated by my lack of empathy with their traditions: the servants and relatives in the hospital, and the caste system, which was evident in the duties assigned to the punes. Because the ward was slack, I was unable to use my technical skills and knowledge of nursing procedures. Therefore, I was uncomfortable. I was not learning new skills. I was a staff nurse and I had no authority to initiate my ideas, although I thought them worthwhile. I wanted to feel that I was a success and that I was needed on the ward. No one filled that need, so I was insecure and unhappy.

My second experience was in the postoperative cardiothoracic intensive care unit. I was placed in charge of the unit. In the beginning the chief of surgery was an American, and later and Indian doctor who had recently returned from the States. I was told to organize the nursing staff and the room, and to order new equipment as needed.

The work was difficult. The equipment was in ill repair, and quite often it took a long time to get the equipment. I worked with five competent Indian nurses, and together we set up new routines and procedures. We worked hard as a team, and we became friends. Along with the doctors, we fought for the lives of our open heart surgery patients. We were scolded for our errors, challenged to do better, and praised for our good work.

I was challenged and interested. I had been working with my Indian colleagues to give all around nursing care.

In analyzing my reactions to my second experience, many factors come into play. A year had passed, and I was more accustomed to the land. The relatives were no longer a frustration, for I began to appreciate their apprehension, and to make use of their willingness to aid their loved ones. The caste system began to take on parallels to our society. The work was challenging and difficult. I was able to make use of my technical skills. I was learning a great deal about a fascinating field of surgery. I had been placed in a position of authority, and was able, therefore, to initiate action.

I was praised for my work, and I was made to feel welcome. I was comfortable and happy.

In this case, the nurse describes overcoming her fear and threatened self-image to offer constructive help and moral support. The ratio of *came to terms with own feelings; was able to enter into patient's prob-*

lem is highest where Cultural Adaptation, Unmarried Mothers, and Adolescence are involved.

This situation occurred while I was working on an Indian reserve in Northern Alberta—I live and work in a nursing station. We are responsible (there are usually two nurses) for the physical and mental health for all living in that area. This includes evaluation of a patient and initiating primary emergency care—an overwhelming job at times.

How I Helped

There had been a fatal shooting of a 19-year-old boy, John; he had been shot while breaking into a white teacher's home. It was the reserve's first violent death. It was the first time a patient had died while directly under my care. It was an earth-shattering event for the family, community, and myself—and it was my duty to go and give the family, chief, and his council the news.

Before I left John's room so many thoughts went screaming through my head: John can't be dead—things like this just don't happen. Could I have done more and saved his life? Am I responsible in some way for his death? I'm frightened, I'm white, and a young Indian boy is dead. What's going to happen? Will there be retaliation? The teacher who shot John is a friend. What really happened? What will happen to her?

With this jumble of confusing thoughts I went to face the Indian tribe with tears in my eyes and an ache in my heart; I was just waiting to be scalped. I don't remember what I said, but before I knew what was happening we were all crying, holding on to each other, giving comfort, mourning together for the life that had been taken and taking comfort from those who gave it. At that moment we forgot the Indian-white conflict; we forgot why John had been killed. All we realized was that a death had occurred and we were all deeply sad and groped for each other and for warmth and understanding.

I gathered the immediate family together and took them to my sitting room so they could be together, hoping they would gain strength from each other. I tried to meet their immediate needs by being there, listening, and accepting the anger, disillusionment, and grief, and by giving direct nursing care and counseling when necessary.

The clinic area was now another center of activity—the reserve elders had gathered to chant and pray for John, keeping away the evil spirits so he might rest in peace. The chief understood that the mourning in the nursing station could only last for so long—because we again had to prepare the clinic and deal with the sick—and he took the responsibility of moving his people when the time came.

Relatives and close friends of John's began to arrive to kiss him good-bye and wish him a safe journey. This presented another small problem: the body was supposed to be locked away until mounted police could arrive to handle the situation. We held another quick meeting and decided to put a respected elder on guard and allow one person in at a time to pay his last respects; everyone went along with this and no confusion or resentments were aroused.

Because of the way John's death was handled I felt I accomplished the following:

1. Aid was given to the family to help them cope with this traumatic situation—just being there, accepting, and understanding meant so much.
2. By accepting the Indian Culture and beliefs and allowing these to be expressed at the mourning ceremony in the nursing station, I felt I acted as a buffer and cut down any resentment that might have been present, and it allowed people to work out their feelings.
3. It helped me adjust to the fact that John was dead and I had done all I could. It also made me realize I wasn't a doctor and as long as I worked in the north in a nursing station, situations like this would happen again—and I must learn to accept whatever might happen.

I'll never forget the words the chief spoke to me when he left: "Mary, we know you tried and did your best. We don't want you to feel responsible for John's death. It was just one of those crazy things no one can really explain or understand fully."

Here, the nurse describes *treated the condition, overlooking the patient* as related to not wanting to appear inadequate to professional colleagues.

On a Tuesday last August, Mike, a ward of the Children's Aid Society, came to the medical clinic for a camp and annual checkup. His departure for camp was booked for the following Tuesday. On examination he was found to be a handsome, well-developed, 14-year-old Canadian Indian boy in good health. However, his urine showed 4 + albumen. The attending physician felt that further investigation was necessary before Mike could leave for camp.

It was explained to Mike very carefully that adolescents who are very active might have a condition called orthostatic albuminuria, which is not a disease, but the doctor had to be quite sure before he signed the camp medical. We asked Mike to bring an early morning specimen the next day. After Mike got dressed I gave him the sterile specimen bottle and explained again the procedure used to collect the morning specimen.

Mike informed me that he would not be able to bring the specimen because it would take him 2 hours to come to the clinic. When asked for his address Mike stated that it was at Main and Ryan streets. I said that it would take him about 7 minutes by subway. Mike replied, "Oh, I also work." I suggested that he might place the specimen in the refrigerator and bring it to the clinic after work as the clinic was open until 5:00 P.M., or he could leave it with the night watchman.

During the morning Mike's foster mother, Mrs. C, phoned, blasting me in a very snappy British accent about keeping children too long at the clinic and being disorganized. She extended her criticism not only to the clinic but to the agency. I told her that Mike was on his way home. The noises in the waiting room were such that I did not attempt to explain about Mike's morning specimen.

In the afternoon Mrs. C phoned again; she was upset and very cross. She said she knew all along that the agency discriminated against Indians and not only the agency but all Canadians discriminate against the native people, etc. I explained to her about Mike and asked her to cooperate in obtaining the specimen, as the doctor would not be able to sign the camp form without being sure that Mike was really in good health. Mrs. C started on another barrage of insults, saying that it was obvious that even the doctor was against Mike and did not want him to go to camp and so it went on and on. Finally, she agreed to send Mike down to the clinic the next morning with the urine specimen. Mike did not appear the next morning or the following morning.

Thursday afternoon I phoned Mrs. C. She was quite vague but suggested that they, the C's, might take Mike to their private doctor to obtain the camp medical. Friday, just before I left the clinic, I phoned again and this time I reached Mr. C, who sounded very reasonable. He promised to bring Mike and the specimen on Monday morning. Monday morning Mr. C and Mike, with specimen, arrived. The doctor had found out in the meantime that Blackfoot Indians, and Mike was one, are prone to this kidney condition (which is not pathological). The camp form was signed and Mike pronounced fit and ready for camp.

In the course of the morning I found out that:

1. Mike did not want to go to camp.
2. Recently Mike had shown an interest in girls and kept late hours, much to Mrs. C's annoyance. The C's came from England, were very strict, and were unable to tolerate such behavior in a 14-year-old boy. As a deterrent, Mrs. C talked a great deal about VD to Mike, and as a result Mike was terrified of contracting VD. By not really understanding what was said in the clinic, Mrs. C and Mike both concluded that our interest in Mike's urine could be nothing other than the result of Mike's late hours.

3. Mrs. C really felt that all social workers handle Mike differently from other children; her relationship with the present worker was very strained. (Mrs. C used to be a foster parent in England, but Mike was her first and only foster child in Canada.)

In a purely technical sense the case was solved satisfactorily. Mike had his camp and annual checkup completed. In analyzing my behavior and my interaction with Mike, the foster parents, and the doctor, I was quite ineffectual.

I let myself be irritated by Mrs. C's rudeness and lack of willingness to understand our problems at the clinic. I reacted by being as snappy as she was, not even attempting to understand her point of view or to find out the cause of her animosity.

In dealing with Mike, I just saw a sullen, uncooperative teenager with a urinary problem. I did not consider the difficulties, the agonies of adolescence, his relationship with his foster parents and the agency, his status as a ward of the agency or that of an Indian boy living with an English new-Canadian family.

What Should I Have Done?

1. At the first sign of difficulty I should have phoned the caseworker and asked for a consultation. I hope I would have gained understanding and insight.

2. The caseworker and myself should have tackled the problem in the best possible way, maybe even with outside help (school, YMCA, Scouts, etc.). We should have talked with Mr. and Mrs. C regarding adolescents, sex, discrimination, and the damage they might inflict by fostering resentment in Mike due to his Indian background.

What I Did Wrong

I failed to ask for a consultation because I felt that the caseworker might be resentful, feeling that the clinic nurses were unable to handle a small problem by ourselves. I failed to deal with the patient as part of a family. I failed to consider Mike as a total person and concentrated only on his urinary problem. To sum up my failure, I showed lack of insight, and irritability.

The result was Mike was in deeper trouble than before with his foster mother and she was more resentful to both Mike and the agency.

Actually, both Mike and his foster parents were trying to "break into" Canadian culture. This could have been used as an effective tool in counseling and could have constituted a real bond.

As noted, Cultural Adaptation shared the highest rating among all Conditions in *avoided needs of family members.*

Several years ago on an Indian reservation a 2-year-old lad was very ill. When the grandmother called me to her home I saw before me a child sick with fever and I made an initial diagnosis of bronchitis. The child had been ill for more than a day and, although there were three adults in the house, nothing had been done for the child to relieve his fever or discomfort. I explained the necessary actions to take when a child felt ill and feverish. I showed them how to give a tepid sponge bath to bring down the fever. I treated him with the necessary antibiotics and antifever medications and asked the grandmother to sponge bathe the child every 1 to 2 hours. I assured her I would return and decide if the child needed to be evacuated.

When I returned the grandmother had done absolutely nothing but sit by the child's bedside. She told me she was too busy cleaning the house to attend to her grandson. Her house was not only messy, it was filthy, but this was not unusual. However, I was enraged with her because she had done nothing, had not told me that she would do nothing, and the child had not improved. I minced no words and told her how filthy her house was and that she had not cleaned it for weeks, let alone today. I reminded her she was a horrible housekeeper and that I was upset with her for not doing anything for the child.

Being the only nurse on the reservation at any time and the hospital 200 miles away, I had to weigh my evacuations carefully. At times it is very difficult to make the decision and one is apprehensive. I felt a bit helpless, as the station was very poorly equipped for emergencies. So I let off some steam. The fact that her house was dirty should have been no concern of mine at that particular time. Other problems were much more important. Following my scene the grandmother followed my instructions very well. The child recovered very well a few days later and the grandmother was grateful for my part.

I believe that the grandmother loved the boy very much. She had her own way of showing concern and that was by remaining at his bedside. Her excuse about cleaning was to have satisfied me. Indian parents usually do not force their children to do things they do not like doing. The child did not want to drink fluids nor be disturbed and so she did what she could by staying with him. She had confidence that I would be returning shortly to look after her sick child. She could not understand what had happened to the usually pleasant nurse. She felt very guilty.

I suppose I could chuck the whole thing to cultural misunderstanding, but I know better. I admit I was shocked at her not having sponged the child at the time. But it was no time for lessons on housekeeping. She was coping as best she knew how and I was not helping. I think someone should have told me about the ways of the Indians before I went to nurse them. However, I was in the wrong. I was projecting my feelings of possible failure and inadequacies onto the one person available. I was too ready to judge her on my values and beliefs and gave her no credit for what, she felt, was doing her duty.

Frequently, anxiety causes a person to make judgments not therapeutic to oneself or others. This is often an unconscious act. We rationalize that it is someone else's fault when it really is not a matter of fault but of circumstances. I wanted to be effective and help the child recover from his illness. I needed help to achieve this goal. I did not consider that my instructions perhaps were not as important to the grandmother as they were to me. It was not only unnecessary to reprimand her, it was also a very immature thing to do. Had I been patient and understanding I would have accomplished the task as well and on a happier note.

Not all problems of Cultural Adaptation involve persons of differing racial or ethnic origin. Here the nurse describes her rejection of a lower-class family with all the prejudicial stereotyping that can be involved in entering another "culture."

I wish to discuss two visits that I made to the home of Mrs. O and her six children as a student public health nurse (with my R.N.). The children ranged in age from 12 years to 7 months and the family resided in a slum-type rooming house downtown, where they occupied three attic rooms and shared a washroom on the floor below with approximately 10 other people.

The main health problem for which I was visiting concerned Mary, a 4-year-old girl who had her right eye enucleated in December of last year for bilateral retinoblastoma. I had a great deal of difficulty locating the family, as they were very transient and had been evicted from their former residence by the sheriff. I had formed a rather negative opinion of this family by the time I was able to visit them and was actually afraid to meet them or go into their home.

As I went into this house on my first visit I felt as though I were entering a different world. It seemed cold, dirty, foul-smelling, and so dark that I could barely find my way along the hall and up the stairs to their flat. When I arrived and met Mrs. O, a small woman in her mid-30s who was not the least bit impressed by my arrival, I was shocked to see the condition of the home. I was really shaken by the whole atmosphere and could not imagine how people lived in such conditions. The floors were dirty and cluttered, the walls badly soiled and the furniture sparse and beyond repair. There had been no heat that day, even though it was cold; the mother had the burners on the stove turned on high to try and keep the kitchen warm. Two of the younger children, including Mary, were running around dirty, barely dressed, and in bare feet. I reluctantly accepted a chair as Mrs. O motioned from the kitchen but refrained from removing my coat for fear I would dirty my clothes.

I felt, as I unenthusiastically began to pursue a rather formal and impersonal conversation with this mother, that I was being rather benevolent in giving some of my time to help this unfortunate, underprivileged, and rather scruffy group. Mrs. O commenced to tell me about her infant's feeding problem, which I felt was rather insignificant in comparison with what I considered to be a rather catastrophic situation. Instead of attentively listening to Mrs. O, and respecting and recognizing what she felt was a very real problem, I proceeded to pick out the flaws in her use of the English language and recalled the family's recent eviction from their former residence as well as all the accusations the landlady made against them. I also thought about the many common-law husbands this woman had obviously had and wondered which one she was living with at the moment, if any. This woman's conversation seemed so incongruent in these circumstances. She did not measure up to my standards of what I thought a mother should be and I felt that she must be handing me a line and attempting to discuss the topics that I would consider most acceptable. I sensed that she distrusted me but did not look to myself for the reason.

Mrs. O then took me into the bedroom and showed me her 7-month-old baby girl, Elizabeth, lying quietly on a rather dirty and dishevelled bed. The room smelled stale and musty and the baby appeared underdeveloped physically and rather pale and listless. I had never seen a baby so inadequately provided for and felt a great urge to take some immediate action.

I seemed to sense a difference in this mother as she picked up her baby. She obviously had a great deal of love and affection for this little child and she seemed to lose the hardened look that struck me so visibly when I first arrived.

In the midst of your negativism here, it was good that you were open to seeing this.

Mrs. O then began to discuss her other children, who attended school, and the progress they were making. I had not met these children but I visualized in my mind what I thought they would be like (which, incidentally, was a very negative impression). The mother told me how well these children were doing in school and how eager they were to learn. Instead of encouraging and supporting this mother, who was truly concerned about her family's welfare, and recognizing the difficult task she had of rearing children in this environment, I made no recognition of her efforts and went on to discuss something else. I did not realize how much this woman needed encouragement and recognition of her efforts as a mother. I could not see how desperately she was trying to seek my approval. I did not see her or treat her as an equal human being, or listen attentively or acceptingly to her conversation.

Mary had been in the hospital that particular day for an eye examination under anesthetic to check the progress of the tumor in the left eye. It never occurred to me to consider that Mrs. O was concerned over the results of Mary's eye examination and might have benefited from some reassurance and support. I also never realized at the time that the house was probably more untidy than usual because the mother had spent most of the morning with Mary at the hospital. I lacked real consideration and empathy for this mother, and could not see past the living conditions to realize that she was another person just like myself, with wants, needs, and fears and with every right to human dignity and respect.

Before I left that day I asked the mother in a slightly condescending manner if the children needed any warm winter clothing. I realize now that, due to my lack of concern for this woman's pride and self-respect, I did not give her the opportunity or the right to broach this subject herself. I guess I was so shocked by the lack of facilities by my standards that I felt compelled to rush in and make immediate improvements. I was in fact questioning this mother's ability to provide for her children and had failed to realize the many strengths and resources present in this family, for they were really functioning adequately in their present limited circumstances and with a little support and guidance could cope with many of their problems themselves.

During my next couple of visits to this family my attitude began to change. I began to realize the great privilege and responsibility that a public health nurse assumes on entering a home, regardless of the economic or cultural status of its members. I began to feel progressively more at ease in this situation and developed a great deal of admiration and respect for this mother. Mrs. O is the real strength and unifying force in this family and both mother and children enjoy a close and mutually supportive relationship with each other. I began to shed my outer covering of reservation and professionalism and started conversing with her as an equal, listening with intent and acceptance to her conversation.

Actually this is real *professionalism.*

She began to talk more freely and earnestly and revealed her difficulties to me without fear of judgment or disapproval.

Mrs. O now takes great pride in telling me of small accomplishments she has made and of her children's progress in school. I can now appreciate that she is attempting to elevate the children's standards and values beyond her own. These children are neat, polite, and considerate and one cannot help but be impressed by the tremendous job this mother is doing in raising these children in this environment. Mrs. O has needed someone to understand how difficult a task she has in raising these children, to give her a little support and encouragement, and to show some recognition of her accomplishments. A great deal of attention up until now has been focused on Mary, who has made an admirable adjustment to her disability, but little concern has been shown for the mother's anxiety and inability to accept Mary's deformity.

I believe this family and I have given each other something very special. Many encouraging results are beginning to emerge from our relationship. It amazes me how small thoughts and suggestions carefully planted can blossom into real results when one least expects it. Mrs. O took my suggestion about obtaining some clothing for the children. She took the initiative and was able to obtain clothing for both her children and herself. During the first visit, as I mentioned previously, Mrs. O had discussed the difficulty she was having with the baby, in that she would not take any solid food or tolerate her formula well. I subsequently made a few grudging suggestions but at the time I had no confidence in the mother's ability to carry them out. During my next visit Mrs. O informed me that she was now giving the baby both vegetables and fruit and she was tolerating her feeding very well. I cannot describe the pleasure and pride on her face as she described these daily accomplishments to me for my approval. I felt wonderful just to see how pleased and proud she was in having succeeded at mastering this problem herself.

I believe this mother sensed my increasing confidence in her ability as a mother and value as a person. I realize now how perceptive people are, and the disapproval that I felt on the first visit was as easily conveyed as my subsequent change of attitude.

I have gained real respect for this family through working with them. I am sure life will never change dramatically for these people, but with support and intervention during crises I am sure this family can sustain itself. I believe any deviance in their behavior is overshadowed by their great drive and motivation to better themselves.

I think this is a family you will never forget. The benefits to them and you of redirecting your attitudes and thus your use of self will be lifelong and far-reaching.

14
DEATH/DYING

Of the 550 cases in the study, 14% focus on Death/Dying. Of the 78 cases that focus on Death/Dying, 49% are described as Helpful, 51% as Unhelpful.

COMPARISON WITH ALL OTHER SITUATIONS

Helpful Factors

Highest Rating

- Helped family members deal with the situation.

Unhelpful Factors

Highest Rating

- Felt inadequate to enter into patient's problem because had not personally resolved the issue.
- Incapacitated by own fear of death.
- Felt guilty but could not communicate.
- Felt pressured (within self) into doing things rather than coping with feeling elements (tension present).
- Avoided needs of family members (same rating as Cultural Adaptation and Alcoholism).

Helpful Factors	% of Cases in Which Cited
1. Gave moral support	66
2. Helped family members	63
3. Helped patient express feelings	53
4. Was a sounding board	53
5. Came to terms with own feelings; was able to enter into patient's problem	37
6. Wanted to understand how patient felt	32
7. Took time to explain	29
8. Nonjudgmental	29
9. Used physical closeness	26
10. Looked beyond patient's outward response/behavior to underlying causes	26
11. Positively identified with patient due to similar life/professional experience	21
12. Liked the patient	18
13. Was honest with patient/relatives	13
14. Not unduly influenced by negative opinions of other staff regarding the patient's personality	11
15. Initiated referral to another profession/resource	8
16. Made this case the basis for overall policy change/improvement	3
17. Had received training in recognizing social-emotional needs of patients	3
18. Was trying to prove self to senior staff members	0
19. Discussed religion with patient	0
20. Used innovative rehabilitative procedure	0

Unhelpful Factors	% of Cases in Which Cited
1. Felt inadequate to enter into patient's problem because had not personally resolved the issue	70
2. Felt guilty but could not communicate	53
3. Treated the condition, overlooking the patient	43
4. Avoided needs of family members	40
5. Self-image was threatened	40
6. Felt pressured (within self) into doing things rather than coping with feeling elements (tension present)	38

7.	Incapacitated by own fear of death	38
8.	Purposely disregarded significant cues in patient's statements/behavior	30
9.	Rationalized actions and thoughts	28
10.	Felt guilty but still would not communicate	18
11.	Lacked training in recognizing social-emotional needs of patients	15
12.	Lost professional role: patient became friend	15
13.	Short-staffed; too little time to devote to the patient	10
14.	Did not want to understand	10
15.	Was disapproving, judgmental	10
16.	Failed to look beyond initial negative impression of patient's personality	10
17.	Prejudiced toward group of which patient was a member	10
18.	Overidentified due to being similar age to patient	10
19.	Breakdown of interprofessional communication/cooperation	8
20.	Negatively influenced by opinions of other staff members regarding personality of the patient	8
21.	Afraid would break down and cry in front of patient	8
22.	Disregarded own judgment because wanted approval of senior staff members	8
23.	Failed to seek authoritative advice regarding innovation	5
24.	Disliked patient	0

In 70% of the Unhelpful cases, the nurse describes herself as *felt inadequate to enter into patient's problem because had not personally resolved the issue.* She was, therefore, able to be of little or no help in the nurse-patient relationship. This is the highest rating of this response among all problem situations.

My job was to care for Miss Y on the evening shift along with one other patient, which was to enable me to give her the attention she required. This young woman had been in and out of hospitals for several years with her illness but this time she seemed to know that the prognosis was poor. I was aware that she would need much comforting, both physically—and probably more—emotionally. I didn't know how I was going to deal with the latter.

When I entered her room, a private one, she looked very uncomfortable and I felt quite panicky. I had never cared for a young girl who was dying. I introduced myself and told her that I was going to try to make her more comfortable. She was under regular sedation, but she was still alert, looked terribly anxious, and was having difficulty breathing, even though she was in an oxygen tent. I felt adequately competent to care for her physical needs and to check the equipment but I felt at a loss when trying to help her emotionally. She was continually crying out things like "I'm dying, aren't I?" or "I don't want to die . . . please help me!" I couldn't answer and I couldn't wait to leave the room. I was in and out of the room several times to do things but never just to sit with her.

I was feeling very guilty about my inability to face the situation and was quite happy when her parents arrived a little later in the evening. Even so, I sent them out of the room a number of times so that I could putter around and satisfy myself that I was nursing her. She seemed a little more relaxed when they were there, talking to her quietly or just listening to her, holding her hand.

When I returned to the room at one point, I found a number of relatives gathered around the bedside crying and praying. I was horrified at this! I didn't think this would be good for her; besides, the hospital rule allowed only two visitors at one time. I felt that I was justified in sending them out. She was less alert by this time, and did not seem to have been upset by all the visitors. She still had some difficulty breathing. I gave her the sedation ordered and a sponge bath because she was perspiring and again changed the linen. I left that evening feeling very dissatisfied with myself, even though her parents seemed quite grateful that I had done my best for her.

Analysis

Although Miss Y had required a fair amount of physical care, I felt that I had overdone this aspect to make up for my inability to deal with her emotional needs. Miss Y was very close to me in age and I was anxious myself when I pictured myself in her shoes. I was so concerned with my own feelings and fears of dying, that I was unable to help her with her needs.

In the first few hours when we were alone, I didn't really have to answer all her questions. I could have just sat by her side and listened, talked a little, and simply given her the comfort of having a human being close at hand. Had I not been thinking of myself and my need to do something tangible (e.g., change the bed) I would have allowed her parents to be with her longer in her last hours. She needed them more at this time than a straightened sheet.

By the time that the relatives were in the room Miss Y was less alert, so I don't think their presence helped her, but it also did not hurt her. The crying and praying were their ways of expressing their sorrow and their desire to help her according to their cultural pattern; I think it would have been more helpful to them had I allowed them to stay at least a little while. I could only think about how I wouldn't like people gathered around my bedside in that fashion and that the hospital rule limited the number of visitors. However, hospital regulations were flexible and had I been more aware of the needs of the family to express their feelings, I would have been more helpful.

I was not professional in this situation—I was me-centered and not patient-centered. The next day, I was informed that Miss Y had died during the night and although no one could have saved her life, I did not feel that I had done my best.

*   *   *   *

Jim S, a 13-year-old boy, died 4 months after he was admitted to the floor on which I was working as a general duty nurse. His official diagnosis was leukemia, but he was told that he had a blood dyscrasia, the general term we used for all children suffering from this fatal illness. When Jim pressed the medical and nursing staff for more details about his condition, he was told that he just needed to be built up.

During the day, there were usually three R.N.s on the floor, and one during the evening. The nursing students were rotated quite often, so it was with the R.N.s that Jim became most familiar and to whom he posed his questions. I, therefore, was confronted with his questions and doubts almost every day I worked, as were the other nurses.

When Jim had been on the floor for about 2 months, another boy of his age was admitted, with the same diagnosis. The two boys became friends, but Jim's chum went downhill rapidly and died within 2 weeks of his admission. Jim began questioning the nurses about this, asking if he, too, was going to die, since he had the same diagnosis. We all brushed off this question with the explanation that there are several kinds of blood dyscrasias, and that he was suffering from a different type than his friend. Here too, I failed to see the need to sit down with Jim and listen to him in order to give him reasonable reassurance and hope. In fact, I really didn't want to discuss it with him at all, which Jim probably sensed, and this heightened his anxiety.

By the end of his third month in hospital Jim was quite ill. Transfusions, painful tests, and treatments added to his discomfort. He soon started to confront me (and the other staff members) with "I am going to die soon, aren't I?" I brushed this off, telling him that the treatments would soon start to work.

When Jim seemed to be particularly low emotionally, the head nurse would telephone his mother, and she would come and spend the day with him. She, too, continued the charade until Jim lapsed into unconsciousness and died.

We all failed Jim, perhaps for different reasons. We answered none of his questions with any kind of sensitivity, and were unsuccessful in giving him reasonable reassurance or hope. He was never given the opportunity to discuss his fears about his illness or about death.

Social

I was brought up as an only child in an isolated nuclear family. Edgar Jackson [1967] brings out how this can affect one's attitude toward death. He states that in a multigenerational family living together death was never remote, and both the event and the accompanying feelings could be dealt with realistically.

With the advent of the nuclear family, the basic family unit is broken only by the death of one of the members. With this threat, members of the family pretend that this catastrophe will never happen to them, making the members extremely vulnerable, unable to contend openly and honestly with the fact of their own and other people's death [Jackson, 1967, p. 176].

Robert Fulton brings out the fact that in Western societies, emerging attitudes are reflected in death suppression, making this an unpleasant topic—one to be avoided if at all possible [Fulton, 1964]. This, too, characterizes the way death was treated by those around me as I grew up.

Philosophical

The thought that I will die, and with my death my life as I know it will cease, frightens me. Theological explanations of the nature and purpose of human life are explicitly and implicitly challenged by medical and social science. Since I cannot really accept the inevitability of my own death, I do not like to be confronted with it in other people.

Professional

In her book, *On Death and Dying*, Dr. Kübler-Ross [1969, p. 10] has brought out very clearly the attitude of people in the healing professions toward death. Because we are involved in trying to save and prolong life, we tend to deny death exists—to ourselves and to our patients—particularly those who are dying. We are often uncomfortable in the presence of death.

In this case, the nurse realizes too late that she has not been willing to let her patient go.

Before many days Mrs. P was put into an oxygen tent. When her face became quite expressionless and she was going semiconscious, I tried to stimulate her with encouragement but she'd only turn her head from side to side and perhaps a tear would run down her face. I talked into her ear and her eyelids would flicker and she would squeeze my hand. She knew she was going to die. Her daughter had discussed this in the beginning, and I had only said, "I hope we can make her well again." Mrs. P was really very strong emotionally. She knew she wasn't going to get better and had come to terms with it. I should have let her tell me; she seemed to want to, but I didn't want to let her go.

An important insight.

When I did realize what she was trying to tell me, she was much more relaxed and actually more comforted.

That both nurse and family become caught up in asking the patient to hold on is clearly described below.

Ricky, a 17-year-old boy, was found to have cancer of the lung 3 months prior to his death. He was told by his parents the nature of his illness but also that it would be able to be successfully treated in hospital, although they knew that Ricky would only live for a few months.

I first met Ricky on his third hospital day. He was a cheerful and likable boy and soon became the favorite patient on the floor. His condition deteriorated gradually. His parents told him that his not feeling well was due to the side effects of radiation. On this third admission to the hospital Ricky was a very sick boy, but he still had his little smile for everyone.

His mother was almost constantly at his bedside and we got to know her well. One day I asked her if Ricky knew how sick he was. She told me that he had asked her just a few days ago if he was going to die, which she had denied. She told me that had she told him the truth, he would not have been able to hold on, and she continued, "We love him so much and we want him to hold on."

I looked after Ricky the day he died. He required continuous oxygen and was given large doses of morphine, for which his parents had asked as they did not want him to suffer. Ricky was still conscious but he dozed on and off between the injections, which he required every 1 ½ hours. As the family did all the care for him, there did not seem to be anything left for me to do, but I had the feeling that they wanted me to be there, and I came as often as I could.

When I returned with another needle I noticed a great change in Ricky. I knew that, if I administered the morphine, his life might come to a quick end. When I explained this to the family, they asked me if Ricky would experience pain during semiconsciousness, which I was unable to answer. Thereupon Ricky's mother said, "We don't want him to have any pain, but we leave it to you, nurse."

I believe this decision was the hardest one I ever had to make. This woman, who had wanted him to hold on, was giving up her son out of pity and love. How could I hold on to my ethics when she was giving up her child?

Ricky died soon after the injection. It was heartbreaking to see the family's grief, yet I felt that I had made the right decision.

I wonder what she meant by "holding on." There are times when to deny the truth to someone is really preventing them from feeling the peace that can come from facing and walking this road together, i.e., Ricky may have most of all wanted to share his fear and even the truth within the very love his parents had for him. Perhaps his parents were saying that they couldn't control themselves if they admitted the truth. Then the focus for everyone becomes self-control, rather than how the family could be close to each other, even in this.

Here a nurse discusses her philosophy concerning talking to patients and families about death.

I realize that not telling patients has some advantages but it also has disadvantages. Dying patients fear death probably because they are incapable of imagining a state of nothingness. Fear probably comes from what one projects into the unknown of death, and this projection takes place on the unconscious level. A person can have faith in God, and an afterlife, but when you are entering something you know nothing about, naturally you are afraid. Will the unknown be a physical world like ours with seasons and night and day? Will we ever see our loved ones again?

Some doctors feel a patient does not want to know if he is going to die. They feel that denial enables the patient to see hope where none exists and takes away mental suffering by eliminating reality since the reality of one's own death is impossible to grasp. Such doctors feel evasiveness supports the natural defenses in a patient. They feel that since death is something beyond comprehension, it should be denied and avoided by silence. But what about the fears caused by the imagination—sometimes unrealistic fears? Does denying these fears erase them from mind? I hardly think so.

I strongly believe that these fears should be talked through instead of being repressed and stimulating all sorts of weird things in the unconscious.

A young graduate describes her way of coping.

I remember one dying old gentleman on a surgical floor. He had been granted the dignity of a private room, but it was still a noisy, busy place. His wounds were open and suppurative—he had cancer, but the resident surgeon was determined to treat. Although my personal feelings distinctly flavor my words I felt that the medical staff were prolonging an inevitable death.

That man must have been in agony. I requested to nurse him as much as possible. His eyes said that he knew he was dying, and when the "men in white" gave new orders, and came into the room to poke and probe his gaping abdomen, shouting encouraging words at him (for some reason we think all old people are deaf) I took his hand and tried to show him that I understood how he felt.

When his dear little wife came to visit each day the nursing staff would disappear mysteriously. (For some reason nurses find it difficult to really face death, although they can certainly handle the bodies of the dying and dead.) Mrs. K would cry on my shoulder (literally) and ask me for encouragement. I couldn't give her any. She would reminisce about their life together and I would listen, perhaps cutting the time that should have been spent with my other patients. A few backs were not rubbed during those few weeks before he died.

When Mr. K finally did die, in spite of all that medical science could do for him, it was to me that his little wife came again, to pour out her grief and even to thank me. I felt so inadequate. I had not been able to stop his torture.

In retrospect though, I can see that just because I took the time when others would not, and because I touched his hand when others would not look him straight in the eye, and because I was listening instead of running away, I was in some way able to help this couple through their crisis.

Even if the help was ever so slight, and if perhaps my young ways were immature—I could not find many words—I was willing to become involved with them.

The pain of becoming involved in another's pain is described below.

Chris S was a 9-year-old boy who suffered 79% body burns during a fire at summer camp. Ordinarily he would have soon died, but because medical care had been started almost immediately, he was brought to the unit completely conscious. Chris's mother, a widow, was engaged to be married, and Mrs. S and her husband-to-be required a lot of emotional support.

When I first heard about Chris, I was horrified at the extent of his burns, and did not think I would ever be able to look after him. My attitude was very common among the staff, although the fact that we worked in pairs with Chris decreased our anxiety a little. It was not uncommon for someone to come to work, telling of the bad dream she had had the night before, involving Chris.

My turn to look after Chris (who was being nursed in isolation to minimize possibilities of infection) came within a week. I entered the room and said hello to the bundle of dressings lying on the bed in the midst of numerous machines and pieces of equipment. Although I had been told Chris was conscious, I was completely unprepared for the nodding of his head and the gasping sounds from the respirator. From that moment on I had no trouble accepting the fact that Chris was a previously normal 9-year-old boy who had been burned.

When Chris's mother visited a few hours later she said that she hadn't any idea of how we could work with and talk to Chris as we did. I realized that this must have been a big worry to her—she had taken almost a week to approach her son and talk to him in a normal voice, and I don't really think she expected that we would be able to accept Chris at all. From that time on my relationship with Mrs. S and her fiance was very open and honest. Almost all of the other nurses developed as good if not better relationships with these parents, and Mrs. S quickly developed confidence and trust in us.

A great deal of nonverbal communication went on and I found out that Mrs. S wondered if it would be better if Chris had not been so well cared for at the beginning of his illness. I secretly agreed with her but felt that since Chris was with us he deserved the best care I could give him and should be kept as comfortable as possible. I communicated this verbally, although not as bluntly, to his mother. I tried to involve Mrs. S in Chris's care by suggesting she read to him, bring in his radio, etc. The other nurses also did this, and I think Mrs. S felt part of the team caring for her son. I know that she felt free to talk to us about her frustrations when Chris was particularly demanding, and we tried to make her feel that it was permissible to get annoyed with him at times.

I wish this story could end happily, but it didn't. Chris died 3 months after his admission after a long fight full of pain and frustration. As his mother had feared, his initial survival had spared him for a more lengthy death after he had undergone still more suffering.

I will remember this family for a very long time, and keep in mind that the nurse is in a position to make a tremendous contribution to families in a crisis, if she will allow herself to become involved.

And if she will allow herself to remain involved in subsequent situations—for in such cases, the nurse becomes a lifeline emotionally as well as physically. You have been a part of a great deal of suffering for your age. This has deepened your willingness to give, and in this you will also share in the heights that people experience. This is the pain and the joy of service.

In 53% of the Unhelpful cases the nurse describes *felt guilty, but could not communicate.* This is the highest rating of this Response among all Situations.

My patient, Mrs. M, age 26, had three children (ages 10, 7, and 4). She was admitted with terminal carcinoma, severe metastasis, and a pregnancy of 30-weeks gestation. Her malignancy was first diagnosed when she attended a prenatal clinic in a small town. Mrs. M was escorted by a nurse who just gave her report and left. Mrs. M's husband could not afford the time off work that day.

On admission to the obstetrical floor Mrs. M appeared pale, tired, and above all, there were obvious signs of fear and anxiety in her eyes. She was placed in a private room on the labor floor. Her prognosis was poor and the staff knew she was going to die at any time. Due to her poor general condition, she would not survive a caesarean section, leaving a postmortem caesarean section as the alternative to saving the baby. With this in mind, the room was prepared with the emergency caesarean section set, baby's resuscitator, and the premature nursery and anesthetist were alerted. Throughout all this, Mrs. M was informed by the obstetrician exactly what was happening. She gave the impression of acceptance, but said very little—just a faint smile occasionally.

It became necessary for Mrs. M to have a special nurse, and due to seniority I was designated. I performed my nursing duties efficiently but found it impossible to communicate with her verbally. I bargained with myself—I could not say "Good morning"; what was good about it for her? I could not ask how she was feeling. I knew how—she was dying. What else could one say to a dying person? I felt dumb and helpless, as often I could see and feel her eyes following me around the room. It made me very uncomfortable, but I kept busy. I thought to myself, Why should she, so young, pregnant, and with a young family, die? Then I reflected upon my past nursing experience, when I avoided dying patients and left them to the older nurses.

I consoled myself with the fact that her husband visited quite often, so all I was supposed to do was continue to administer good nursing care and ensure that she remained comfortable. I specialed her from 8–4 for 5 days and spoke to her only when absolutely necessary; I did not even speak to her husband. I had an awful feeling of guilt, but due to pride I mentioned it to no one.

Mrs. M died at noon on the fifth day. She struggled, but without pain, while I stood at the other end of the room and watched. To me it was a frightening experience. When she was pronounced dead, the operation was performed, and a live male child was extracted, which survived only 2 hours.

The following case illustrates the range of coping mechanisms employed due to *felt guilty but could not communicate: treated the condition, overlooking the patient* (43% of cases); *felt pressured (within self) into doing things rather than coping with feeling elements (tension present)* (38% of cases); *purposely disregarded significant cues in patient's statements/behavior* (30% of cases).

That these Responses in the face of death are not peculiar to the young or inexperienced nurse is illustrated in this supervisor's account.

The most frustrating experience of my nursing career was my inability to comfort a dying patient.

This patient was a 48-year-old orderly who had undergone chest surgery for bronchogenic carcinoma. Several days after surgery he was successfully resuscitated following a cardiac arrest. After this, he became very depressed and frequently asked why he had been resuscitated. "Why didn't you let me go?", he said, "I'm done for." These were remarks that he repeated constantly. As he had not yet been told the prognosis of his disease, I endeavored to reassure him that this was not so. However, I soon began to have feelings of guilt in following this course of behavior. There were several reasons for my guilt complex.

In the first instance, I felt that my brisk, cheerful, optimistic manner was an insult to his intelligence. He had worked in the intensive care unit for several years and had a fairly good knowledge of the reasons for such drastic surgery.

Secondly, he was beginning to distrust me. I evaded his inquiries by always initiating the conversation and keeping up a running commentary of hospital news and gossip. In fact, I became quite adept at exiting from the door of his room at the exact moment that I finished my daily news bulletin. I could not bring myself to lie to him, so I ignored the issue.

Thirdly, I began to find excuses for not visiting him daily. I rationalized that so many staff members visited him that he would not remember if I, the supervisor, had been in every day. My own feelings of helplessness and inadequacy led to this withdrawal from the situation. Rather than run the risk of betraying my own emotions, I betrayed his trust of me.

A very honest self-appraisal.

The following cases focus on what is obviously seen as a key Response in both Helpful and Unhelpful cases. *Helped family members deal with the situation* is cited in 63% of the Helpful cases and *avoided needs of family members* is cited in 40% of the Unhelpful cases. In both instances, this is the highest rating of these Responses among all Situations.

A nonhelpful situation I was involved in took place in a suburban hospital where I was the head nurse of a surgical unit. The patient concerned was a

Jewish lady in her late 50s. She had had a successful mastectomy for carcinoma 7 years previously. On this occasion she was admitted with acute abdominal distress and a queried perforated ulcer. Emergency surgery was performed a few hours after her admission and at the operation she was noted to have widespread carcinoma of the abdominal cavity. The ulcer was patched and a permanent colostomy performed to bypass an inoperable condition.

Her convalescence was slow and hindered by the usual postoperative discomforts, which seemed to last longer than in normal postsurgery situations. This was difficult for the family to realize and accept. The patient realized she was not progressing satisfactorily but never openly stated the realization that she had a reoccurrence of her past cancerous condition. I felt she knew she had a terminal illness, however.

During this crisis, her family was summoned and told by the attending doctors of her terminal condition. Her husband and son, though stunned and saddened, quietly accepted the news. Her daughter was a potential problem immediately. She was a psychology major, teaching at a university, and dressed unusually for a person in her 20s and married. Nothing about her mother's hospital care satisfied her. She continually had the patient, her roommate, the special duty nurses, the doctors in attendance, my staff nurses, and myself in an emotional, tense uproar. For example, as her mother's condition worsened to a comatose state, she would not leave the now private room; she whispered sweet nothings repeatedly in her mother's ear (to which the dying woman could not respond, of course) and even cut locks of her mother's hair for each family member. Her attitudes and ways were unbelievable to all concerned. At last, after many harrassing and sad episodes, the patient expired and we, as a staff, were thanked by this daughter for "helping to murder" her mother.

Description and Analysis of Situation

Neither my staff nurses nor I broached this subject of dying on our own with the patient but we did with the family. Perhaps this was due to the fear of not knowing how to direct conversation along this vein with the patient or how to allay her fears of a terminal illness. Old-school professional ethics reminded us to only answer questions asked and not to initiate conversation on this subject.

I employed every method I could think of in dealing with this unusual daughter. I felt that my staff and I gave the patient excellent nursing care. We tried in vain to help this daughter but did we really exist to help the daughter or the patient?

Can you really separate them?

I did not feel we failed the dying patient then, but now looking back I wonder if we could not have talked her terminal illness over with her. Then she, in turn, might have gained enough insight and strength to help her family, especially her daughter. The unanswerable question still to me is to what degree was this girl my responsibility? Except for her involvement with the patient, perhaps none. To help her accept or deny the impending death appeared a gigantic task and much beyond my scope. Even after the death, which she was present for, she had to be taken to the morgue to verify her mother's death. During this crisis period I showed sympathy, antipathy, astonishment, rebellion, and other ploys toward this daughter.

Now looking back I realize that she was in the shock and/or denial stages of this family crisis before the actual death took place. In her nonacceptance of the situation I paralleled myself with her as I was still going through the stages of grief crisis. Her retort to this was that I had half a heart. I became angry with her, threatening to remove her 24-hour visiting privileges, but hostilities were only aroused and this solved nothing. The patient was still my main concern. The nursing office supported me in all the methods I employed. In the end analysis I felt that I had failed in not being able to enlighten or improve this deplorable situation for the patient, her family, my staff, myself, and above all, the mixed-up daughter. It was indeed a strange situation and 4 years later I am still trying to analyze it.

Could other resource people have helped?

*   *   *   *

I was involved as a private duty nurse caring for a young married man in the latter stages of leukemia in the hospital. His very attractive wife, Mrs. M, was 8 months pregnant at the time and he had two preschool children. She wanted to come to the hospital to see him every day, but his sister and brother insisted that two or three times a week should be the limit because of her pregnancy. Brother and sister were very attentive in visiting every day. As time went on, Mrs. M's visits seemed to be less frequent. Occasionally the patient mentioned this to me, but I suggested that perhaps she might be in later, or she might not be feeling well enough to come that day.

Most of the time, the patient was heavily sedated, so that many days his wife just sat in the room while he slept, although sometimes he would awaken to carry on a short conversation with her. After each visit she would become emotionally upset, but she never did cry in front of her husband. She would break down in the lounge and his family felt that this was detrimental to her health.

As the time of death grew very near, the patient's family advised Mrs. M not to come at all. They felt that his appearance alone would be something she would never forget. As a result, I last saw her about 3 days before the patient died.

In this case, I felt I should have interviewed Mrs. M at greater length to let her express her feelings about visiting her husband. I should have perhaps tactfully told the brother and sister not to interfere with Mrs. M but to encourage her to visit if she so wished. I should have told Mrs. M that her husband did ask for her when he woke, indicating that her presence was a comfort in itself to him. Then she would have derived a great deal of satisfaction in being with him, even though she could not do anything to help his condition; thus she might have felt that she was doing her part as his wife.

I should have pointed out to her that in a situation such as this, we should disregard our own feelings and make more of an effort to console or comfort the dying. This would not involve crying or whispering in low tones in front of the patient but being calm and talking in normal tones. Near death, the dying might feel very lonely and frightened, so that if they rallied long enough to see their loved ones near them, they would be comforted and feel less alone. I accepted the patient and his wife as individuals but I considered the wife's feelings and physical condition in preference to the dying patient's feelings or needs.

I failed, also, in reassuring the patient that his wife had visited him while he was asleep. I might have passed on to him the information she had given me about his children, their quotable sayings and their amusing actions. These family details would have been of interest to him and would also have made him feel closer to his family. These details would have given comfort and made him feel less alone and cut off from his family.

As you say, their needs were actually quite similar—to be together; perhaps even to speak together about what was happening. At the right time, it can be a real release and relief to both patient and family to share the fact that death is coming. The spoken can be less frightening than the unspoken.

In this case the nurse describes how difficult it is for the healing team to admit that medicine has so many limitations. In their unwillingness to accept these inevitabilities, patient and family are often pulled into a circle of false hopes.

To use yourself effectively in any relationship you must be aware of your innermost thoughts and feelings and how you convey them both verbally and nonverbally. You must actively listen to your patient and take in what his words are saying as well as what his actions and expressions are saying. There have been few occasions when I have truly felt useful in helping a patient or family resolve some inner conflict. So often on a busy, active floor there just isn't enough time or staff (a very convenient excuse for the nurse who cannot handle her own feelings regarding the problem and is, therefore, unable to cope with the patient's feelings).

I worked on a neurosurgical floor where the problems rarely seemed to be minor to anyone, staff included. So often we had to deal with impending death. It never seemed to be an elderly person who had lived a full life, whose death you could view as a relief from pain, but always a young person with a young family and so much to live for. That kind of death seems so much harder to understand, to accept, and to deal with.

If the patient is unconscious it is the family who suffers alone. Nursing staff can deal with the unconscious patient with little problem. The patient is not asking threatening questions, or is not aware that the doctor is quickly passing his room while making rounds. The patient is not questioning his treatment or in any other way making the nurse uncomfortable. It is the family who is doing all of these things.

Although we understand their worry, concern, and grief, we fail to deal with it. We hate to admit that medicine has so many limitations. So often in reference to an unconscious patient you hear the nurses and physicians say to the family, "We don't know how long he will be unconscious. It's a slow healing process. These things take time." Always the positive statement "Yes he will get well, we just don't know when" is heard by the family and they cling to this hope, often a false hope.

Such was the case with Mrs. B. Her husband Louis was 33. They had two young children. Louis had had major surgery for the removal of a fast-growing malignant brain tumor. At first it was hopeful that Louis would regain consciousness, but after many weeks of being in a comatose state, and many serious setbacks, it became evident to all staff that his prognosis was indeed poor. No one, however, was able to convey this to the family.

Their endless questions continued to be answered with hopeful stock phrases. The nurses felt that it was the doctor's place to level with the family, but the doctor involved just wasn't prepared to do this. It didn't seem fair to me that the family was caught in the middle of this conflict.

Every day Mrs. B would arrive at the hospital with her sister-in-law and Mr. B's brother. Although they too were very upset, they seemed to provide a great deal of support for Mrs. B. Every day the same questions were asked and the same noncommittal answers were given by every staff member.

One day Mrs. B came alone. I was going off duty and poked my head in the room on my way out, just to make sure everything had been done. She trapped me: "How's Louis today? Is he any better?" I felt she deserved an honest ear and this time I had all the time in the world. She began to weep quietly as she had done so many times before, so I suggested that we go down to the sunroom, where we could talk more privately. She readily agreed. When I suggested coffee she accepted, saying she hadn't had any lunch. So I left her alone with her thoughts while I went to get some coffee. On returning I found her exactly as I had left her, sitting forward in her chair, hands tightly clasped, eyes red-rimmed, and her face very drawn and tense. As she took a sip of coffee she seemed to relax a bit, and settling back in her chair she lit a cigarette. Not knowing where to start I asked her how things were going at home. Everything seemed to be as well as could be expected. Her friends and relatives were very helpful; there was always someone willing to care for the children while she was out. She confronted me again, "What's happening with Louis?" Not meaning to hedge I asked her what the doctor had told her.

She seemed to know a great deal about her husband's illness. I was able to clarify a few things she was uncertain about. Her questions flowed freely as we discussed the course of her husband's illness and what the many setbacks indicated. I tried to explain that everything humanly possible had been done, and it was no longer in our hands. She pondered this for a minute and then very calmly asked me how long I thought her husband would live. This seemed to be the first time that she felt free to admit to herself or anyone else that her husband was dying.

Also the first time the staff had been able to admit it.

This was by no means acceptance but it was a recognition of the possibility of death. She almost seemed relieved that it was out in the open.

Trying to be honest I told her that no one knew how long Louis would live: it could be 2 days, it might be 2 weeks.

We talked a little longer and then Mrs. B went back to sit a little longer with her husband. She assured me that someone was coming to pick her up and her sister-in-law lived nearby if she needed anything.

I never saw Mrs. B again—Louis died 2 days later and I was on my day off.

This was one situation in which I felt helpful to Mrs. B. I recognized her need to talk privately where she would not have to be embarrassed about showing her emotions and where she did not have to worry about having her private feelings broadcast to all of the visitors in the room. I had brought myself a coffee too, trying to let her know that I had all the time she needed. I sat down very near to her and pulled my chair so that it was facing hers. I tried to do more listening than talking. When I did talk I was trying to help her verbalize her thoughts and direct her questions rather than give reassurances or solutions. I felt that I did not bluntly tell Mrs. B that her husband was going to die, but rather let her express what she had probably known for a long time without being afraid of being reprimanded for giving up hope.

In this case, the nurse helps the mother express her need to move out of the mourning role.

Jamey was a 7-year-old who had been in the hospital for over 4 months, dying of Wilm's tumor. He had been ill for 3 years, and had required many lengthy and costly hospitalizations. This week, the most critical, his parents were keeping a 24-hour vigil, as it was expected that he would die at any moment. There were three other children in the family, including a month-old baby.

I had known the family for about a year at this time, due to Jamey's frequent admissions. I really admired Jamey's mother, Mrs. R, as she was always so kind and patient with Jamey, who could be quite obnoxious and demanding at times. She could always think up new stories and songs for him, and just never seemed to tire under the strain. She appeared very mature and self-sufficient.

One evening I saw Mrs. R sitting alone in the cafeteria, and decided to join her. I cannot remember the exact conversation, as it continued over the entire supper period. I remember that I remarked that she looked particularly tired that evening, and asked her if she thought she was getting enough sleep. She answered that she was tired and that she had had difficulty sleeping the last few nights. I suggested I would ask one of the interns to order her a sedative if she wished. She thought that would be a good idea, as she was exhausted, and would appreciate a good night's sleep.

I then asked her about her other children, who was looking after them at home, that she must miss them, and that they probably missed her. She said that she was astonished by my questions, as no one had ever asked her about the rest of her family—all they talked about was Jamey.

She said that she loved Jamey very much, but that she also loved her other children, and that her main concern now was not how to handle her grief when Jamey died, for in fact she had really thought of him as having died 4 months ago, and had gone through this whole process then. She said that she was much more concerned now with how Jamey's death would effect her husband, as he still clung to the hope of recovery, and how it would also affect the two older children. She said her main aim was to hold the family together, and develop an optimistic outlook, especially for the children's sake. She said she hoped the new baby would be a help to her in this purpose.

She told me that she was glad I didn't expect her to be the grieving mother, and had recognized that she had a life outside of the one she showed in hospital. She said that it was so hard to keep up this role, as she was really finished with her mourning, and all that was left was fatigue. She was very saddened by Jamey's condition, but said that they all had to go on living in spite of it.

On the way back to the floor, she thanked me for letting her express something she had not dared speak of even to her husband. She said she wished Jamey would die soon, so that she could get back to her family, as she was finished mourning.

Influence of the "Self" Factor

There already existed in this situation a certain degree of rapport. In other words, there existed mutual feelings of trust, acceptance, and respect. I liked her and genuinely wanted to help her, and I was not seeking approval. I did not try to change her point of view.

You demonstrated the sensitivity and ability to appreciate this woman as a total person, not simply the mother of your patient and, further, to verbalize this, and thereby actually free her to keep on coping.

By contrast, in the following case, the nurse attempts to direct the patient as to how she should be reacting to her grandmother's death.

Mrs. G, a 30-year-old energetic multigravida in the 20th week of her third pregnancy always seemed very happy and really enjoying her present condition. She was a prenatal patient attending a midwife's clinic where I was one of the midwives on staff.

Mrs. G always kept her appointment so when she failed to attend I decided I would visit her at home the following day. When I arrived at the home and knocked on the door, Mrs. G answered. She appeared rather dishevelled, hair uncombed, housedress torn and unbecoming, and her slippers were very shabby. She invited me in but I detected that she did this rather reluctantly; she then made excuses for the appearance of the living room. When I entered I could understand the reason for her reluctance: the living room was in a state of complete disorder.

We spoke generally for a few minutes and I inquired about her two boys, who were at school. I told her I had come to do the routine monthly tests because she did not keep her appointment of the previous day, and to find out the reason for her absence.

When the test was completed she told me that she was very upset because her grandmother had just died. I asked the age of her grandmother. She told me and I commented that she had outlived her allotted life span—three score years and ten; she was in fact 79 years old. I encouraged Mrs. G to resume her former social activities, which she usually enjoyed, and regain her self-composure. I asked of her brother and how he was reacting to the death of his grandmother. She said that he seemed to have recovered from the shock. I told her she should try behaving like her brother because that was much better. If she did, soon she would be happier. She became very silent and withdrawn and from then on there seemed to be a barrier between us.

I feel I was not helpful in the situation because I visited her at home without making an appointment. I invaded her privacy at a time when she may not have been ready for outside contact. I caused her embarrassment because of her personal appearance and attire and the disorderly state of her living room. Had I made an appointment she would have been ready for my visit. I made Mrs. G feel guilty by referring to the appointment she did not keep and implying that she should have cancelled the appointment or informed the clinic that she would be unable to attend, and then my visit would not have been unheralded.

I conveyed to Mrs. G through my attitude that I wasn't too disturbed about her grandmother's death because she had lived her life, ignoring that an elderly person can find meaning in living.

I tried to cheer her up by thrusting gaiety on her, not realizing that she should be allowed to suffer her loss and grieve over it. Grief and bereavement is a normal process that is necessary for continued health and it should not be interrupted. Scientifically it is known that when a loved person is lost through death, certain mental processes go into operation, processes that take time to work out. The attitude I displayed to Mrs. G was not what she expected, that of warmth, caring, interest, and respect. Instead I appeared, to her, to be very removed and disinterested.

I attached values to the reaction of her brother and herself—her brother's being good and hers bad. Here again I failed to realize that no two people react identically to the same situation.

Also, perhaps you were somewhat thrown by the very different way in which she presented herself that day. Inadvertently, you were trying to cheer her back to the self that was familiar to you. A very common error, I think, as we tend to label people and don't like to allow them to jump to another pigeonhole!

That very little can be done for the dying patient may be one of the most difficult realities for the nurse. Even when she sees herself as being helpful in death, she does very little at the verbal level by way of *took time to explain* (29%); rather, she *gave moral support* (in 66% of cases), *was a sounding board* (in 53% of cases), and *helped patient express feelings* (in 53% of cases). It would seem that explanation is directly related to the nurse's perception that she has something helpful to say. Here a nurse discusses her conflicts about listening and finally questions whether it is good enough to simply be a sounding board.

This was a man of 39 years of age and dying of cancer. He was married with two small children and another due any day. He had deteriorated very rapidly. Numerous treatments had been attempted, including a course of nitrogen mustard therapy, all with no apparent results.

This man was quite verbal and bitter. I guess he was angry, afraid, and frustrated. He was in a semiprivate room. It was summer but he kept the windows shut and the curtain drawn between the beds. It became hot and stuffy in the room so it was almost impossible to have another patient in the room with him. He had considerable physical pain, although usually the sedation was adequate to control this. At this time it had been increased to ½ gr. morphine. He was difficult to nurse because it hurt and frustrated me to hear him and see him—since there did not appear to be even the chance of a remission.

When I entered the room I would be the recipient of such remarks as "Why don't you give me an extra shot, no one would know," and "Well, if you ever wanted to see a dying man, you're looking at one now." In such situations I usually attended to his physical needs and asked him if there was anything else he would like. I usually tried to take time then to just sit quietly in a chair beside his bed so he would not always be so alone. Sometimes I would do this if I had free moments through the day. I do not feel that he expected any answer to his questions but at least it was a form of release for him for his anger and frustration. I suppose he was using the defense mechanism of substitution. I don't really know what answers could have been given, for he would know that I couldn't give him an extra shot. As for the second statement, I don't really believe he felt I wanted to see a man die. Maybe he was hoping for denial but I find this difficult to believe too, as he knew as well as or better than I that he was going to die. I feel that to have made a pretense of anything else would have been letting the patient down. I think he would have felt he couldn't trust me to be honest with him and that I was shutting him off from venting his feelings. I did not resent being asked these questions or having been placed in that situation, although I can't say that I would have chosen to be in such a situation either then or now.

I had resentment at moments that this should happen to someone so young and with a lovely family. Somehow it never seems right even though I know it has to happen and that there must be a reason somewhere. I suppose I reached an internalized acceptance of death. It is a part of life.

The question is whether I could have done more to help him. Should I have encouraged him to talk about it? I sat with him and talked or chatted about things if he wished but I did not actively encourage him or lead him to continue to talk about death. Rather, I let him lead the conversation where he wished, but he may have been wanting some encouragement or sign that I was willing to talk about death also. Usually he had very little to say about anything and seemed quite content just to have someone sitting there. Possibly this is rationalization on my part as I find it difficult to express my own intimate views even though as a nurse I know this may be helpful at times. I find it difficult just to express myself and I don't even know whether I would be able to do so on this subject.

I think you are right to ask yourself what you might have done to help this man move beyond knowledge of his dying. You faced the fact of impending death, but in a sense, you were both stopped there. Even though you didn't feel ready to express your own views about death, he probably wasn't wanting this; perhaps he needed an opportunity to talk out his fears, doubts, plans, etc. I think we all too often steer clear of such situations, feeling we will have to announce our own conclusions—when really what is required is to offer openings so that patients may share their fears of the unknown and the unmentionables, and at least not have to be embarrassed or left alone with them. Yours is a sensitive self-appraisal.

Of all patients, it is often those who are themselves doctors or nurses who may feel the most alone and helpless as they face their own death.

Last year, I nursed a dying doctor, a specialist in malignant neoplasm dying of the same disease. Her condition was deteriorating very speedily and she was quite aware of her impending death. She was very pleasant and considerate when first admitted, but as her illness progressed she became very difficult and demanding. Her symptoms of the disease had not developed until a few months prior to admission and were misdiagnosed. As soon as she learned about the positive results of various tests, which confirmed that she was filled with cancer, her attitude was changed completely. She talked to herself very often and once I heard her muttering, "No, not me, it couldn't be me. I'm not ready yet. I still have a lot of things to do, a lot of patients to look after. My husband died of cancer: why is it I have to die of cancer too? Life is too tough, too unfair." Even though she was already told by her doctor about the positive results of the tests, she still asked every health worker who entered her room what the results were and whether she was going to live. Actually her own medical knowledge would have been able to tell her what her prognosis would be like. This shows that she was at the denial stage of "not me."

Later on she became very withdrawn and quiet. She would not let any visitor see her and sometimes pretended to be asleep if anyone went into her room. She even refused to see the minister who came to visit her. I understood that she used to be a very devoted Anglican, and participated in many church activities; yet her refusal to encounter the clergy demonstrated her anger at God and she had entered that "why me?" stage. She then became very nasty, more difficult, and obnoxious. I was doing a night shift at that time and the floor was pretty heavy, as I was the only nurse on duty. She was a staff doctor of the hospital and understood how difficult it was for one nurse to run the whole floor, yet she was ringing her bell constantly for no apparent reason. For instance, she asked for a drink of orange juice, but by the time I brought the orange juice in as requested, she wished for apple juice instead. After another couple of minutes she would ask for orange juice again or just test the bell.

On one hand I was quite exhausted because of the frequent back-and-forth trips to her room and also the intensive care needed for other sick patients; on the other hand I realized she required attention and company as she was haunted with fear, despair, and restlessness. She had good reason for being inconsiderate at that point and was taking every opportunity to express her anger, but was apologetic for being difficult because of her educational background and her professional training. I reassured her that her behavior was normal and sat down by her bedside and encouraged her to talk.

She was quite reluctant to talk at first, but later she just poured it out. She cried heartily and at the same time expressed her anger, fear, and despair. Like some health workers, I had made the mistake of avoiding talking about the patient's own death before, not because of superstition, or because the subject was too gloomy, morbid, and depressing, but because I was afraid it was not good for the patient's morale. Such expression is touchy, sentimental, and melancholy, but fulfills the needs of dying patients.

After the relatively long stay in her room, she appeared more comfortable and relaxed. She fell into deep slumber not long after and did not ring again for the rest of the night.

Actually, what I did was just hold her hand, loan her my ears, and act as a sounding board and listener. I was amazed how effective that was, just encouraging her and giving her the opportunity to express her feeling and emotions, instead of her suffering like a stoic by suppressing them. Also, she was no longer left alone in her suffering.

In 40% of the Unhelpful cases, nurses point to the fact that their *self-image was threatened*. Sometimes this is related to going along with the opinions of other staff members in order to be acceptable to them rather than to the patient.

Mr. B was brought into Mercy General Hospital with 30% burns to his body and died 2 days later. His wife was notified immediately upon his admittance, but because of poor weather conditions, it took her almost 2 days to arrive.

The doctor in charge had talked to Mrs. B twice on the phone and assured her that her husband was in satisfactory condition and she was not to worry. She arrived rather anxious but also very unsuspecting of the seriousness of his condition; he died 2 hours later.

Mrs. B's first reaction was shock. She appeared unable to see, hear, or speak and was generally unresponsive. Shortly afterward she broke into tears and her whole body went into tremors. I was called to special her as we decided to keep her in the hospital overnight as a guest, rather than a patient.

I found it difficult to talk to her at first because everything we talked about related to her husband. The doctor came in with a needle and after drawing it up in front of her he administered Valium intravenously. She looked terrified and said, "This isn't going to put me asleep is it?" Both the doctor and I said no, knowing that she would be asleep in 30 seconds. I felt so deceitful and guilty and I wondered if she would ever trust me.

The doctor heard from a relative by phone that Mrs. B was close to becoming an alcoholic and he decided to order an ounce of vodka every 4 hours. This became a big joke with the floor nurses, probably because they couldn't cope with Mrs. B or the needless death of her husband. I didn't think it a joke; however, I did encourage her to take the liquor without giving her a choice or letting her ver‑ balize her own feelings on the matter. Here was a woman completely alone, lost and insecure, and totally embarrassed regarding her drinking problem in front of many strangers. Yet we were pouring liquor into her while not having any par‑ ticulars of her background. However, I unquestioningly went along with the doc‑ tor, despite all the negative implications.

That evening I went back to visit Mrs. B and help her pass the time, as she was alone until the next morning, when she was to fly out with her husband's body. She remarked that I was the only one who seemed to sympathize with her and that the evening nurses were very rude and made her feel like she had done some‑ thing terribly wrong. I made up some excuse for the nurses to the effect that they were very busy and didn't have time to spend with her. This was most definitely a cop-out on my part, which I probably did to stay on good terms with the nurses I had to work with. I also think I was covering for the nurses and doctors because having worked in a burn unit for a year I knew that Mr. B's death was needless in that there was no justification for it.

While I was visiting, Mrs. B asked me if I would phone her sister for her, be‑ cause she was afraid she would break down again if she phoned. We went to the nurse's station together and the nurse in charge said that Mrs. B was to phone herself, because the doctor had left an order that it would help Mrs. B to take on some of her own responsibility. I was quite sure that this wasn't so, but didn't want to start an argument with Mrs. B standing there, so I said to her, "Why don't you try making the call yourself?" She said she would and asked if she could have her ounce of liquor beforehand. The nurse in charge said she had to wait half an hour and that then she should probably wait another half an hour for it to take effect. With this I really felt like asking the nurse in charge to justify her reasoning, but instead we walked back to her room. Mrs. B said, "You see what I mean? They tease me with the liquor and I'm sure they are laughing behind my back." I said that it would be a lot simpler if she listened to them and did what they asked because she would be leaving in the early morning anyway. This was another cop-out, which meant that this woman would spend a miserable night not even feeling comfortable with the nurses and doctors.

Because I was not on duty I left the floor without confronting the nurses in order to avoid another conflict of opinions, of which we seemed to have many. Nurses so often forget that patients are human beings with feelings and emotions and I think that a helpful way to relate to difficult situations is to place yourself in the exact same situation. I know that I would have a great deal of difficulty cop‑ ing in Mrs. B's position. I wonder how many of the nurses on the floor would have put up with what she put up with.

Besides talking to the nurses I should have confronted the doctor and ques‑ tioned his order if, in fact, there was such an order, and I'm sure he would have consented to let Mrs. B generally do what she pleased, since she wasn't even an admitted patient.

Everyone feared for his position, including myself, and refused to even acknowledge any true feelings. No one was completely honest with himself and
unfortunately this all took place at the expense of another person's feelings and
pride. I'm sure Mrs. B could hardly wait to get out of that town and has no pleasant memories of her stay. As I accompanied her to the escort plane she said to
me, "I think I can believe that you wanted to help me. Thank you for that and
good-bye." That hit the nail right on the head and drove it home. It taught me
that in order to really help someone and be successful you should be able to look
at the situation afterward and say that, whatever the outcome, you did everything humanly possible to help.

Breakdown of interprofessional communication/cooperation is cited as
one factor in this patient's death.

Lorna was a 27-year-old, ungainly, unattractive spinster. She had spent most of
her childhood in a boarding school convent. When she was 16 she discovered that
the aunt with whom she had lived and who was responsible for her upbringing
was in truth her own unwed mother. Lorna was extremely intelligent and later
graduated from the university and went on to obtain her master's degree. At the
completion of this she had bought a car and with a friend was traveling from
California to New York. Her friend was driving when they had a bad accident.
Lorna had a fractured back and leg. The friend had not been injured and continued on her way, leaving Lorna in the hospital and to face the ensuing court action over the accident. Two people in the car involved had been killed. She never
heard from this friend directly again.

When I met Lorna she had returned home and was admitted to a convalescent
hospital for further rest. I was on night duty, and did not see her often. She had
bathroom privileges and on several occasions got up and fell en route. She said
that she felt this was a mild epileptic seizure and had been experiencing this type
of thing since the accident. She was not on any medication that would indicate
that her doctor felt that this was so and inquiries to him did not substantiate her
explanation. The second time that I saw this happen, I felt sure that it was a drug
reaction, and reported this in the morning. Investigation proved that she did
have her own supply of pills and this indeed was what was happening.

The result was that Lorna became very upset with me because I had discovered
the truth and the nights became almost intolerable. Her doctor made an appointment with a psychiatrist for her, which she refused to keep. With only the
normal amount of sedation ordered, she did not sleep, was noisy and trouble-
some. She insisted on smoking in bed, which was not allowed at night. I asked
her repeatedly to come to the desk, or said that I would stay with her in her room
if she wanted to smoke, but she refused. I had no alternative but to again report

this because she was careless and had burned the sheet, and the other patient in her semiprivate room was in a full body case and was terrified. The result of this was that she refused to stay, signed herself out, and by dinner time the following day had committed suicide in her apartment. One of the nurses on the day staff who was worried about Lorna had persuaded her to meet her for dinner. Her failure to appear led to the discovery of her death.

This case has bothered me considerably for a long time. Could I have done something that might have avoided this tragedy? I don't know. I am convinced that I, as a member of the medical team, failed this girl. Because of her argumentative, uncooperative attitude and my limited time, I failed to see how absolutely desperate she was. I was not there at the time that she was allowed to leave but apparently her doctor was notified and said to let her go and he would see her at her apartment the following day. He obviously did not realize the seriousness of or the depth of her depression. I feel that I should have tried harder to understand the problems this girl had, and realized that by her behavior she was actually calling for help.

Much of this history I was not aware of until after her death, and I feel that case histories such as hers should accompany patients to give us a better understanding of their problems.

What a painful and difficult experience. There was a long build-up here of Lorna feeling that people were deceiving her—you might have attempted to get her to tell you about the drugs that night by opening up with "I think you're awfully worried or sad about something—sometimes it helps to share it." As you point out, there was a combination of several factors here concerning history, team communication, etc. I think every professional carries at least one of these experiences in his/her past. Your willingness and ability to face any part you had in this situation is very good insurance for your future as a very self-aware and therefore helpful professional.

Overidentified due to being similar age to patient and *lost professional role: patient became friend* each hold the second-highest rating vis-à-vis Death/Dying as compared to all other Situations.

On a November afternoon, a couple of months after I started to work in the emergency department of a large hospital, a 3-year-old child was brought in in critical condition. She had been hit by a train. I did not see the child but although these accidents are always a shock I feel that I probably could have handled that particular situation. There would have been different procedures that had to be performed and performed quickly.

Rather, I was sent into the quiet room with this little girl's mother. Mrs. C was

7 months pregnant. The family was Jamaican and had moved to our city only 3 weeks prior to this. The husband had gone out for the day to buy a car and Mrs. C did not know where to reach him.

This woman was absolutely beside herself with grief, worry, fear, probably guilt, and goodness knows how many other feelings. She was crying, calling out, sitting down, standing up, pacing, wringing her hands and putting them over her head and ears. All this was really very understandable. I didn't know whether I wanted her to sit down or whether I wanted to pace with her.

I tried to get Mrs. C to calm down. Although I knew that the doctors hadn't been able to save her little girl, I told her that the doctors were doing everything possible to try and save her. It was perfectly understandable that Mrs. C would be reacting in this way. Although not forceful, I tried to persuade Mrs. C to sit still. I sent someone for a doctor to come and talk to her and possibly order a sedative. When the doctor came he told her that their attempt to save her little girl had been unsuccessful. This seemed to be almost more than she could bear. Although this situation had upset me from the beginning, I was afraid at this time that my emotions would get the better of me. The doctor did order a sedative for Mrs. C, which I immediately went to get. This opportunity to get away provided me with enough relief that I finally broke down.

When I got to the medication room I started to cry. The nurse in charge came in and said that I would have to get hold of myself. I tried to, and took the medication in, and with some difficulty finally convinced the woman to take it. Although I wasn't crying at this point I felt afraid that I might again and didn't want this to happen in front of the patient. By this time the priest, doctor, supervisor, police, and others had converged on the scene. I felt that I wasn't able to cope with the situation so I left.

This woman had the right and the need to react the way she did under the circumstances. Her daughter had been killed tragically and suddenly, and she was there alone to face and cope with these facts. I had really been no help to her. The fact that she was alone to face this and in an advanced state of pregnancy compounded the situation greatly in my mind.

I had just recently had a baby of my own and had had quite a personal traumatic experience to deal with. I also was alone and although my situation was quite different from Mrs. C's I seemed to identify with her. I feel that a great deal of self-pity mixed with my feelings of inadequacy in the situation; my sympathy for Mrs. C in this dreadful experience ruled my emotions at this critical time and rendered me ineffective in this particular situation.

On the other hand, in the following instance, it is because of similarity of experience that the nurse describes herself as being able to use herself positively.

At first I was hesitant to approach the man who was to spend the night in the hospital to be near his dying mother. I knew only too well what it was like to sit by, waiting and watching someone you love dying, as my own mother had died a short time before this. I was able to identify with what this man was feeling. I could understand his wanting to be near his mother in her final hours on the chance that she might somehow know that someone who loved and cared about her was there with her.

I observed that he was hesitant to enter her room at times. I remembered that I had felt the same fear of finding my mother dead. Each time I checked on his mother I tried to report to him and offered to go with him into her room but he said that wasn't necessary. I did everything I could to make her as comfortable as possible and gave her sedation to prevent restlessness, knowing that this would ease his suffering also. I tried to make him as comfortable as possible in the lounge and encouraged him to try to get some sleep, reassuring him that I would wake him if necessary. In this manner I was able to express my sympathy and concern for both him and his mother. I understood the loneliness he was experiencing and was able to show him that he was not alone in his feelings.

Before I went off duty that morning I knew that this short relationship had been a helpful one when he thanked me for my understanding and kindness. Then he told me that he knew that someone close to me had died recently and asked me if it had been my mother. At that moment I knew how completely transparent, sincere, and real the messages in our interaction had been and that we had really communicated with each other.

By drawing on my own life experiences to show empathy to this man I was able to help him through that long, lonely night (which was his mother's last) and make it more meaningful to both of us. This gave me confidence in my own ability to be of help in similar situations in the future.

Here the nurse describes how, due to experiences in her own family, her prejudice about the hopelessness of cancer affects her judgment.

The use of self in nursing practice is influenced by all the factors that have gone into making you the person you are when you start functioning as a nurse. The area where I feel my perspective has affected my professional ability is in the care of cancer patients. In my family over the last 10 years I have lost two uncles and two aunts from my maternal side to cancer. From my paternal side I lost my father and uncle. Two other maternal aunts so far have survived radical mastectomies. My husband's mother died of cancer. Cancer has become associated in my mind with grief and hopelessness.

When I started working last year with the home care program as a relief hospital coordinator I dreaded the day they would call and tell me to go and relieve someone at Sloan-Dixon (cancer hospital) while the coordinator was on vacation. To be an effective home care coordinator you have to feel within yourself that the person being assessed by you for discharge has a future goal. This positive feeling enables you to approach the patient and family with success in your mind as a goal. This feeling you hope to transmit to the patient and family, who are often apprehensive and fearful about this next step on the road back from illness.

This assessment and discharge planning prior to hospital discharge is the stage in which the nurse encourages the patient and family to assume the responsibilities again for the activities of daily living. The safe cocoon of the hospital must be shed either willingly or with assistance from the health care professionals.

My feelings on my first relief assignment at Sloan-Dixon were ambivalent. My nursing background told me that cancer can be cured or controlled. Unfortunately within me wrestled the 10 years of family cancers and deaths. This negative feeling I felt dominated my responses. I walked into the hospital with my inner voice saying "All hope abandon, ye who enter here."

Unfortunately I was greeted my first morning with a home care referral that reinforced my sense of foreboding. Mrs. B had bony metastasis from her original breast cancer. When I started to work on this referral instead of looking for the positive aspect of getting this patient home with her family I only thought of the negative problems she faced. After reading the history and social service report and because of my own experiences, I rejected this referral, claiming the problems were too complex to be managed at home. I am ashamed to say I did this without even discussing it with her family, as is the normal procedure. I let my prejudices influence home care assessment technique.

The hospital's social worker dropped in for a visit of welcome and to discuss the pending discharges. She asked my opinion concerning Mrs. B's discharge to home care. I told her that I hesitated to send Mrs. B home even with home care help because the problems she presented seemed overwhelming. The social worker then spoke at length with me about the philosophy behind the sending home of terminally ill patients to their family, which is one of avoiding the isolation a terminally ill patient may experience in the hospital. The isolation is felt because dying can be a lonely experience if those around are having trouble accepting their own feelings of mortality. She felt that when possible cancer patients should be at home for as long as they can be safely managed by their families.

I sat back after she left the office and tried to put my thoughts and feelings in perspective. Had I treated this referral for Mrs. B as a professional home care coordinator, or as a reaction to past experiences?

I then took this referral and reread the information, weighing the positive factors against the negatives. The patient and her family were consulted and the referral proceeded through the normal home care assessment plan.

This hospital is still an intimidating place for me. I do not feel I function at my best level there but at least I am beginning to have some insight and have tried to remedy my failings. When I go to that hospital now I try to read the available positive research to counteract my negative responses.

Across all Situations, *felt pressured (within self) into doing things rather than coping with feeling elements (tension present)* is highest in Death/Dying.

Usually on my floor there was one graduate nurse and one nursing assistant, depending on the census. Since this particular night we had only 13 patients, the nursing office had decided to take away my assistant. Realizing that most of my patients were not sick I was still quite annoyed that I was the only staff nurse. I still had toddlers to feed and bathe plus be ready to give medications and deal with any emergencies that might arise. On top of all that one of my patients was very ill with a brain tumor and was expected to die at any time. Fortunately I had a special nurse to stay with him.

When I had sent the relief nurse to supper it was up to me to stay with Peter (the terminal patient). His mother was in the room and had been in the city for the previous 2 weeks that he had been with us. It was impossible for the father to come because of the distance. He had suffered a coronary not a month before and it was advised that he stay home as long as possible. However, in the last 24 hours it was obvious that Peter was not going to live much longer. A call was sent home earlier that day requesting that the father come to the hospital. He had not arrived at the time I came on duty. While I was in the room with him, Peter was showing signs of death. His mother was not ignorant and by seeing the mottling of his skin knew that Peter was approaching the end.

Great anxiety was evident in the mother because she wanted more than anything for the father to arrive before Peter died. Peter went into Cheyne-Stokes respirations, where he would breathe but then not take another breath for a minute, maybe more. This breathing went on for at least 15 minutes, but during that time the father had come into the room.

I had experienced deaths before on previous shifts so I felt that I could cope effectively. I left the parents in privacy and allowed relatives to go in after a while; there were two couples who had come with the father. Peter died.

My first concern was for the calmness of the rest of the unit. I had to get the body ready and have it taken away in a manner that would not be too obvious for other parents and children. I also had to deal with the routine floor duties and have the doctor come up. Being the only nurse on the ward at the time I could feel myself getting panicky. It was just the time when the other patients needed attention, either in medication or immediate physical care (e.g., an ulcerative colitis toddler needing perineal cleaning).

Once the parents had left the room and had gone down the hall to see the doctor, I thought the way was clear to prepare the body for the morgue. My relief nurse had come back so the two of us went in and cleaned and wrapped the body. I took all of Peter's belongings out of the room and carried them down to the nurse's station.

On coming back down the hall I saw the most pathetic sight. The father was slowly coming out of Peter's room, pausing to look back in with the most disturbed expression on his face. I then realized my unforgiveable mistake.

The one most important thing a nurse must consider in the case of death is the parents. Above all else the child's body must never be moved until the parents have left the hospital. In this situation I allowed my own feelings of anxiety to overpower my empathy for the parents by preparing and wrapping their child while they were still on the floor. With the confusion of the floor, the death itself, and the aloneness I felt in dealing with the parents of Peter and others I felt pressured into doing something concrete. Unfortunately, I chose my priorities in the wrong perspective. I should have left Peter until I had completed my other tasks and the parents had left. The shock that the convalescing father received was that of an everlasting picture of his baby in a white shroud like an inanimate object. It was so unnecessary; I still ask myself how one can allow oneself to become so taken up with routines.

III/CONCLUSIONS

15

DISCUSSION OF FINDINGS

1. There are distinct Helpful and Unhelpful factors that nurses themselves identify as regularized responses when they are in interaction with patients and colleagues.
2. There are distinct Situation factors that nurses themselves identify as regularized settings for their responses.
3. When the Situation factors cited by nurses are cross-tabulated with the Helpful and Unhelpful Response factors cited by nurses, regularized Situation-Response patterns may be identified.

Tables 2.1, 2.2, 2.3, 2.4 (pp. 27, 32–35) prove the validity of hypotheses 1–3. As noted earlier, the fact that the final categories of Helpful and Unhelpful cases, each involving 275 cases, confirmed the initial categories of the pilot study, which involved 25 cases each (see appendix 1) is an indication of the reliability of these categories during the period of 5 years of collected assignments. The 70% interjudge agreement that was required on coding of the data is a further test of the construct validity and reliability of the findings.

HYPOTHESES 4 AND 5

4. The subjectively described thought and feeling processes of nurses prior to and simultaneous with their actions in the nurse-patient relationship will not include the Response factor of affective neutrality.

5. The preceding hypothesis will apply equally whether the nurse is describing a Situation in which she perceives herself as being Helpful or one in which she perceives herself as being Unhelpful.

When all the Response factors—both Helpful (20) and Unhelpful (24)—are examined, no nurse describes herself as being either helpful or unhelpful due to not being emotionally involved, or affectively neutral. The section that follows pursues further analyses and summary of the findings.

MOST HELPFUL AND MOST UNHELPFUL SITUATIONS

Twelve Situations emerged from the data as regularized settings for nurse-patient interaction. In analysis of these Situations across 550 cases, nurses describe themselves as more likely to be Helpful in the Professional/Personal Relationship, Psychiatric, and Pregnancy/Birth Situations. Conversely, they are more likely to be Unhelpful in the Cultural Adaptation, Adolescence, Unmarried Mothers, and Colleague Relationship Situations. Table 15.1 condenses Table 2.2, p. 27 and plots in descending order those Situations where the ratio of Helpful to Unhelpful cases indicates a marked difference.

We may ask what, if any, factors can be identified that account for this

TABLE 15.1
**Ratio of Helpful to Unhelpful Cases
in Descending Order**

Situation	Ratio of Helpful to Unhelpful Cases
Professional/personal relationship	2:1
Psychiatric	3:2
Pregnancy/birth	3:2
Colleague relationship	2:3
Unmarried mothers	2:3
Adolescence	1:2
Cultural adaptation	3:7

data? Are the reasons unique to each of the Situations or are there Response factors that are common to some of these Situations that might point to causal linkages?

The Professional/Personal Relationship has the highest ratio of Helpful cases across all Situations (2:1). This is important in view of the well-known dictum that the professional relationship does not mix well with a personal relationship: helping professionals should not treat members of their own family or friends. Being forewarned, as it were, and therefore aware of the potential dangers involved, nurses may, in fact, make a more conscious effort to succeed in these cases. *Gave moral support,* while ranging from 50% to 80% in all Helpful cases, is highest in the Professional/Personal Relationship and this may be a reflection of knowing the patient as a personal friend.

At the same time, the ambivalence toward knowing the patient as a friend is very evident when one examines those Professional/Personal Relationships that are described as Unhelpful (approximately one-third of the cases in this Situation). The three Response factors that nurses cite as most relevant to their Unhelpfulness are: *self-image was threatened; purposely disregarded significant cues in patient's statements/behavior;* and *felt inadequate to enter into patient's problem because had not personally resolved that issue.* Each of these has the second highest rating of these three Response factors across all Situations.

Understandably, the Professional/Personal Relationship constitutes a particular tension for the nurse, one in which she perceives the self to be uniquely at issue. Nevertheless, nurses indicate to a limited but also an unprecedented degree relative to all other Situations, that they are not prepared to accept *all* the responsibility when they are Unhelpful in this relationship. At higher ratings than in any of the other Situations, nurses point to educational and organizational factors: *lacked training in recognizing social-emotional needs of patients* and *short staffed, too little time to devote to the patient* as contributing to their Unhelpfulness. Given that nurses describe themselves as Helpful in the Professional/Personal Relationship two-thirds of the time, contradicting the "accepted" dictum, they in turn point a small but nonetheless visible finger at the very educational and organizational systems that may hold to this dictum and, therefore, do not prepare practitioners for this Situation.

The Situation that has the highest ratio of Unhelpful cases is Cultural Adaptation (7:3). *Self-image was threatened* is cited in 7 out of 10 cases and is the highest rating of this response across all Situations. That the concept of self is inextricably related to culture and potentially threatened by cultural differences to this degree points to a critical area for examination in education and practice. Conversely, when Cultural Adaptation is handled Helpfully (in less than one-third of the cases), nurses identify the fact of *came to terms with own feelings to enter into patient's problem* as a key factor to the extent that this Response factor shares the highest rating across all Situations.

In summary, the Situation with the highest ratio of Helpful cases and the Situation with the highest ratio of Unhelpful cases cite, respectively, the second highest and highest ratings of the Unhelpful Response *(self-image was threatened)* and the third highest and highest ratings of the Helpful Response *(came to terms with own feelings to enter into patient's problem)* (see Tables 15.2 and 15.3). These findings press us to look for similar linkages among the other Situations in Table 15.1.

The three Situations with the highest ratio of Helpful cases (Professional/Personal Relationship, Psychiatric, and Pregnancy/Birth) were examined for Response factors that are (1) common to all three and (2) cited in 40% or more cases. One Helpful Response factor emerges: *gave moral support*. Where Professional/Personal Relationships and Psychiatric patients are concerned, three Unhelpful Response factors emerge: *self-image was threatened; purposely disregarded significant cues in patient's statements/behavior;* and *felt inadequate to enter into patient's problem because had not personally resolved that issue.* Table 15.2 plots this data. To facilitate comparisons, the symbol + is used to indicate that the Response factor occurred in 40% to 59% of cases and + + is used to indicate that the Response factor occurred in 60% or more cases.

When three of the Situations with the highest ratio of Unhelpful cases (Cultural Adaptation, Adolescence, and Unmarried Mothers) are similarly examined for common Response factors with 40% or higher ratings, three Unhelpful Response factors are shared (with one exception): *did not want to understand; was disapproving, judgmental;* and *self-image was threatened.* When Helpful Response factors were examined, the reverse of the above Unhelpful factors emerged: *wanted to understand how patient felt; was nonjudgmental;* and *came to terms with own feelings to enter into patient's problem* (see Table 15.3). While it will be recalled that the total number of cases in these Situations does not exceed 20 and, therefore, percentages cannot be considered statistically reliable, this inverse response phenomenon suggests that when these generally problematic Situations are handled Helpfully, there is a compensatory mechanism at work. The findings further suggest that these Response factors are of considerable salience to these Situations in which nurses describe them-selves as more likely to be Unhelpful.

Further pursuing the incidence of Unhelpful Response factors across all Situations, it becomes evident that in a total of five Situations—four of which are cited as more inclined to be handled Unhelpfully—four Re-sponse factors are not only common but also consistently high (see Table 15.4). These findings would appear to indicate a tendency to stereotype those groups that are, in one way or another, different from the practi-tioner (e.g., *failed to look beyond initial impression*). Is there a need to be highly *judgmental, not wanting to understand* in order to cope with this difference and the *threat to self-image?*

One might logically ask why the same Unhelpful Responses are not similarly high where Psychiatric patients are concerned, for they, too, are often perceived as "different." Interestingly, as noted earlier, nurses de-scribe themselves as more Helpful than Unhelpful with Psychiatric pa-tients in the ratio of 3:2. Is this because the difference is perceived in medical rather than social or personality terms, that is, psychiatric pa-tients are perceived as being victims of a medical problem over which they have less control than the groups of patients shown in Table 15.4?

Following this reasoning, one might wonder why alcoholics are not sim-ilarly perceived, since alcoholism is often referred to as an illness. The data does not appear to reflect the internalization of this concept, however. In fact, three out of five cases specifically cite prejudice toward alcoholics as a group. (In the case of Unmarried Mothers, the incidence of prejudice to-ward alcoholics rises to five out of six cases.)

In fact, of those Unhelpful Response factors that are consistently high across all Situations, *self-image was threatened* is the highest. Except in the Situation of Unmarried Mothers, this response is cited in 35% or more of all Unhelpful cases, that is, in more than one out of every three cases, regardless of Situation. We recall that this Response factor provided a highly salient linkage between the two most Helpful and the two most Unhelpful Situations, (see tables 15.2 and 15.3).

Perhaps one of the most striking Response factors that emerged from the study (remembering that all Situations and Response factors were not predetermined by the researcher, but rather identified by the respon-dents) was, on the one hand, *felt inadequate to enter into patient's prob-lem because had not personally resolved the issue* and, on the other, *came to terms with own feelings; was able to enter into patient's problem.* These Responses in their Unhelpful and Helpful forms were cited in every

TABLE 15.2
Most Helpful Situations: Common Response Factors

Ratio of Helpful to Unhelpful	Situation	Helpful Response Factors	Unhelpful Response Factors		
		Gave Moral Support	Self-Image Threatened[a]	Own Feelings Unresolved[a]	Disregarded Cues
2:1	Professional/personal	+	+	+	+
3:2	Psychiatric	+	+	+	+
3:2	Pregnancy/birth	+			

[a]Response factors common to most Helpful Situations and most Unhelpful Situations.
+ Response factor occurred in 40% to 50% of cases (see tables 2.3 and 2.4 for exact percentage).

294

TABLE 15.3
Most Unhelpful Situations: Common Response Factors

Ratio of Helpful to Unhelpful	Situation	Helpful Response Factors			Unhelpful Response Factors		
		Resolved Own Feelings[a]	Nonjudgmental	Wanted to Understand	Self-Image Threatened[a]	Judgmental	Did Not Want to Understand
3:7	Cultural Adaptation[b]	+	+	+	++	++	+
1:2	Adolescence[b]	+	++	++	+	++	+
2:3	Unmarried Mothers[b]	+	++	++		++	+

[a]Response factors common to most Helpful Situations and most Unhelpful Situations.
[b]Total number of cases does not exceed 20 (percent shown for comparative purposes only).
+ Response factor occurred in 40% to 59% of cases (see tables 2.3 and 2.4 for exact percentage).
+ + Response factor occurred in 60% or more cases (see tables 2.3 and 2.4 for exact percentage).

TABLE 15.4

Ratio of Helpful to Unhelpful	Situation	Unhelpful Response Factors			
		Self-Image Threatened	Judg-mental	Did Not Want To Understand	Initial Negative Impression
3:7	Cultural adaptation[a]	+ +	+ +	+	+
1:2	Adoles-cence[a]	+	+ +	+	+
2:3	Unmarried mothers[a]		+ +	+	
4:5	Alcohol-ism[a]	+	+ +	+	+
1:1	Elderly	+	+ +	+	+

[a]Total number of cases does not exceed 20 (percent shown for comparative purposes only).
+ Response factor occurred in 40%–59% of cases (see tables 2.3 and 2.4 for exact percentage).
+ + Response factor occurred in 60% or more cases (see tables 2.3 and 2.4 for exact percentage).

Situation without exception. In fact, this Response factor is notable to the extent that the two Situations that have the highest ratio of Helpful cases point to not coming to terms with their feelings as their highest-rated problem. Conversely, the three Situations that have the highest ratio of Unhelpful cases point to coming to terms with their own feelings as the highest-rated factor in their Helpful cases (see Tables 15.2 and 15.3). Further, the importance of this Response factor is dramatically highlighted in the Situation of Death/Dying. Seventy percent of the cases that were Unhelpfully handled specifically cite *felt inadequate because had not personally resolved the issue.*

It is obvious that nurses are very conscious of the fact that they are personally and individually struggling with fundamental value issues and philosophic questions concerning the quality and meaning of life and suffering in its many forms. Is it as obvious that educational and organizational systems are prepared to address with nurses those issues that are most fundamental to the way in which practice is conducted?

TOWARD A TYPOLOGY OF RESPONSE FACTORS

In the interests of more stringent classification and summarization of the most salient Response factors it is only logical to attempt to classify these factors into, for example, cognitive, affective, behavioral, and situational categories. However, most of the Response factors do not readily fall into one or another of these categories. For example, *wanted (did not want) to understand* has both cognitive and affective dimensions and *felt pressured (within self) into doing things rather than dealing with feeling elements* has both affective and behavioral components. Similarly, to make a distinction between inner and outer Response factors or between visible (to an observer) and nonvisible responses is also inexact. For example, *purposely disregarded significant cues in patient's statements/behavior* and *treated the condition, overlooking the patient* have elements of all four. To impose classifications of this type is to introduce more arbitrary research interpretation of the data than has been the purpose of this study. It is hoped that subsequent research will pursue such categorization, formulating further hypotheses and testing these within a more pre-structured frame.

By the same token, it would be an equal disservice to the data not to point out two classifications for consideration. While not devoid of all ambiguity, they offer an important distinction relative to types of Response factors, and at the least provide a basis for further investigation and theory construction.

Types A and B Response Factors

Type A Response factors may be said to be associated with a primary reaction—not in a conscious or chronological sense, but in the sense of that response being a root cause. Examples of Type A Response factors are *wanted (did not want) to understand how patient felt, was judgmental (nonjudgmental), liked (disliked) the patient.*

Type B Response factors may be said to be associated with a secondary reaction—again, not in a consciously chronological sense, but in the sense of being connected to or emanating from a Type A response. For example, *looked beyond patient's outward response/behavior to underlying causes* and *treated the condition, overlooking the patient* may be said to be manifestations or expressions of a more primary, Type A response such as *liked (disliked) the patient.* In a general sense, Type B Response factors focus on description of feelings and actions, while Type A factors focus on analysis of their root causes.

In order to plot the incidence of Type A responses as distinct from Type B responses, particularly among those Response factors that are most prevalent, the percentage of cases in which each Response factor is cited was determined. Percentages were computed by dividing the frequency of a Response factor (see appendix 2) by 275 (the total number of cases) and multiplying by 100. For example, *helped patient express feelings* was cited in 156 of the 275 cases, or in 57% of the Helpful cases. Tables C and D of appendix 3 list these percentages, ranking them in descending order. For comparative and summary purposes, Table 15.5 condenses this data, rank ordering the seven most prevalent Response factors and plotting each as to Type A or Type B.

Even a cursory glance at Table 15.5 reveals that Unhelpful use of self involves twice as many Type A responses as Helpful use of self. This differ-

TABLE 15.5
Most Prevalent Response Factors: Type A and Type B

	Rank	Response Factor	Type A	Type B
Helpful	1	Gave moral support		✓
	2	Helped patient express feelings		✓
	3	Wanted to understand how patient felt	✓	
	4	Took time to explain		✓
	5	Looked beyond behavior		✓
	6	Was a sounding board		✓
	7	Nonjudgmental	✓	
Unhelpful	1	Treated condition, overlooking patient		✓
	2	Initial negative impression		✓
	3	Self-image threatened	✓	
	4	Judgmental	✓	
	5	Had not personally resolved issue	✓	
	6	Disregarded cues in patient's statements/behavior		✓
	7	Did not want to understand	✓	

ence is borne out when all Response factors are included. Type A responses comprise 50% of the Unhelpful Response factors, whereas they comprise only 30% of the Helpful Response factors (see appendix 3, tables C and D). That is, relative to Unhelpful use of self, nurses are more prone to analyze than describe themselves. Stated another way, nurses pursue their analysis to a more fundamental level (Type A response) when they see themselves as Unhelpful, when it is potentially more threatening for them to undertake this level of analysis. (Clearly, the somewhat popular conception that practitioners tend to credit themselves when they are Helpful and name extraneous factors when they are Unhelpful is not substantiated in this data.)

To what extent are practitioners offered specific and concrete help relative to Type A and Type B responses? A number of key relationship factors such as *treating the condition, overlooking the patient* and *avoided needs of family members* have long received recognition in the literature and in classrooms as being problematic for the nurse and, therefore, important to address. Similarly, educators have emphasized the need to *give moral support* and *help the patient express feelings*. These Type B responses are absolutely vital to address. It must be asked, however, whether educationally and organizationally we are equally prepared to discuss Type A responses—those responses that are related to the root causes of Type B responses.

It would seem axiomatic that unless such fundamental (Type A) Response factors as *disliked (liked) the patient, did not (did) want to understand how patient felt* and *had not (had) personally resolved the issue* are openly recognized and accepted as basic realities in the lives of practitioners, and unless specific and ongoing structures are devised that address these realities, it should not be surprising that many practitioners develop the protective armor discussed in chapter 1. It is important to reconsider our conceptual and practice models in light of these questions.

Conceptual and Practice Models Reconsidered

The study's findings indicate a wide disparity between the concept of affective neutrality and the realism of actual practice, at least from the perspective of the practitioner. In situations where the nurses saw themselves as helpful, it was not because they perceived that they had neutralized their affect but rather because they had directed their (inevitable) affect in a particular way.

It may be argued that where professional practitioners are concerned,

there is some justification for maintaining an "ideal type" concept because of the goal it will encourage practitioners to attempt to achieve:
"Man's reach must exceed his grasp. . . ." However, the concept of emotional noninvolvement cannot be legitimized even on these grounds. For,
as described earlier, it is actually a contradiction of the other qualities of
self-investment that are presently required of the therapeutic function.
To be concerned, sensitive, and caring is not to be affectively neutral. This
then renders the "ideal type" internally inconsistent.

In fact, it is a physiological question as well as a psychological one as to
whether it is indeed possible for a normally healthy individual to be
neutral in his/her affect. It is at least partially to this end that surgical
lobotomies are performed. (That the practitioner may direct or use her affect in such a way as to appear to respond in a neutral fashion to a statement made by a client is a well-recognized therapeutic technique. "On
occasions, there are some very plausible technical reasons why the patient
should be challenged by the stress of having to take a few steps, at least,
without the crutches of the counselor's concern. In this sense the counselor's indifference—seeming indifference—can be described as therapeutic" (Halmos, 1965, p. 82. See also Searles, 1963). But there is every
difference between a neutral response consciously adopted for a particular
therapeutic purpose and a practitioner's initial internal, quite involun-
tary reaction to an individual.)

But perhaps the issue is only semantic, one reasons, as one reaches for
the dictionary. There, under "affect," it cites: "feeling, emotion and
desire as factors in determining thought and conduct" (Webster's New
Collegiate Dictionary, 1959, p. 15). Again, one is reminded of the fact
that thought and conduct are not synonymous: indeed, one may feel one
way and choose to act in another. But even more significantly, one seldom
feels one way. As evident in the study, no Situation, Helpful or Unhelpful, elicited a single Response factor. In fact, the salient factors were sometimes of a conflicting nature: for example, *felt guilty, but would not communicate*. Apparently, depending on which factor(s) is/are given priority
(which in turn is a psychological-sociological-situational decision-making
process) the external response (i.e., the conduct) is constructed, consciously or unconsciously. Rather than setting the practitioner the unrealistic task of neutralizing her affect, a more productive focus would seem to
be to attempt to identify and direct (inevitable) affect in a particular way
—examining the priorities under which one tries to operate when one is
functioning in a professional capacity. For it would appear from the data

of the study that affective neutrality is not even a useful or relevant response to attempt to develop. In fact, there is every evidence from the findings that, at least from the nurses' perspectives, helping relationships emanated from very definite affective Response factors such as *liked the patient* and *wanted to understand how patient felt*.

FRONTSTAGE AND BACKSTAGE

Interestingly, there is no reference in the various professional dictionaries and encyclopedias (general, scientific or medical, including psychology and psychiatry) that lists the concept of affective neutrality. Yet this characteristic has been advanced as one of the hallmarks of a highly professionalized occupation (Blishen, 1969; Friedson, 1970; Parsons, 1951). What does this mean?

In part, it may be that affective neutrality or not becoming emotionally involved is a concept that (some) professionals have used in an attempt to interpret and legitimate their service to the public. For inside, i.e., "backstage," not all professional texts uphold this as a goal in practice. "Midway between acceptance and denial is a kind of neutrality. The caseworker is neither denying nor neutral about the person or his problem. The caseworker wants to understand" (Friedlander, 1958, p. 80).

However, it may be that in order to ensure the public of a standardized product (i.e., one which is not dependent on the practitioner's individual life / world view) professionals have tended to perpetuate this image of the practitioner as emotionally neutral—with at least the more thoughtful among them admitting to their trusted colleagues that this is a patent unreality (Daniels, 1975, pp. 440–445). The irony is that the public has begun to catch them on the horns of their own dilemma. For along with emotional noninvolvement can scarcely go the willingness to care deeply . . . and the myth is wearing thin.

In an occupation that is fraught with emotionally difficult situations, to be able to retreat to the scientific—to reify practitioner affective neutrality—offers a legitimate way of opting out of a great deal of emotional soul-searching. In this way it is another example of how the ideology of an occupation can be constructed and used in order to protect the practitioner from himself and his anxiety. What is proposed as a protection for the patient is in fact a protection for the practitioner.

Not only is the concept of affective neutrality inconsistent with human physiology, but it is also inconsistent with more recent understanding of the therapeutic relationship. This means that the alert practitioner is no longer comforted by this concept on either count. It is neither realistic (something nurses have probably always felt from their own experience) nor (now) helpful.

All of this has valuable insights for research methodology. To date, as mentioned previously, much of the research that has been conducted on the nurse-patient relationship has been based on methods of observation, taping of interviews, etc., with analysis of the interaction made by a third, objective party. Perhaps this particular method of investigation has also helped to perpetuate the myth of affective neutrality. Too often the implicit, if not explicit, assumption has been that if the relationship was unhelpful, it was because the nurse had become emotionally involved. Conversely, if it was helpful, it was because she had not. However, this study—based on nurses' perceptions of their own thoughts and actions and the reasons for these—has revealed very different data. It has revealed that, at least in their view, it is the direction and expression of the practitioner's inevitable affect, in every situation, that differentiates the Helpful from the Unhelpful practitioner response.

IMPLICATIONS FOR ORGANIZATIONAL AND EDUCATIONAL CONTEXTS

These findings would seem to suggest that, from the actor's perspective, to put forward emotional noninvolvement as characteristic of a highly professional occupation is a misnomer, if not a myth. If the qualities of emotional openness, active concern, and personal risk in a relationship are hallmarks of the helping relationship, one is always emotionally involved: the question is how this involvement is directed.

Obviously these findings have enormous implications for all health professionals who consider the practitioner-patient relationship to be a central focus in their practice. They have very specific implications for the way in which student and neophyte practitioners are educated concerning the dimension of total patient care. Not least of all, they impact the way in which health-care institutions structure the organizational context within which the practitioner is required to function.

Increasingly, there is recognition of the need for training programs, administrative changes, and further research in the practitioner-patient relationship.

Nursing educators should formally integrate theory and experience in learning helping skills into their curriculums. Hospital and nursing administrators should be aware of the need to assess levels of empathy of their nursing personnel and incorporate human-relations–modeled in-service programs into their structures. . . . [While our] research documents that the nurses studied were practising with dangerously low levels of empathy . . . a danger in interpreting the results is to blame practising nurses; the human-relations-model of helping, however, should be role modeled by deans, educators, and administrators. Caring needs to become a bond between every person across the organizational structure. No one can maintain a helpful caring attitude in an institution that mitigates against it. (LaMonica et al., 1976, p. 450)

Increasingly, there is recognition of the fact that the question of professional caring and being able to practice it in a conducive environment cannot be left open-ended. Several studies document extremely high attrition rates among graduate nurses for reasons other than marriage and family. For example, in one 2-year study among a group of 220 baccalaureate nurses, most of whom had worked between 1 and 2 years following graduation, 28.9% left nursing practice due to job dissatisfaction (Waters, Chater, Vivier, Urrea, and Wilson, 1972).

It is hoped that more and more readers are turning to Kramer's book, *Reality Shock: Why Nurses Leave Nursing* (1974) and her subsequent work with other nurse educator-researchers, which not only documents real world problems but offers definite suggestions for resolving them (Kramer & Schmalenberg, 1978a, 1978b).

IDENTITY REVISITED

To return to the question of nursing's search for a unique identity, Vollmer and Mills (1966) reiterate the fact that "in the literature on highly professionalized occupations, much is made of professional detachment, of affective neutrality" (p. 225). Accordingly, they are led to ask, "If an integral part of the nurse's role is the overt display of supportive feelings [in order to facilitate] the faster recovery of the patient, [does this mean that] nursing [is] permanently precluded from a high degree of professionalization?" (p. 225). It is for this reason, among others we have discussed, that the one-to-one relationship of professional to patient is often delegated to less qualified persons, if in fact it is specifically delegated at all.

At the same time others would maintain that a high degree of professionalization can only accrue to nursing if it develops a unique body of knowledge and skill as an expressive specialist. Still others contend that even if this model is adopted, nursing's time may have already run out. Psychosocial experts have already made significant inroads into the health-care field in general, and hospital wards in particular.

Psychologists, social workers, and clergy are all claiming permanent places on the treatment team, requesting that they accompany the doctors on rounds in order to spot and treat problems. In these cases, even the reporting and coordinating functions of the nurse are at least potentially threatened. In any event, this model leaves her in the role of generalist humanizing agent, rather than specialist.

On the other hand, if the specific role of expressive generalist or generalist humanizer can be elevated to the status of a specialty—much as general practice is now considered a specialty within medicine—nursing may achieve at least a more consolidated identity. For while general practitioner specialists may not claim equal prestige with their colleagues in the superspecialties, they do command considerable power over them in the area of assessment and referral-giving. Unless the superspecialists respect and include the general practitioner as a colleague among colleagues (i.e., include them in the treatment plan, etc.), the superspecialist can be cut off from the very source of his livelihood.

> Somehow, if nursing is to rise to its potential status in the healing arts, nurses must grow to the point where they become able to establish communicative contact with a broad range of people, because it would seem that such contact is a *sine qua non* for helpful nursing transactions. I am coming to believe that it is the peculiar privilege of nurses to play, not just an important role in healing, but possibly *the* important role. (Jourard, 1964, p. 150)

If—and this is a very problematic if—the humanizing of patient care gains sufficient value on the health market, nurses may, if they have underwritten this investment, find themselves with a highly negotiable currency.

and perceptions of themselves in interaction with patients. In this respect I attempted to offer alternatives to a stereotyped self-image of nurses: to make it no longer necessary for them to deny their real feelings, to deplete their psychic energy in guilt compensation and thus never be able to face or deal with the vicissitudes of the practitioner-patient relationship in a consciously directed purposeful fashion. For example, it is quite understandable, in the sense of normal, to dislike a patient for any number of rational, arational, or irrational reasons. As a teacher, one hopes to demonstrate this as much by one's manner in reaction to students' statements and questions as by actual verbal concept. This involves being ready to expose one's own feelings in a spontaneous manner in order that a bond of being truly human becomes an experience students and lecturer share together. For, not unlike the therapeutic relationship per se, it is the experiencing of the quality of this acceptance from another that creates meaning and makes it possible for the nurse to be real with herself.

On the other hand, I do not concur with those who believe one must become totally submerged with one's students or respondents (i.e., "go native") in order to establish this trust. As Miller (1952) points out, there are significant dangers involved in losing one's identity as a scientist. The classroom orientation in the present study was not such that new freedom to accept her feelings as natural thereby released the nurse from further expectation of herself in professional relationships with patients. It is this latter orientation that is implicit in the assignment's requirement that the nurse make a distinction between a helpful and unhelpful situation. In effect then, the subjects were not asked simply to describe their feelings and thought processes in relation to their conduct, but also to assess their Helpful/Unhelpful use of self as professional practitioners.

LIMITATIONS OF THE DATA

Any method that is devised to solve the problem of the researcher being a stranger and yet attempts to maximize his/her understanding of a situation and minimize distortion carries with it its own particular costs. The present strategy of inquiry is not without its limitations.

Initial confidence in findings that are elicited from a teacher-student context should be suspect. Ethical and political factors come to the fore when the status of the researcher gives him/her possible control over the career line of the respondent.

In teaching, one can be so doctrinaire as to allow no room for independent response. The same holds true for research and inherent bias in the construction and use of research instruments (Warner & Lunt, 1941; Osgood, Suci, & Tannenbaum, 1957). In either case one endeavors to recognize the fact and influence of one's own predilections and seeks to actively demonstrate and foster conviction concerning the importance of being honest with oneself and others as a base for further operations. Whether or not it is actually possible to ultimately and fully suspend bias and to "surrender" as Wolff (1968, pp. 72–105) suggests, is problematic. What is required is that both teacher, researcher, and in this study, also the nurse, be consciously self-aware of these predilections and be prepared to accept responsibility for taking them into account. In effect this commitment to self-awareness was what I was attempting to communicate conceptually to the nurses as their teacher, as well as to actively demonstrate as a researcher in the actual methodology of the study. In this sense at least the two roles were not as incongruent as might at first appear.

For, while the subjects were asked to describe, assess, and give reasons for their use of self in two situations, neither the criteria for assessing helpfulness and unhelpfulness, nor various categories of behavior, nor possible alternative reasons for it were specified. The nurse was given unlimited scope in accounting for her use of self. The explicit assumption was that helpfulness is not a static feature of personality, but a dynamic one that is dependent upon a number of factors. Emphasis therefore was not on self-blame for its own sake nor upon intrapsychic factors as accounting for all behavior. The significance of this particular teaching orientation to the present research context is that there was every possibility for the nurse to relate in effect, "I was helpful in this situation because I felt nothing either for or against this patient: I was not involved emotionally."

In terms of establishing rapport with respondents, it is questionable whether the nurses would have been as intellectually or emotionally prepared to write this type of analysis without the teaching and supportive process that preceded. It would be instructive in this respect to give this assignment to a random sample of graduate nurses in practice, with no preliminary preparation. However, whether practitioners—even those who were familiar with the self-awareness school—would trust this degree of self-revelation to a complete stranger is questionable. Regardless of whether one is asked to sign one's name to such material or not, there is a reticence about exposing this kind of material about oneself on paper to an absolute stranger. The teacher role afforded me the opportunity to actively build trust in a way that even the in-depth unstructured interview would not. That is, the classroom situation provided a forum for con-

siderable personal interaction without incurring the confidential complications that can accompany the one-to-one intimacy of the researcher-
respondent "friendship." At the same time, I was relieved of the pretense of playing a disguised role as complete participant and being confronted with the contradictory role demands that this incurs. For example,
Gold (1958, p. 219) refers to the complete participant who finds himself
simultaneously responding to the demands of his hidden self, his pretended self, and his self as an observer. Neither was the ambiguity of the
participant-as-observer role involved (Olesen & Whittaker, 1967). This is
significant, for the role that the observer claims—or to which he/she is
assigned by the subjects—is perhaps the single most important determi-
nant of what he/she will be able to learn (Jackson, 1975).

Other than subjectively, it is difficult for me to assess how the nurses
perceived me. Of significance was the fact that, related to my particular
background in hospitals, I could demonstrate a backstage understanding
of the life and activities of a nurse, and from my own direct experience in
working with patients, I was in a position to understand the complexity of
the situational factors involved. The fact that administratively I was an
outside lecturer from the faculty of sociology, not a member of their own
faculty, and not a trained nurse, may have facilitated their responses. Had
I been asking them questions related to the technical mistakes they had
made during their careers, for example, my particular orientation would
have probably constituted a hindrance. This does, however, raise the
question of replicability. Another lecturer might have quite another emphasis and might have elicited somewhat different material.

It may be useful to contrast certain features of the strategy used in this
study with alternative strategies of observation. This method shares some
features with the life history method. In autobiographical materials, for
example, the social scientist is afforded certain opportunities to relate the
actor's subjective thought processes to his conduct. However, considerable difficulty is implicit in this method in that the purpose for which
the writer undertook his autobiography may not be sufficiently consistent
with the social scientist's focus as to lend any more methodological rigor
than other observational studies.

The present strategy of inquiry shares features of the free association
method (Linder, 1956), although the present study involves the nurse's
subjective understanding of her associations; it has some aspects of the
focused interview, the objectifying interview, and the group interview
(Sjoberg & Nett, 1968, pp. 213–218). In more respects this approach ap-
proximates the in-depth interview where the interviewee is prompted to

recall the feelings he/she had in relation to certain behavior. However, in the in-depth interview, the material is elicited in a face-to-face situation and allows for considerably more contamination by researcher bias through the observer's immediate words, gestures, and reactions. In the present study the researcher's influence was distributed among the group as a whole in a classroom setting prior to their writing the material individually.

FURTHER RESEARCH OPPORTUNITIES

While this study deals exclusively with the thought and feeling processes of the practitioner from the stated perspective of the practitioner, and therefore cannot be put forward as conclusive proof of the total fallacy of affective neutrality per se, the findings suggest that a much closer analysis of this concept is essential. Subsequent studies might incorporate both the nurse and the patient, in addition to an observer, each commenting on their individual perceptions of a helpful as opposed to an unhelpful nurse-patient encounter and the criteria or response factors involved.

Further, studies might be conducted across several professions to explore interprofessional differences. In undertaking what Glaser and Strauss (1967) refer to as theoretical sampling when attempting to generate formal theory, this study on affective neutrality has applicability to the study of other interactional relationships, such as that of employer-employee. It has potential for the reconstruction of existing theory concerning role-demand in relation to self-demand, and has connections with how role distance is often regularized and structured. (For example, nurses are rarely assigned to the same patient for many consecutive days.)

Moreover, despite the equalizing effect that the course's conceptual content might exert, obviously responses are effected to a degree by the respondent's past personal and professional experiences, belief systems, social class, social status factors, etc. Subsequent data could explore possible correlations between the biographical characteristics of the individual respondent and the situation and factors she describes. (Is there a correlation, for example, among specific philosophy about death and experience with it, and self-identified Responses in Situations of Death/Dying?) Such a biographical information instrument would obviously be more structured and would lend itself to some forms of quantitative analysis. If this data were matched with case data such as was elicited in the present study, hypotheses that were generated in the foregoing material could be further explored and tested. This dual methodological approach to data collection would represent an attempt to bring to bear various research perspectives upon the subject: to check particular factors against another body of data gathered in a different way. (However, the ethical-political limitations of the teacher-researcher role are a factor here. It will be recalled that in this study my primary role was one of teacher, and the assignment—though later analyzed from a research perspective—was totally appropriate to this role. In a biographical study, my role would have been primarily researcher and as such—in combination with the evaluative aspect of the teacher role—would have posed certain ethical questions for me and limitations on the data collection. I would not have felt justified, for example, in asking the students to append their names to highly personalized data, which I could have then matched with the data from their individual assignments. I may have been overcautious but I did not feel that on the basis of my administrative links with their faculty and their potential vulnerability as students that I should require this type of private disclosure to facilitate my own research purposes. Had I been a thoroughly independent researcher, I would have coded the twin studies. But then, as discussed earlier, I question whether the same material would have been forthcoming.)

For researchers such a dual methodological approach could provide very useful insights concerning the differential and simultaneous use of quantitative and qualitative research methodologies in the same project. Rather than lining up adherents to one method as opposed to another, with too little readiness to admit the limitations of each, or the potential for cooperative perspectives, it could happen that this type of study would encourage a restructuring of closed methodological thinking and categorization.

To date, existing social systems and symbolic interaction approaches have apparently engaged in either raising issues or using methods that have not seriously examined the concept of affective neutrality. This raises the question of how many other dimensions of reality are similarly effected. It is only as theory is opened to a wide range of research methodologies that may refine it, and only as these methodologies become open to each other, that the real world may ever emerge.

APPENDIX 1

APPENDIX 1

THE PILOT STUDY

As indicated in Chapter 2, page 24, a pilot study involving 50 of the 550 cases was undertaken in order to determine the feasibility of a larger study. The following data list the categories that emerged from the pilot study, any additional factors that emerged when all the cases were coded, and any categories that were collapsed.

Problem Situations

1. Death/Dying
2. Interpretation of Condition
3. Convalescence
4. Unmarried Mothers
5. Elderly
6. Psychiatric (includes suicide)
7. Cultural Adaptation
8. Colleague Relationship
9. Professional/Personal Relationship
10. Alcoholism
11. Birth of child
12. Preoperation
13. Adolescence
14. Pregnancy

Only 1 category was added to the original 13: that of Pregnancy. In this category 9 cases were involved. However, as the ratio of Helpful to Un-helpful cases and the distribution in cross-tabulation of Situation and Response factors paralleled those of Birth, these two categories were collapsed into the category of Pregnancy / Birth. Similarly, the previous Situation of Preoperation (total of 11 cases) paralleled the Situation of Interpretation of Condition to the extent that Preoperation was included in the latter category.

These changes resulted in a final total of 12 Situations.

Helpful Response Factors

1. Took time to explain.
2. Was a sounding board.
3. Gave moral support.
4. Came to terms with own feelings; was able to enter into patient's problem.
5. Initiated referral to another profession / resource.
6. Helped patient express feelings.
7. Liked the patient.
8. Not unduly influenced by negative opinions of other staff members regarding the patient's personality.
9. Nonjudgmental.
10. Helped family members deal with the situation.
11. Wanted to understand how patient felt.
12. Looked beyond patient's outward response / behavior to underlying causes.
13. Made this case the basis for overall policy change / improvement.
14. Was trying to prove self to senior staff members.
15. Discussed religion with patient.
16. Used innovative rehabilitative procedure.
17. Used physical closeness (e.g., held patient's hand).

Three additional factors emerged when the 275 Helpful cases were coded: (1) positively identified with patient due to similar life / professional experience; (2) had received training in recognizing social-emotional needs of patients; (3) was honest with patient / relatives.

These changes resulted in a final total of 20 Helpful Response factors.

Unhelpful Response Factors

1. Felt inadequate to enter into patient's problem because had not personally resolved the issue.
2. Felt guilty but could not communicate.
3. Treated the condition, overlooking the patient.
4. Breakdown of interprofessional communication/cooperation.
5. Short-staffed; too little time to devote to the patient.
6. Purposely disregarded significant cues in patient's statements/behavior.
7. Felt pressured (within self) into doing things rather than coping with feeling elements (tension present).
8. Negatively influenced by opinions of other staff members regarding personality of the patient.
9. Lacked training in recognizing social-emotional needs of patients.
10. Did not want to understand.
11. Afraid would break down and cry in front of patient.
12. Was disapproving, judgmental.
13. Failed to look beyond initial negative impression of patient's personality.
14. Avoided needs of family members.
15. Prejudiced toward group of which patient was a member.
16. Overidentified due to being similar age to patient.
17. Incapacitated by own fear of death.
18. Failed to seek authoritative advice regarding innovation.
19. Disregarded own judgment because wanted approval of senior staff members.

Five additional factors emerged when the 275 Unhelpful cases were coded: (1) rationalized actions and thoughts; (2) self-image was threatened; (3) disliked patient; (4) lost professional role: patient became friend; (5) felt guilty but still would not communicate.

These changes resulted in a final total of 24 Unhelpful Response factors.

APPENDIX 2

TABLE A
Cross-Tabulation of Problem Situations with Helpful Response Factors: Frequencies

	Pregnancy/ Birth	Adolescence	Interpretation of Condition	Professional/ Personal	Psychiatric	Unmarried Mothers	Convalescence	Alcoholism	Elderly	Colleague Relationship	Cultural Adaptation	Death/ Dying	Total
Took time to explain	21	3	29	9	10	3	27	0	8	9	0	11	130
Was a sounding board	7	4	12	6	9	2	18	0	6	7	2	20	93
Gave moral support	20	4	31	12	15	2	39	3	9	11	2	25	173
Terms with own feelings	6	3	14	5	8	2	18	1	3	3	2	14	79
Initiated referral	11	2	18	6	6	1	26	0	4	3	0	3	80
Helped patient express	17	5	28	5	17	3	35	3	11	11	1	20	156
Liked patient	1	0	6	1	6	1	7	0	5	0	1	7	34
Not influenced	3	2	2	0	3	0	13	0	1	3	0	4	31

Nonjudgmental	11	3	15	1	8	4	18	2	2	7	2	11	84
Helped family members	7	0	15	6	2	0	16	1	4	2	1	24	78
Wanted to understand	15	4	27	4	12	4	34	1	11	10	2	12	135
Looked beyond behavior	10	5	21	2	12	1	31	3	6	5	1	10	107
Basis for policy change	3	0	4	2	1	0	2	0	0	1	0	1	14
Prove self to senior staff	0	0	1	0	0	0	1	0	0	1	1	0	4
Discussed religion	0	0	0	1	1	0	2	1	0	0	1	0	6
Innovative procedure	1	2	12	1	5	0	7	1	4	5	3	0	41
Physical closeness	5	2	7	1	4	3	2	0	2	0	1	10	37
Positively identified	4	2	4	2	2	1	7	1	4	5	0	8	39
Had training in needs	0	1	1	1	0	0	3	0	1	1	0	1	9
Honest	1	0	3	1	4	0	2	1	3	1	0	5	21
Total number of cases	30	6	50	15	27	4	63	4	16	18	4	38	275
Total number of responses	143	42	250	66	125	27	308	18	84	85	20	186	1354

TABLE B
Cross-Tabulation of Problem Situations with Unhelpful Response Factors: Frequencies

	Pregnancy/ Birth	Adolescence	Interpretation of Condition	Professional/ Personal	Psychiatric	Unmarried Mothers	Convalescence	Alcoholism	Elderly	Colleague Relationship	Cultural Adaptation	Death/ Dying	Total
Inadequate, hadn't resolved	8	3	17	3	8	1	15	1	3	6	3	28	96
Guilty, couldn't communicate	5	2	9	2	2	2	6	0	3	8	2	21	62
Treated condition, not patient	10	4	24	1	9	3	36	3	5	7	3	17	122
Breakdown of communication	8	3	7	0	2	1	5	1	4	6	1	3	40
Short-staffed; too little time	0	1	8	1	2	0	7	0	1	1	0	4	25
Disregarded cues	7	3	15	4	11	2	20	1	6	6	2	12	90
Doing rather than coping	2	3	9	2	1	2	7	0	2	2	1	15	46
Influenced by other staff	3	2	10	1	0	0	10	0	3	3	0	3	35
Lacked training in needs	7	3	8	3	5	0	7	0	1	4	3	6	47

													Total
Didn't want to understand	5	7	20	2	6	3	21	2	8	7	5	4	90
Afraid would cry	0	0	1	0	0	1	2	0	0	0	0	3	7
Judgmental	8	8	28	1	7	5	25	4	10	7	7	4	112
Initial negative impression	11	5	30	2	10	2	31	2	8	11	5	4	121
Avoided needs of family members	2	1	9	1	0	1	8	2	2	0	4	16	46
Prejudiced	2	2	8	0	3	5	7	3	2	2	2	4	38
Overidentified	0	0	1	1	0	0	1	0	0	0	0	4	7
Incapacitated by fear of death	1	0	1	0	0	0	1	0	0	0	0	15	17
Failed to seek advice	0	1	1	0	1	0	4	0	1	4	1	2	15
Disregarded own judgment	1	2	1	0	2	0	1	0	0	3	0	3	12
Rationalized	9	2	15	1	5	1	6	1	5	4	2	11	62
Self-image threatened	8	6	21	4	8	1	22	2	7	10	7	16	112
Disliked patient	0	2	7	0	2	1	13	1	6	3	1	0	36
Lost professional role	0	0	4	1	4	0	2	0	1	1	0	6	19
Guilty, would not communicate	1	0	3	0	5	0	7	1	1	3	0	7	28
Total number of cases	21	12	62	7	19	6	53	5	15	25	10	40	275
Total number of responses	98	58	259	30	93	31	264	24	79	98	49	208	1289

APPENDIX 3

APPENDIX 3

TABLE C
Helpful Response Factors: Percentages and Type

% of Cases in Which Cited	Rank	Helpful Response Factor	Type A	Type B
63	1	Gave moral support		✓
57	2	Helped patient express feelings		✓
49	3	Wanted to understand	✓	
47	4	Took time to explain		✓
39	5	Looked beyond patient's behavior		✓
34	6	Was a sounding board		✓
31	7	Nonjudgmental	✓	
29	8	Initiated referral		✓
29	9	Came to terms with own feelings	✓	
28	10	Helped family members		✓
15	11	Innovative procedure		✓
14	12	Positively identified	✓	
13	13	Physical closeness		✓
12	14	Liked patient	✓	
11	15	Not influenced by other staff opinions		✓
8	16	Honest with patient, family		✓
5	17	Basis for policy change		✓
3	18	Had training in needs	✓	
2	19	Discussed religion		✓
2	20	Prove self to senior staff		✓

TABLE D
Unhelpful Response Factors: Percentages and Type

% of Cases in Which Cited	Rank	Unhelpful Response Factor	Type A	Type B
44	1	Treated condition, overlooking patient		✔
44	2	Failed to look beyond initial negative impression		✔
41	3	Self-image was threatened	✔	
41	4	Judgmental	✔	
35	5	Had not personally resolved issue	✔	
33	6	Purposely disregarded cues		✔
33	7	Did not want to understand	✔	
23	8	Guilty, could not communicate		✔
23	9	Rationalized actions and thoughts		✔
17	10	Lacked training in recognizing social-emotional needs	✔	
17	11	Avoided family members		✔
17	12	Doing things rather than dealing with feelings		✔
15	13	Breakdown of interprofessional communication		✔
14	14	Prejudiced toward group	✔	
13	15	Disliked patient	✔	
13	16	Negatively influenced by other staff		✔
10	17	Guilty, would not communicate		✔
9	18	Short-staffed, too little time	✔	
7	19	Lost professional role	✔	
6	20	Incapacitated by own fear of death	✔	
5	21	Failed to seek advice		✔
4	22	Disregarded own judgment	✔	
3	23	Overidentified: similar age		
3	24	Afraid would cry		✔

REFERENCES

REFERENCES

Aiken, L., & Aiken, J. A systematic approach to the evaluation of interpersonal relationships. *American Journal of Nursing,* 1973, *73*(5), 863–867.

Barrett-Lennard, G. T. Significant aspects of a helping relationship. *Canada's Mental Health,* July-August 1965, pp. 1–5 (Suppl. 47).

Becker, H. S. Performing arts—music. In H. M. Vollmer and D. L. Mills (Eds.), *Professionalization.* Englewood Cliffs, N.J.: Prentice-Hall, 1966.

Becker, H. S., Geir, B., Hughes, E. C., & Strauss, A. *Boys in white.* Chicago: University of Chicago Press, 1961.

Berne, E. *Games people play.* New York: Random House, 1978.

Blishen, B. *Doctors and doctrines.* Toronto: University of Toronto Press, 1969.

Brown, E. L. Nursing and patient care. In F. Davis (Ed.), *The nursing profession.* New York: Wiley, 1966.

Bruce, S. J. Reactions of nurses and mothers to stillbirths. *Nursing Outlook,* February 1962, *10,* 89–90.

Bullough, B., & Bullough, V. L. Sex discrimination in health care. *Nursing Outlook,* 1975, *23*(1), 43.

Carkhuff, R. R. *Helping and human relations: A primer for lay and professional helpers* (Vol. 1). *Selection and training.* New York: Holt, Rinehart & Winston, 1969.

Churchill, L. Ethical issues of a profession in transition. *American Journal of Nursing,* 1977, *77*(5), 873–875.

Cicourel, A. V. *The social organization of juvenile justice.* New York: Wiley, 1967.

Cothell, L. S. Jr., & Dymond, R. F. The empathic responses: A neglected field for research. *Psychiatry,* 1949, *12*(4):355–359.

Daniels, M. J. Affect and its control in the medical intern. In T. Millon (Ed.), *Medical behavioral science.* Philadelphia: W. B. Saunders, 1975.

Davis, F., Olesen, V. L., & Whittaker, E. W. Problems and issues in collegiate nursing education. In F. Davis (Ed.), *The nursing profession.* New York: Wiley, 1966.

Deutscher, I. *The evaluation of nurses by male physicians.* Kansas City, Mo.: Community Studies Inc., 1955. (Publication No. 93)

Dickinson-Taylor, C. *Sociological sheep-shearing.* Unpublished manuscript, College of Nursing, University of Florida, 1960.

Duff, R. S., & Hollingshead, A. B. *Sickness and society.* New York: Harper & Row, 1968.

Edwards, W. Don't let sympathy cloud your judgment. *Nursing Times,* April 1957, *53,* 395.

Etzioni, A. *The active society.* London: Collier-Macmillan, 1968.

Friedlander, W. A. *Concepts and methods of social work.* Englewood Cliffs, N.J.: Prentice-Hall, 1958.

Friedson, E. *Profession of medicine.* New York: Dodd, Mead, 1970.

Fulton, R. Attitudes toward death: An emerging health problem. *Nursing Forum,* 1964, *3*(1), 106.

Glaser, B. G., & Strauss, A. L. *The discovery of grounded theory.* Chicago: Aldine, 1967.

Goffman, E. Characteristics of total institutions. *Symposium on Preventive and Social Psychiatry,* April 1957, pp. 46–47.

Goffman, E. *Relations in public.* New York: Harper & Row, 1971.

Gold, R. L. Roles in sociological field observations. *Social Forces,* 1958, *36,* 217–223.

Gow, K. M. Public health nurses and social workers: Partners or adversaries? *Canadian Journal of Public Health,* 1968, *59*(2), 75–81.

Gow, K. M. Resolution of a revolution. *American Journal of Nursing,* 1967, *67*(3), 578–582.

Gramzow, C. J. An uncaring attitude taught me nursing. *R.N.,* 1976, *39*(12), 35–37.

Hall, J. E., & Weaver, B. R. *Nursing of families in crisis.* Philadelphia: J. B. Lippincott, 1974.

Halmos, P. *The faith of the counsellors.* London: Constable, 1965.

de Hartog, J. *The hospital.* New York: Atheneum, 1964.

Jackson, B. An experience in participant observation. *Nursing Outlook,* 1975, *23*(8), 552–555.

Jackson, E. The theological, psychological and philosophical dimensions of death in protestantism. In E. A. Grollman (Ed.), *Explaining death to children.* Boston: Beacon, 1967.

Johnson, M. M., & Martin, H. W. Nursing. In H. M. Vollmer and D. L. Mills (Eds.), *Professionalization.* Englewood Cliffs, N.J.: Prentice-Hall, 1966.

Jones, C. P. We used paperwork to hide from our patients. *R.N.,* 1978, *41*(4), 50–52.

Jones, E. M. Who supports the nurse? *Nursing Outlook,* July 1962, *10,* 476.

Jones, R. K., & Jones, P. A. *Sociology in medicine.* London: The English Universities Press Ltd., 1975.

Jourard, S. M. *The transparent self.* New York: Van Nostrand, 1964.

Jourard, S. M. *The transparent self.* New York: Van Nostrand, 1971.

Kalisch, B. J. What is empathy? *American Journal of Nursing,* 1973, *73*(9), 1548–1552.

Katz, F. E. Nurses. In A. Etzioni (Ed.), *The semi-professions and their organization.* New York: Free Press, 1969.

King, A. P. Speak out: Can I love them all? *Journal of Practical Nursing,* 1978, *28*(12), 22.

King, E. S. Should we get emotionally involved? Hell yes. *R.N.,* 1977, *40*(6), 49–53.

Kramer, M. *Reality shock: Why nurses leave nursing.* Saint Louis: C. V. Mosby, 1974.

Kramer, M., & Schmalenberg, C. Bicultural training and new graduate role transformation. *Nursing Digest,* 1978a, *5*(4), 1–47.

Kramer, M., & Schmalenberg, C. The first job—A proving ground basis for empathy development. *Nursing Digest,* 1978b, *5*(4), 75–82.

Kübler-Ross, E. *On death and dying.* New York: Macmillan, 1969.

Lambert, V. A., & Lambert, C. E., Jr. *The impact of physical illness and related mental health concepts.* Englewood Cliffs, N.J.: Prentice-Hall, 1979.

LaMonica, E. L., Carew, D. K., Winder, A. E., Haase, A. M. B., & Blanchard, K. Empathy training as the major thrust of a staff development program. *Nursing Research,* 1976, *25*(6), 447–451.

La Sor, B., & Elliott, M. R. *Issues in Canadian nursing.* Scarborough, Ontario: Prentice-Hall, Inc., 1977.

Lewis, G. K. *Nurse-patient communication.* Dubuque, Iowa: Wm. C. Brown, 1973.

Linder, R. *The Fifty Minute Hour.* New York: Bantam Books, 1956.

Lovegrove, B. Nurse, could you care more? *Nursing Times,* 1979, *75*(7), 272.

Maslach, C. Burned-out. *Human Behavior,* 1976, *5*(9), 16–22.

Matthews, B. P. Measurement of psychological aspects of the nurse-patient relationship. *Nursing Research,* 1962, *11*(3), 154–162.

Mehrabian, A., & Epstein, N. A measure of emotional empathy. *Journal of Personality,* 1972, *40*(4), 525–543.

Merser, L. S., & O'Connor, P. *Fundamental skills in the nurse-patient relationship.* Philadelphia: W. B. Saunders, 1974.

Miller, S. M. The participant observer and over-rapport. *American Sociological Review,* 1952, *17*(1), 97–99.

Mulligan, J. E., & Casse, G. E. Clearance rates of 131 iodine in mechanically injured and normal muscle tissue. *Nursing Research,* 1965, *14*(2), 126–131.

Olesen, V. L., &ₗWhittaker, E. W. Role making in participant observation: Process in the research-actor relationship. *Human Organization,* Winter 1967, *26,* 273–281.

Olesen, V. L., & Whittaker, E. W. *The silent dialogue.* San Francisco: Jossey-Bass, 1968.

Osgood, C. E., Suci, G. J., & Tannenbaum, P. H. *The Measurement of Meaning.* Urbana: University of Illinois Press, 1957.

Parsons, T. *The social system.* Glencoe, Ill.: Free Press, 1951.

Peitchinis, V. A. Therapeutic effectiveness of counselling by nursing personnel: Review of the literature. *Nursing Research,* 1972, *21*(2), 138–148.

Peplau, H. E. Professional closeness. . . . *Nursing Forum,* 1969, *8*(4), 343–360.

Pickering, E. A. *Report of the Special Study Regarding the Medical Profession in Ontario.* A report to the Ontario Medical Association, Toronto, April 1973.

Purtilo, R. *The allied health professional and the patient.* Philadelphia: W. B. Saunders, 1973.

Reich, W. *Character analysis.* New York: Orgone Press, 1948.

Ross, A. D. *Becoming a nurse.* Toronto: Macmillan, 1961.

Saupe, P. How do you feel, nurse? *American Journal of Nursing,* 1974, *74*(6), 1105.

Schwartz, L. H., & Schwartz, J. L. *The psychodynamics of patient care.* Englewood Cliffs, N.J.: Prentice-Hall, 1972.

Searles, H. F. The place of neutral therapist responses in psychotherapy with the schizophrenic patient. *International Journal of Psychoanalysis,* 1963, *44*(1), 42–56.

Shockley, J. S. Perspectives in femininity: Implications for nursing. *Nursing Digest,* 1975, *3*(6), 49–52.

Sjoberg, G., & Nett, R. *A methodology for social research.* New York: Harper & Row, 1968.

Sklar-Mathie, L. Do I still care? *Canadian Nurse,* 1978, *74*(4), 33–35.

Solley, C. M., & Murphy, G. *Development of the perceptual world.* New York: Basic Books, 1960.

Strauss, A. The structure and ideology of American nursing: An interpretation. In F. Davis (Ed.), *The nursing profession.* New York: Wiley, 1966.

Travelbee, J. *Interpersonal aspects of nursing.* Philadelphia: F. A. Davis, 1971.

Truax, C. B., Altmann, H., & Millis, W. A., Jr. Therapeutic relationships provided by various professionals. *Journal of Community Psychology,* 1974, *2*(1), 33–36.

Vollmer, H. M., & Mills, D. L. *Professionalization.* Englewood Cliffs, N.J.: Prentice-Hall, 1966.

Wallston, K. A., Cohen, B. D., Wallston, B. S., Smith, R. A., & De Vellis, B. M. Increasing nurses' person centeredness. *Nursing Research,* 1978, *27*(3), 158.

Warner, W. L., & Lunt, P. S. *The social life of a modern community.* New Haven, Conn.: Yale University Press, 1941.

Waters, V., Chater, S., Vivier, M. L., Urrea, J., & Wilson, H. Technical and professional nursing: An exploratory study. *Nursing Research,* 1972, *21*(2), 124–131.

Webster's New Collegiate Dictionary. Toronto: Thomas Allen, 1959.

Wolff, K. H. Beginning: In Hegel and today. In K. H. Wolff and B. Moore, Jr. (Eds.), *The critical spirit: Essays in honor of Herbert Marcuse.* Boston: Beacon Press, 1968.